Occupational Medicine

Health Hazards of Farming

Guest Editors:

D. H. Cordes, MD, MPH
Chief, Section of Preventive and Occupational Medicine

and

Dorothy Foster Rea, MA
Consultant

Department of Family and Community Medicine
University of Arizona College of Medicine
Tucson, Arizona

Volume 6/Number 3
HANLEY & BELFUS, INC.

July–September 1991
Philadelphia

STATE OF THE ART REVIEWS

Publisher: HANLEY & BELFUS, INC.
210 South 13th Street
Philadelphia, PA 19107

OCCUPATIONAL MEDICINE: State of the Art Reviews is included in *Index Medicus, MEDLINE, Bio Sciences Information Service, Current Contents* and *ISI/BIOMED.*

OCCUPATIONAL MEDICINE: State of the Art Reviews   **(ISSN 0885-114X)**
July-September 1991   **Volume 6, Number 3**   **(ISBN 1-56053-076-6)**

OCCUPATIONAL MEDICINE: State of the Art Reviews is published quarterly by Hanley & Belfus, Inc., 210 South 13th Street, Philadelphia, Pennsylvania 19107. Second-class postage paid at Philadelphia, PA and at additional mailing offices.

POSTMASTER: Send address changes to OCCUPATIONAL MEDICINE: State of the Art Reviews, Hanley & Belfus, Inc., 210 South 13th Street, Philadelphia, PA 19107.

The 1992 subscription price is $74.00 per year U.S., $84.00 outside U.S. (add $40.00 for air mail). Single copies $36.00 U.S., $38.00 outside U.S. (add $10.00 for single copy air mail).

CONTENTS

(For article summaries, see pages 331–333)

CONTRIBUTORS

Kenneth Abrams, MD
Fellow, Department of Dermatology, University of California, San Francisco, School of Medicine, San Francisco, California

Aaron Blair, PhD
Chief, Occupational Studies Section Environmental Epidemiology Branch, National Cancer Institute, National Institutes of Health, Bethesda, Maryland

W. Danny Brown, PhD, MD
Regional Occupational Physician, U.S. Public Health Service, Federal Employee Occupational Health Program, Region X, Seattle, Washington

D. H. Cordes, MD, MPH
Chief, Section of Preventive and Occupational Medicine, Department of Family and Community Medicine, University of Arizona College of Medicine, Tucson, Arizona

Clifton D. Crutchfield, PhD, CIH
Director, Industrial Hygiene, Division of Community and Environmental Health, University of Arizona, Tucson, Arizona

Jennifer Lowe Ellis, MD
Resident, General Preventive Medicine, Department of Family and Community Medicine, University of Arizona College of Medicine, Tucson, Arizona

Thomas Ferguson, MD, PhD
Occupational & Environmental Medicine Fellow, Division of Occupational & Environmental Medicine, University of California, Davis, School of Medicine, Davis, California

Thomas E. Gamsky, MD, MPH
Department of Pulmonary Medicine, Veteran's Affairs Medical Center, Martinez, California

Paul R. Gordon, MD
Assistant Professor, Department of Family and Community Medicine, University of Arizona College of Medicine, Tucson, Arizona

Leslie V. Boyer Hassen, MD
Fellow in Clinical Toxicology and Assistant Clinical Lecturer in Pediatrics, Section of Emergency Medicine, University of Arizona Health Sciences Center, Tucson, Arizona

Daniel J. Hogan, MD
Associate Professor, Department of Dermatology and Cutaneous Surgery, University of Miami School of Medicine, Miami, Florida

Paul A. James, MD
Assistant Professor of Family Medicine, Department of Family Medicine, East Carolina University School of Medicine, Greenville, North Carolina

Evan W. Kligman, MD
Assistant Professor, Department of Family and Community Medicine, University of Arizona College of Medicine, Tucson, Arizona

Ricky Lee Langley, MD, MPH
Assistant Professor of Preventive Medicine & Public Health Policy, Department of Preventive Medicine & Public Health Policy, East Carolina University, Greenville, North Carolina

Howard I. Maibach, MD
Vice Chairman and Professor, Department of Dermatology, University of California, San Francisco, School of Medicine, San Francisco, California

Joel S. Meister, PhD
Research Assistant Professor, Southwest Border Rural Health Research Center, Department of Family and Community Medicine, University of Arizona College of Medicine, Tucson, Arizona

James A. Merchant, MD, DrPH
Professor of Preventive and Internal Medicine, Department of Preventive Medicine and Environmental Health, and Department of Medicine; Director, Institute of Agricultural Medicine and Occupational Health, University of Iowa College of Medicine, Iowa City, Iowa

Wayne F. Peats, MD, MPH
Clinical Lecturer, Section of Preventive and Occupational Medicine, Department of Family and Community Medicine, University of Arizona College of Medicine, Tucson, Arizona

Dorothy Foster Rea, MA
Consultant, Department of Family and Community Medicine, University of Arizona College of Medicine, Tucson, Arizona

Marc Schenker, MD, MPH
Associate Professor and Division Chief, Division of Occupational & Environmental Medicine, University of California, Davis, School of Medicine, Davis, California

Caryl Smith Shaver, MD
Chief Resident, Section of Preventive and Occupational Medicine, Department of Family and Community Medicine, University of Arizona School of Medicine, Tucson, Arizona

Stephen T. Sparks, MD
Medical Director for Occupational Health, H.C.A. Wesley Medical Center, Wichita, Kansas

Theodore G. Tong, PharmD
Professor of Pharmacy Practice, Pharmacology and Toxicology, University of Arizona College of Pharmacy, Tucson, Arizona

Shelia H. Zahm, ScD
Occupational Studies Section, Environmental Epidemiology Branch, National Cancer Institute, National Institutes of Health, Bethesda, Maryland

PUBLISHED ISSUES, 1988–1990
(available from the publisher)

1991 ISSUES

**Prevention of Pulmonary Disease
in the Workplace**
Edited by Philip Harber, MD, MPH
University of California, Los Angeles
and John R. Balmes, MD
University of California, San Francisco

Health Hazards of Farming
Edited by D. H. Cordes, MD, MPH
and Dorothy Foster Rea, MS
University of Arizona College of Medicine
Tucson, Arizona

The Biotechnology Industry
Edited by Alan M. Ducatman, MD
and Daniel F. Liberman, PhD
Massachusetts Institute of Technology
Cambridge, Massachusetts

The Nuclear Energy Industry
Edited by Gregg S. Wilkinson, PhD
University of Texas Medical School
   at Galveston
Galveston, Texas

1992 ISSUES

Occupational Lung Disease
Edited by William S. Beckett, MD
Yale University School of Medicine
New Haven, Connecticut
and Rebecca Bascom, MD
University of Maryland School of Medicine
Baltimore, Maryland

Ergonomics
Edited by J. Steven Moore, MD
Medical College of Wisconsin
Milwaukee, Wisconsin

Unusual Occupational Disease
Edited by Dennis J. Shusterman, MD,
   MPH
Berkeley, California
and Paul D. Blanc, MD, MSPH
University of California, San Francisco
San Francisco, California

Occupational Skin Disease
Edited by James R. Nethercott, MD
The Johns Hopkins University
   School of Hygiene and Public Health
Baltimore, Maryland

Additional 1989 special issue:

**Occupational HIV Infection:
Risks and Risk Reduction**
Edited by Charles E. Becker, MD
University of California, San Francisco,
California

Special issue prices:

$18.00—subscribers (add to 1991
   subscription rate)
$36.00—nonsubscribers

Ordering Information:
Subscriptions or full year ($74 U.S., $84 outside U.S.) and single issues
($36 U.S., $38 outside U.S.) are available from the publisher—
Hanley & Belfus, Inc., 210 South 13th Street, Philadelphia, PA 19107.
Telephone (215) 546-7293; (800) 962-1892.

PREFACE

This issue of *OCCUPATIONAL MEDICINE: State of the Art Reviews* is particularly timely. To quote from a *Wall Street Journal* article of July 20, 1990, "Farming is America's most dangerous line of work. Agriculture has eclipsed mining as the occupation with the highest death rate."

Death and disease on the farm have gone too far—and a movement has begun to try to control the problem. Much of the impetus for the movement has come from the National Institute for Occupational Safety and Health (NIOSH) and from the Office of the U.S. Surgeon General. The NIOSH 1990 Agricultural Initiative was set in motion over 1 year ago with the establishment of new Agricultural Health and Safety Centers and the awarding of academic grants for applied research in intervention methods. The Surgeon General's Conference—Agricultural Safety and Health—was held in April of this year. It is hoped this issue of *OM:STARs* will further increase awareness by detailing some of the areas of farm safety and health in need of attention. And with this issue of *OM:STARs* we hope to join and stimulate the movement to reduce accidents and illness on the farm. Our emphasis is on prevention, because it is only through knowledge and implementation of preventive measures that the movement can succeed.

We wish to thank the authors of the articles in this issue for their contributions. In addition, we thank the external reviewers who critiqued the content of this issue before publication and helped improve both focus and content:

Peter J. Attarian, PhD
Family and Community Medicine
University of Arizona

W. D. Brown, PhD, MD
Regional Occupational Physician
Public Health Service
Seattle, Washington

Anthony Camilli, MD
Internal Medicine
University of Arizona

Richard C. Dart, MD, PhD
Director, Clinical Toxicology
Emergency Medicine
University of Arizona

Joel Meister, PhD
Rural Health
University of Arizona

Ronald E. Pust, MD
Family and Community Medicine
University of Arizona

Joseph Rea, MD
Medical Director
Texas Eastman Company
Longview, Texas

Janet Senf, PhD
Family and Community Medicine
University of Arizona

Caryl Shaver, MD
Family and Community Medicine
University of Arizona

Mark Van Ert, PhD
Division of Community
    and Environmental Health
University of Arizona

The Hanley & Belfus staff was cooperative and supportive. We appreciate their offering us the opportunity to organize and contribute to this issue, and then helping us in our efforts to accomplish the task. We wish also to acknowledge especially the library research, word processing, and office support of Alison Pearson, MA and Beulah Blunt, Administrative Secretary, of the University of Arizona.

D. H. Cordes, MD, MPH
Dorothy Foster Rea, MA
GUEST EDITORS

D. H. CORDES, MD, MPH
DOROTHY FOSTER REA, MA

FARMING: A HAZARDOUS OCCUPATION

From the Section of Preventive
and Occupational Medicine
Department of Family and
Community Medicine
University of Arizona College
of Medicine
Tucson, Arizona

Reprint requests to:
D. H. Cordes, MD, MPH
Chief, Section of Preventive and
Occupational Medicine
Department of Family and
Community Medicine
University of Arizona
Tucson, AZ 85724

The farming work force does not consist of readily countable employees, as do work forces of other industries and businesses. The latest figures indicate there are 4,951,000 people living on 2,197,000 farms in the United States.[2] However, the size of the farm population and the number of people working on farms have always been difficult to determine because of problems of definition. In the aforementioned figures the smallest farms are not counted, nor are unpaid family members who worked on the farm less than 15 hours during the survey week.

Although it is impossible to count accurately the number of family members, young and old, experienced and inexperienced, who accompany the principal farmer into the farm work environment, it is important to be aware that a family is often the occupational unit on the farm, rather than a single worker. When considering the health hazards of farming, we must take into account that the entire family is exposed to the work environment.

Seasonal workers, migrant workers, and hired hands are also difficult to enumerate. The U.S. Department of Agriculture reports there are 1,037,000 hired workers on farms.[2] But, migrant workers are not counted separately by the Agricultural Service, and their reported number in the U.S. ranges from as few as 300,000 to as many as 1.5 million.[4] Migrant workers, by their itinerant nature and sometimes undocumented status, are virtually impossible to count.

The size of the population at risk that is involved in farm work, based on all figures, is a minimum of 6.5 million people in the U.S., and includes farm managers, farm operators, farm families, seasonal or occasional workers, and migrant workers and their families. Estimates indicate that 25% of the agricultural work force is comprised of children under 16 years of age.[4] Also, many people engage in part-time farming activities, such as gardening or raising animals, and are exposed to some of the same hazards. These people are also never tallied as part of the farm work force.

Farming as an occupation, especially on a family farm, is distinctly different from other occupations, and when considering the health risks of farming, it is important to understand the characteristics that set it apart. These characteristics can be put into three categories: (1) worker traits and behavior, (2) the work setting, and (3) organizational structure.

CHARACTERISTICS OF FARM WORK

Worker Traits and Behavior

Farmers have traditionally been viewed as being staunchly independent and resourceful. Unlike other categories of workers, farmers tend not to work in groups. The typical family farmer spends the day alone or with one or two other workers or family members, whereas workers in other occupations tend to spend the workday in small-to-large groups. Even when working with a co-worker or hired hand, the farmer may be occupied in one section of the farm while the co-worker is in a completely remote area.

Farmers are generalists, of necessity. One farmer must have selected skills of a carpenter, mechanic, veterinarian, laborer, manager, agronomist, horticulturalist, and animal tender, to name a few of the many requirements of the job. The various tasks in which the farmer is engaged depend on the geographic location of the farm and on the crops or livestock raised.

These traits figure largely in the success of the farmer, but they also can lead to particular health problems and social maladaptation due to the inherent stresses caused by isolation and continual overreaching of capacities.

Work Setting

The work setting also is an important determinant in the health and safety of the farmer. The work environment of the farm is not static. Work takes the farmer into barns, sheds, grain enclosures, silos, animal confinement buildings, fields, woods, and towns, all of which are affected by varying climatic and other conditions, some severe. The accompanying physical, chemical, and biological hazards are diverse and numerous. Other workers are more likely to spend the day under one roof, where workplace hazards are predictable and measurable.

Statistics make the health risks of farming evident. The facts of illness, injury, and death connected with farm work are startling. According to the National Safety Council, the accidental-death rate of agriculture, 48 per 100,000 workers, has eclipsed mining as the occupation with the highest death rate. The Bureau of Labor Statistics estimates the incidence of injury and illness in 1988 in agricultural production alone was 10.9 per 10,000 workers. This rate placed agriculture as the third most hazardous occupation, outranked only by the construction and manufacturing industries. Disabling injuries totaled 120,000 in agricultural occupations in 1989.[1,2]

Agriculture had the second highest incidence rate for occupational illness in 1988, with 48.8 per 10,000 full-time workers, second only to manufacturing. However, agricultural workers had the highest incidence of all industry divisions for skin diseases and for poisoning. The incidence rate of 48.8 consisted of: skin diseases and disorders (30.8), disorders associated with repeated trauma (3.7), poisoning (3.2), disorders due to physical agents (2.7), respiratory conditions due to toxic agents (2.1), and all other occupational diseases (5.8). (Components do not add to total due to rounding.)

One of the major causes of accidents involves tractors. In 1989, there were 7.2 deaths per 100,000 tractors, with overturns accounting for 55% of all tractor fatalities on the farm. Other tractor-related deaths mainly occur due to tractor run-overs and power-takeoff accidents. An estimated 320 tractor-related deaths occur annually on the farm nationwide. Other causes of deaths on farms are reported as machinery, drowning, firearms, falls, struck by object, fires, electricity, animals, poisoning, suffocation, and lightning.[2]

Childhood farm accidents are yet another aspect of death and injury on the farm, because children under 16 are not counted in occupational morbidity and mortality statistics. Children play a significant role in work on the farm and face similar risk of injury and illness. A 1985 review indicated that 300 children and adolescents die each year of farm injuries and 23,500 suffer nonfatal trauma.[3] The same source revealed that more than half of these victims die without reaching a physician. In addition, 19% die on the way to the hospital. The most common cause of both fatal and nonfatal injuries is farm machinery. No statistics are available on agriculture-related illness in farm children.

The farm environment is a workplace as well as a home for many farmers, and work exposures, therefore, do not stop at the end of the day. With work and home in one place, spouse and family are likely to experience the same exposures as the principal worker. The family not only lives on the farm, but works there as well, unlike other occupations where work and home environments do not typically coincide.

Probably no other occupation encompasses a greater variety of health risks than farming. An estimated 6% of farmers work with a disability; this is more than in any other industry,[3] and is evidence of the inherent dangers of the job.

Organizational Structure

Perhaps the greatest distinction between the farmer and many other work groups involves the organization of farm work. The typical small family farm and even some corporate agribusinesses are not organized to provide workers a hierarchical structure, administrative support, collective bargaining, benefits, safety regulations, sponsored personnel development and training, or stable and flexible financing.

There is seldom a supervisor for worker training, observation, and checking of the work product. Farmers are usually self-taught, rather than formally trained or exposed to programmed instruction, even when confronting new or unfamiliar equipment.

There is no union to act as a control on workplace needs and to provide avenues of communication for improving conditions, hours, wages, and safety standards. The farm workplace is, to a large extent, an unregulated work setting. There are few Occupational Safety and Health Administration (OSHA) regulations that apply to farming, and OSHA, in general, does not oversee or collect data on places of employment with fewer than 11 workers. Not many family farms are large enough to qualify. In contrast, most workplaces of other occupations are regulated by OSHA and subject to OSHA inspections and data collection.

Whereas many city workers have medical care at the work site, or are at least in close proximity to it, the farmer still usually lives and works in a medically underserved area and must drive to urban areas for routine health care. The farm might also be quite distant from emergency medical care.

As self-employed individuals, farmers may feel financial stress more than other workers. They have no large corporation or other financial entity backing them and are one of this country's lowest income groups.[2] Financial downturns caused by crop failure, a small harvest, bad weather, or low market prices cannot be absorbed as easily as they can by industry or other large business. Other workers, while certainly not immune from financial stress related to work, frequently have some shelter because they work for someone else.

Farmers rarely work a 40-hour week. Rather, they work until the day's task is done, and there is no additional pay for overtime. They do not receive payment for their work in the form of hourly wages or salary. They are paid for a product, after it has been delivered for sale. This uncertainty can be another source of financial stress.

Farming is not the peaceful occupation in a pastoral setting it is sometimes pictured to be. Country life and outdoor work might seem the ideal setting for healthy, independent living, but that is hardly the case. The articles in this issue will attest to that. Each article is intended to draw your attention to one of the major hazards of agriculture. They are summarized below under their respective topical headings and authors. The issue cannot possibly cover every aspect of all occupational agricultural hazards. Appendix I is included to indicate further readings on agricultural safety and health for the practitioner with rural patients. Appendix II is a separate listing of resources from the National Institute for Occupational Safety and Health (NIOSH).

OVERVIEW OF TOPICS

Cancer (Blair and Zahm)

Agents known or suspected as carcinogens are part of the daily routine of farming. These include pesticides, fertilizers, paints, solvents, engine exhausts, and fuels. Farmers may even experience exposures heavier and of longer duration than the general population. Studies have begun to identify types of cancer found in farm populations and have indicated elevated risks for leukemia, Hodgkin's disease, non-Hodgkin's lymphoma, multiple myeloma, and cancers of the lip, stomach, skin, prostate, testis, brain, and connective tissue.

Noise and Vibration (Crutchfield and Sparks)

Noise from farm machinery poses a risk of hearing loss for farmers. But farm workers are more difficult to study than workers in industry, and measurement and compliance to decibel level limits on farms are difficult. The same machinery that produces excessive noise can produce hazardous levels of vibration. Tractor driving and other farm operations produce whole-body vibration, and use of hand-held tools produces localized vibration.

Heat and Cold (Brown)

Although they work outside much of the year, winter and summer, farmers may not be acclimatized when rapid seasonal changes occur, or after absence from their work environment. Therefore, each year, vigorous outdoor work in the heat and prolonged work in the cold bring on additional risks.

Chemical Hazards (Shaver and Tong)

In addition to pesticides farmers are exposed to chemicals such as fertilizers, petroleum products, and those in grain storage and animal confinement structures. Potential health effects of fertilizers, solvents, and other petroleum products are similar to pesticides. Pulmonary effects are the main concern in grain storage and animal confinement work.

Pesticides create toxic exposures through inhalation, dermal contact, and ingestion. Through these routes, the home and family can be subject to both acute and prolonged exposure. Using pesticides as an example, the risk of the work environment coinciding with the home environment is underscored. Concerns of low-level exposure stem from dermatitis and neurologic, pulmonary, and behavioral problems. Health effects of prolonged exposure relate to carcinogenicity and mutagenicity.

Respiratory Risks (Schenker, Ferguson, and Gamsky)

Agricultural processes and the farm environment generate dusts, molds, pollens, toxins, and gases that are potential respiratory irritants or health risks. Acquired sensitivity results in allergic reactions, with symptoms such as cough, dyspnea, fever, malaise, myalgia, arthralgia, and weight loss. The illness can become disabling and can lead to asthma and pulmonary fibrosis.

Occupational Infections (Kligman, Peate, and Cordes)

Agricultural occupational infections cause disease and, sometimes, disability. Farmers are at risk for infection through soil handling, animal tending, wild animals, and insects. Susceptibility is increased by stress, fatigue, temperature extremes, dust exposure, and contaminated water supplies.

Venomous Agents (Boyer Hassen)

Farmers are subject to envenomous bites and stings from reptiles and arthropods. They need to know when prompt medical attention is needed, and physicians in rural areas should be cognizant of the array of creatures of concern in their area.

Dermatoses (Abrams, Hogan, and Maibach)

One of the greatest risks connected with pesticide use in agriculture is dermatitis. Occupational skin disease accounts for approximately 70% of all occupational disease in agriculture in California, and pesticides as a cause are second only to poison oak. Other risks include solar effects of outdoor work and other skin infections.

Mental Health (Ellis and Gordon)

Farm family mental health is an issue centering on physical and mental stresses of farming, the physical isolation, the rapid economic and technological changes farming has undergone, and powerlessness to control external factors.

Migrant Workers (Meister)

Seasonal and migrant workers are perhaps at greatest overall risk because their work is concentrated in high-risk crops and activities. In many cases, they also live in or next to the fields or orchards where they have been employed to work, thus literally eating and sleeping with any toxic substances. Inadequate housing, nutrition, or water supply, where these are problems, exacerbate exposures.

Agricultural Health Education (James and Langley)

The Cooperative Extension Service in North Carolina plays an important role in communicating farm safety, nutritional counseling, and health access information to the agricultural and rural population. Through the extension network, local concerns reach university specialists, with lay leaders as the link. Recent grants from the National Institute for Occupational Safety and Health (NIOSH) have provided funding to develop an Agricultural Health Promotion System and to initiate a reporting system for agricultural injuries and illnesses in North Carolina.

Accidents (Merchant)

According to the National Safety Council the highest work-related death rates occur in agriculture, including agricultural services. Accidental deaths among agricultural workers comprise 15% of all occupational fatalities.[1] This extreme extends to children, as evidenced by the high number of accidents and fatalities among children and adolescent groups each year. And, at this point, occupational farm illnesses are not even being estimated among children.

Legislation and Prevention (Cordes and Rea)

Preventive measures are clearly the key to curbing the high accident and mortality rates associated with agricultural activities. Legislation and educational outreach are part of preventive efforts for the future to reduce the hazards of this dangerous occupation.

SUMMARY

Physicians with patients who work in rural areas need to be aware of the potential for illness and injury and be well-versed in preventive measures necessary to help keep these patients well. Physicians also need to be aware that the family's principal worker is not the only one exposed to the work hazards. The family joins in the duties of the farm and shares the risks. Physicians can play an important role in reinforcing the need for safe agricultural work practices.

APPENDIX I: RECOMMENDED READING: HEALTH AND SAFETY IN AGRICULTURE*

1. Adams RM: Occupational Skin Disease, 2nd ed. Philadelphia, W.B. Saunders, 1990.
2. AMA Handbook of Poisonous and Injurious Plants. Chicago, American Medical Association, 1985.
3. Arena JM: Poisoning: Toxicology, Symptoms, Treatments, 4th ed. Springfield, IL, Charles C Thomas, 1979.
4. Association of American Colleges and The W.K. Kellogg Foundation: Rural Health: A Challenge for Medical Education. Acad Med 65(Suppl):S1–S130, 1990.
5. Cordes DH, Rea DF: Health hazards of farming. Am Fam Phys 38:233–244, 1988 (69 refs.).
6. Coward RT, Lee GR (eds): The Elderly in Rural Society: Every Fourth Elder. New York, Springer-Verlag, 1985.
7. Coye MJ, Fenske R: Agricultural workers. In Levy BS, Wegman DH (eds): Occupational Health: Recognizing and Preventing Work-related Disease, 2nd ed. Boston, Little, Brown, 1988, pp 511–521.
8. Donham KJ, Horvath EP: Agricultural occupational medicine. In Zenz C (ed): Occupational Medicine: Principles and Practical Applications, 2nd ed. Chicago, Year Book Medical Publishers, 1988, pp 933–957.
9. Dosman JA, Cockcroft DW (eds): Principles of Health and Safety in Agriculture. Boca Raton, FL, CRC Press, 1989.
10. Goldfrank LR, et al (eds): Goldfrank's Toxicologic Emergencies, 4th ed. Norwalk, CT, Appleton & Lange, 1990.
11. Kasdan ML: Occupational Hand & Upper Extremity Injuries & Diseases. Philadelphia, Hanley & Belfus, 1991.
12. Kuehl A (ed): EMS Medical Directors' Handbook. St. Louis, C.V. Mosby, 1989.
13. Lipton M, deKadt E: Agriculture-Health Linkages. Albany, WHO Publications Center, 1988.
14. Morgan DP: Recognition and Management of Pesticide Poisonings, 3rd ed. United States Environmental Protection Agency. Washington, D.C., Superintendent of Documents, 1982.
15. Proctor NH, Hughes JP: Chemical Hazards of the Workplace, 2nd ed. Philadelphia, J.B. Lippincott, 1988.
16. Rosenblatt RA, Moscovice IS: Rural Health Care. New York, John Wiley, 1982.
17. Rust GS: Health status of migrant farmworkers: A literature review and commentary. Am J Public Health 80:1213–1217, 1990 (35 refs.).
18. Smith M, Andrews R: Farm injuries. In Hafen BQ, Karren KJ: Prehospital Emergency Care and Crisis Intervention. Englewood, CO, Morton Publishing Company, 1989.
19. Stueland D: Respiratory Problems Associated with Farming (videotape). Secaucus, NJ, Network for Continuing Medical Education, 1991.
20. Terho EO, Husman K, Kauppinen T: Proceedings of the International Symposium on Work-related Respiratory Disorders Among Farmers. Eur J Respir Dis 71(Suppl 154):1987.
21. U.S. Office of Technology Assessment: Health Care in Rural America. Washington, D.C., Government Printing Office, 1990.
22. Wilk VA: The Occupational Health of Migrant and Seasonal Farmworkers in the United States. Washington, D.C., Farmworker Justice Fund, 1986.
23. Wodarski JS: Rural Community Mental Health Practice. Baltimore, University Park Press, 1983.
24. World Health Organization: Public Health Impact of Pesticides Used in Agriculture. Albany, NY, WHO Publications Center, 1990.

*See Appendix II for NIOSH publications.

APPENDIX II: NIOSH Publications: Agricultural Safety and Health

Publication	Title	Availability
76-191	Pesticide Residue Hazards to Farm Workers: Symposium	*NTIS PB-86-152-980/A12
77-106	Criteria Document: Methyl Parathion	NTIS PB-274-191/A09
77-107	Criteria Document: Carbaryl	NTIS PB-273-801/A10
77-150	Occupational Health and Safety for Agricultural Workers	NTIS PB-274-760/A07
77-180	Agriculture Chemicals and Pesticides: A Subfile of Registry of Toxic Effects of Chemical Substances	NTIS PB-274-748/A12
78-183	Supplement and Index to Grain Dust Fire and Explosion Bibliography	NTIS IS-EMR-R17/A06
78-184	The Rural Health Study in Minnesota: A Comparison of Hospital Experience Between Farmers and Nonfarmers in a Rural Area of Minnesota (1976–1977)	NTIS PB-297-770/A05
78-200	Special Occupational Hazard Review for DDT	NTIS PB-81-226-656/A10
78-201	Special Occupational Hazard Review for Aldrin/Deildrin	NTIS PB-297-769/A08
79-118	Bis(Chloromethyl)Ether Formation and Detection in Selected Work Environment	NTIS PB-83-174-102/A08
79-120	Working Safely with Anhydrous Ammonia	NTIS PB-80-184-427/A03
86-110	NIOSH Alert—Request for Assistance in Preventing Occupational Fatalities in Confined Spaces	NTIS PB-86-205-754/A02
86-118	NIOSH Alert—Request for Assistance in Preventing Fatalities Due to Fires and Explosions in Oxygen-Limiting Silos	NTIS PB-87-111-399/A02
86-119	NIOSH Alert—Request for Assistance in Preventing Grain Auger Electrocutions	NTIS PB-87-105-599/A02
88-102	NIOSH Alert—Request for Assistance in Preventing Entrapment and Suffocation Caused by the Unstable Surfaces of Stored Grain and Other Materials	**NIOSH
87-115	NIOSH Publications Catalog	NIOSH
89-126	Health Hazards of Storing, Handling, and Shipping Grain	NIOSH
099-74-0110	Planning Report for an Epidemiological Study of Agricultural Workers Exposed to Noise	NTIS PB-83-234-989/A03
210-76-0153	A Comparison of Workers' Compensation Agricultural Data and the Farm Accident Survey in California	NTIS PB-83-127-530/A05
210-77-0110	An Analysis of Workers' Compensation Data in Agriculture	NTIS PB-80-193-915/A10

* National Technical Information Service, Park Royal Road, Springfield, VA 22161, 1 (703) 487-4650.
** NIOSH, DSDTT. Att: Publications, C-13, 4676 Columbia Parkway, Cincinnati, OH 45226-1998, 1 (513) 533-8287.

REFERENCES

1. Accidents claim 96,000 lives, but rate declining for some types. JAMA 262:2195, 1989.
2. National Safety Council: Accident Facts. 1990 edition. Chicago, National Safety Council, 1990.
3. Rivara FP: Fatal and nonfatal farm injuries to children and adolescents in the United States. Pediatrics 76:567–573, 1985.
4. Statistical Abstract of the United States, 1990. National Data Book and Guide to Sources, 110th edition. Washington, D.C., U.S. Department of Commerce, Bureau of the Census, 1990, pp 637–638.
5. U.S. Bureau of Labor Statistics Handbook of Labor Statistics. Washington, D.C., U.S. Government Printing Office, 1983.
6. Wilk V: The Occupational Health of Migrant and Seasonal Farmworkers in the United States, 2nd ed. Washington, D.C., Farmworker Justice Fund, 1986.

AARON BLAIR, PhD
SHELIA HOAR ZAHM, ScD

CANCER AMONG FARMERS

From the Occupational Studies
  Section
National Cancer Institute
Rockville, Maryland

Reprint requests to:
Aaron Blair, Ph.D.
Occupational Studies Section
National Cancer Institute
Executive Plaza North, Room 418
Rockville, MD 20892

The lifestyle of farmers is considered by many to be remarkably healthful due to hard physical work, fresh air, and consumption of home-grown foods. Although this perception is true to a considerable extent, the evidence has been increasing that farmers experience elevated risks for certain cancers. Consequently, a growing number of recent epidemiologic investigations have been designed to evaluate the risk of cancer among farmers.[14] This interest is warranted for several reasons. Although the proportion of farmers in the United States labor force has declined from approximately 40% in 1900 to 2% in 1980, it still represents one of the largest occupational groups in the United States with over 3 million persons in 1988. Cancer risk among farmers is, therefore, an important public health issue. In addition, there exists a large number of dependents of farmers who may also experience argriculture-related exposures. Farmers may come into contact with potentially hazardous agents as they apply pesticides and other agricultural chemicals, handle livestock, and operate and repair machinery. Some of these agents are known or suspected carcinogens.[12,14,109] Many of these exposures (e.g., pesticides, paints, solvents, engine exhausts, and fuels) may also occur among the general population and, thus, investigations of farmers, who may experience exposures that are heavier and of longer duration, may help identify environmental factors that affect cancer rates in the general population.

COHORT STUDIES AND DESCRIPTIVE
OCCUPATIONAL SURVEYS

Over 20 cohort studies of farmers and broad surveys of occupations, each evaluating risks from several diseases, have been conducted. These have included farming populations from many locations (i.e., United States, England and Wales, Australia, Denmark, Sweden, Canada, Finland, Iceland, and New Zealand), have employed different epidemiologic designs (i.e., proportionate mortality, cohort, and case-control), and have typically compared the risk of disease among farmers with the risk in the general population. Summaries of the results from these investigations are displayed in Table 1. Overall, farmers appear quite healthy. They are at lower risk for most major causes of death than the general population. Nearly all surveys show significant deficits for death from all causes combined, heart disease, and cancer. Relative risks for cancer of the esophagus, colon, bladder, and lung are also consistently depressed, with no studies showing significantly elevated excesses for these tumors. For cancers of the rectum, liver, pancreas, testis, kidney, and nose and naval cavities, relative risks greater than one occurred in some studies, but they were seldom statistically significant. On the other hand, a few cancers are often excessive among farmers. The cancers often occurring in excess include leukemia, non-Hodgkin's lymphoma, Hodgkin's disease, multiple myeloma, and cancers of the lip, stomach, skin (both melanoma and other skin cancers), prostate, brain, testis, and connective tissue. The low rates for most diseases but high rates for a few cancers are an unusual pattern that may be due to certain environmental exposures or lifestyle characteristics of farmers.

Epidemiologic research on farmers has tended to seek explanations for diseases that are in excess, whereas little attention has been paid to the deficits. Despite this focus on excesses, we should not lose sight of the fact that, with regard to health habits, farmers must be doing many things right. The deficits for all causes, heart disease, all cancer combined, and cancers of the esophagus, bladder, kidney, and lung may be partially or substantially due to the low prevalence of smoking observed among farmers in many countries around the world.[35,36,96,104,136,145] For example, the prevalence of smoking among farmers is often sufficiently lower than that of the general population to produce, by itself, a relative risk for lung cancer of about 0.6 compared to the general population.[7] A relative risk of 0.6 is approximately the midpoint of the range observed in the epidemiologic surveys summarized in Table 1. Physical activity may also contribute to lower mortality rates for some diseases. Farming is a physically demanding occupation, and physical activity has been inversely associated with a number of diseases, including some cancers.[5,26,58,62,142] Other factors including diet, living in relatively unpolluted areas, and selective migration of individuals with disease from the rural to urban areas, may also be involved, but information is not available to evaluate the effects of these factors on disease risks among farmers.

It is important to attempt to identify factors in the agricultural environment that might contribute to cancer excesses among farmers. Many agents in this environment have been suggested as potential risk factors for the excesses noted. Farmers typically perform many tasks, including machinery and engine repair, welding, painting, carpentry, operation of heavy equipment, truck driving, applying pesticides, and handling grains and livestock. These activities may result in exposure to pesticides, fuels and oils, solvents, engine exhausts, organic and inorganic dusts, metal fumes, paints, sunlight, electromagnetic radiation, and zoonotic viruses, microbes, and fungi.[43,50] Exposure to pesticides has received the

TABLE 1. Summary of Results from Descriptive Surveys of Disease Among Farmers*

Cause of Death/Disease	No. of Studies	Range of Relative Risks	No. of Risks > 1.0	No. of Signif. Elevated Risks	No. of Signif. Depressed Risks
All causes	13	0.6–0.9	0	0	13
Heart disease	19	0.6–1.0	1	0	13
All cancer	23	0.6–1.0	1	0	16
Specific cancer sites					
Lip	9	1.3–3.1	9	5	0
Esophagus	18	0.4–1.2	5	0	4
Stomach	23	0.5–1.7	12	8	2
Colon	18	0.4–2.3	4	0	8
Rectum	15	0.8–1.2	6	1	1
Liver	11	0.5–1.4	4	0	3
Pancreas	20	0.5–1.4	9	1	2
Melanoma	12	0.5–6.3	8	3	2
Other skin	8	0.8–1.8	7	3	0
Prostate	24	0.9–2.0	17	10	1
Testis	9	0.6–2.0	4	0	1
Bladder	22	0.5–1.1	2	0	8
Kidney	13	0.5–1.8	6	0	2
Brain	20	0.7–6.5	15	2	0
Nasal	6	0.6–1.8	2	0	0
Lung	26	0.4–0.9	0	0	21
Connective tissue	9	0.9–1.5	6	0	0
Non-Hodgkin's lymphoma	21	0.6–2.6	11	3	1
Hodgkin's disease	13	0.6–1.5	10	1	1
Multiple myeloma	16	0.4–3.1	12	4	0
Leukemia	21	0.3–2.0	12	3	0

* Data from refs. 23, 28, 29, 39, 41, 42, 47, 59, 61, 67, 80, 96, 98, 115, 119, 120, 123, 132, 134, 135, 143, 147, 150, 152.

most attention in epidemiologic studies and reviews of cancer among farmers.[6,14,109] However, evaluations are needed on other factors in the agricultural environment with carcinogenic potential.

INVESTIGATIONS OF SELECTED CANCERS

In addition to the availability of occupational surveys of cancer and other diseases that were summarized in Table 1, many investigations specifically designed to evaluate risk of specific cancers among farmers have been completed over the past decade. Results from investigations providing information on the 11 cancers often displaying excesses among farmers are presented in Table 2. Most of these studies were of a case-control design, but they varied widely in their focus. Some evaluated cancer risks only in regard to farming as an occupation, others focused on commodities produced, and a few have assessed exposure to specific substances, particularly to pesticides.

Leukemia

Two of the earliest investigations of cancer risks among farmers focused on hematopoietic and lymphatic cancer.[54,97] Nearly all studies of leukemia listed in Table 2 reported excess risk among farmers (32 of 39 comparisons), but only 10 were statistically significant. For all types of leukemia combined, these excesses

TABLE 2. Epidemiologic Studies of Selected Cancers Among Farmers

Author (Reference)	Location	Relative Risk	95% CI	Comments
Leukemia				
Blair[15]	Nebraska	1.2	(1.1–1.5)	All leukemia
Blair[17]	Nebraska	1.3	(NA)	ALL
		1.7	(NA)	CLL
		1.2	(NA)	AML
		1.1	(NA)	CML
Linos[89]	Minnesota	0.7	(0.3–1.2)	
Donham[44]	Iowa	1.5	(NA)	ALL in heavy dairying counties
Blair[16]	Wisconsin	1.1	(0.9–1.4)	All leukemia
		0.9	(0.4–2.1)	ALL
		1.2	(0.8–1.8	CLL
		1.1	(0.7–1.7)	AML
		1.8	(1.0–3.3)	CML
Burmeister[31]	Iowa	1.2	(1.1–1.4)	
Oleske[106]	Chicago	2.9	(0.8–9.9)	Hairy cell leukemia
Pearce[111]	New Zealand	1.2	(1.0–1.6)	All leukemia
		1.3	(0.6–3.0)	ALL
		1.1	(0.7–1.7)	CLL
		1.2	(0.8–1.9)	AML
		1.1	(0.6–2.2)	CML
Flodin[55]	Sweden	1.8	(1.0–3.1)	CLL
Fasal[54]	California	1.1	(NA)	Men
		1.1	(NA)	Women
Giles[63]	Tasmania	1.6	(NA)	AML among men
		2.5	(NA)	AML among women
		2.0	(NA)	CLL among men
		3.7	(NA)*	CLL among women
Milham[97]	Oregon	1.4	(NA)*	
	Washington	1.4	(NA)*	
Brownson[24]	Missouri	0.9	(0.5–1.6)	All leukemia
		2.8	(0.7–12.1)	ALL
		0.8	(0.4–2.0)	CLL
		0.6	(0.2–1.9)	AML
		1.5	(0.4–5.4)	CML
Brown[21]	Iowa/Minnesota	1.2	(1.0–1.5)	All leukemia
		1.2	(0.8–1.8)	AML
		1.1	(0.6–2.0)	CML
		0.9	(0.3–2.5)	ALL
		1.4	(1.1–1.9)	CLL
		0.8	(0.5–1.4)	Myelodysplasias
Hodgkin's Disease				
Matthews[92]	Australia	1.8	(0.7–4.0)	
Bernard[11]	England	1.7	(NA)	Not significant
Brownson[24]	Missouri	1.3	(0.4–4.5)	
Milham[97]	Oregon/Washington	1.1	(NA)	
Giles[63]	Tasmania	2.3	(NA)	Men
		4.0	(NA)	Women
Hoar[78]	Kansas	0.8	(0.3–1.9)	
La Vecchia[86]	Italy	2.1	(1.0–3.8)	
Fasal[54]	California	1.1	(NA)	Men
		0.5	(NA)	Women
Pearce[113]	New Zealand	1.1	(0.6–2.0)	Aged 20–64
		0.2	(0.1–1.4)	Aged 65+
Persson[114]	Sweden	1.2	(0.4–3.5)	
Dubrow[48]	Ohio	2.7	(NA)	
Balarajan[8]	England/Wales	3.1	(1.9–5.2)	

(Table continued on next page.)

TABLE 2 Epidemiologic Studies of Selected Cancers Among Farmers *(Cont.)*

Author (Reference)	Location	Relative Risk	95% CI	Comments
Multiple Myeloma				
Boffetta[20]	United States	3.4	(1.5–7.5)	
Cantor[34]	Wisconsin	1.4	(1.0–1.8)	
Tollerud[139]	North Carolina	0.6	(NA)	
Gallagher[60]	Vancouver	2.2	(1.2–4.0)	
Nandakumar[105]	Australia	1.4	(0.8–2.5)	
Steineck[133]	Sweden	1.2	(1.1–1.3)	
Pearce[113]	New Zealand	2.2	(1.3–3.8)	Aged 20–64
		1.2	(0.8–2.0)	Aged 65+
Burmeister[30]	Iowa	1.5	(NA)*	
Brownson[24]	Missouri	1.0	(0.4–2.3)	
Milham[97]	Oregon/Washington	1.8	(NA)*	
Giles[63]	Tasmania	0.8	(NA)	Men
		1.7	(NA)	Women
La Vecchia[86]	Italy	2.0	(1.1–3.5)	
Fasal[56]	California	1.0	(NA)	Men
		1.0	(NA)	Women
Flodin[56]	Sweden	1.9	(1.1–1.9)	Men and women
McLaughlin[95]	Sweden	1.2	(NA)*	
Cuzick[37]	England/Wales	1.6	(NA)	Risk calculated from percentages in paper
Non-Hodgkin's Lymphoma				
Fasal[54]	California	0.8	(NA)	Men
		0.8	(NA)	Women
La Vecchia[86]	Italy	1.9	(1.2–3.0)	
Hoar[78]	Kansas	1.4	(0.9–2.1)	
Giles[63]	Tasmania	1.8	(NA)*	Men
		1.7	(NA)	Women
Milham[97]	Oregon/Washington	1.3	(NA)	
Pearce[112]	New Zealand	1.1	(0.7–1.9)	ICD 200, aged 20–64
		0.9	(0.5–1.5)	ICD 200, aged 65+
		1.8	(1.0–3.0)	ICD 202, aged 20–64
		1.2	(0.6–2.1)	ICD 202, aged 65+
Brownson[24]	Missouri	1.1	(0.7–1.8)	
Burmeister[30]	Iowa	1.3	(NA)*	
Persson[114]	Sweden	0.3	(0.1–0.7)	
Franceschi[57]	Italy	0.9	(0.5–1.6)	
Pearce[113]	New Zealand	1.0	(0.8–1.4)	
Schumacher[124]	Utah	1.3	(0.9–2.3)	NHL
		1.9	(1.1–3.3)	Lymphocytic lymphoma
		0.9	(0.4–2.3)	Histiocytic lymphoma
Schumacher[125]	North Carolina	0.9	(0.6–1.2)	White men
		0.6	(0.3–1.3)	Black men
Cantor[33]	Wisconsin	1.2	(1.0–1.5)	
		1.4	(1.0–2.0)	Reticulum-cell
		1.2	(0.9–1.6)	Lymphosarcoma
Dubrow[48]	Ohio	1.6	(0.8–3.4)	
Balarajan[8]	England/Wales	1.8	(1.2–2.8)	Lymphosarcoma
Woods[153]	Washington	1.3	(1.0–1.7)	
Zahm[154]	Nebraska	0.9	(0.6–1.4)	
Band[10]	Canada	0.6	(0.4–1.1)	
Lip Cancer				
Dardanoni[38]	Sicily	2.6	(NA)*	
Keller[82]	United States	3.2	(NA)	Risk calculated from percentages in paper
Haguenoer[69]	France	5.3	(NA)*	

(Table continued on next page.)

TABLE 2 Epidemiologic Studies of Selected Cancers Among Farmers *(Cont.)*

Author (Reference)	Location	Relative Risk	95% CI	Comments
Skin Cancer				
Whitaker[147]	England	2.5	(NA)*	Squamous cell risk in 1931
		2.4	(NA)	Squamous cell risk in 1951
Lee[88]	England/Wales	1.1	(NA)	Melanoma in 1966–1967
		1.2	(NA)	Melanoma in 1968–1970
Graham[65]	New York	2.0	(0.4–10.9)	Melanoma
Brain Cancer				
Reif[121]	New Zealand	1.3	(1.0–1.7)	
Musicco[101]	Italy	5.0	(NA)*	
Musicco[102]	Italy	1.6	(1.1–2.4)	Also 1.6 with tumor controls
Preston-Martin[117]	Los Angeles	0.5	(NA)	Gliomas
Thomas[137]	United States	0.8	(0.3–1.7)	In Louisiana, New Jersey and Philadelphia
Brownson[26]	Missouri	1.1	(0.6–1.7)	1.5 for crop farmers
McLaughlin[95]	Sweden	1.1	(NA)	
Soft-tissue Sarcoma				
Smith[131]	New Zealand	0.6	(0.4–1.1)	
Balarajan[9]	England/Wales	1.7	(1.00–2.88)	
Hoar[78]	Kansas	1.0	(0.7–1.6)	
Woods[153]	Washington	1.2	(0.8–1.9)	
Vineis[144]	Italy	2.7	(0.5–14.7)	Female rice weeders
Stomach Cancer				
Burmeister[30]	Iowa	1.3	(NA)*	
Higginson[77]	Kansas	1.6	(NA)	Risk calculated from percentages in paper
Kraus[84]	New York	8.3	(NA)*	Exposed to iron and grain dust
Sigurjonsson[130]	Iceland	1.8	(NA)	Risk calculated from percentages in paper
Armijo[4]	Chile	1.2	(NA)	Risk calculated from percentages in paper
Kneller[83]	China	2.3	(NA)*	4.0 for male grain farmers and 4.1 for female grain farmers
Prostate Cancer				
Burmeister[30]	Iowa	1.2	(NA)*	
Schuman[126]	Minnesota	0.7	(NA)	Risk calculated from percentages in paper
Pearce[110]	New Zealand	1.1	(0.9–1.5)	
Testicular Cancer				
Mills[99]	United States	6.3	(1.8–21.5)	4.6 for crop farmers, 3.6 for livestock farmers
Jensen[81]	Denmark	1.0	(0.6–1.7)	
McDowall[93]	England/Wales	1.9	(1.0–3.6)	
Brown[22]	United States	0.9	(0.6–1.4)	
Haughey[74]	New York	1.5	(0.9–2.5)	Persons exposed to fertilizer
Wiklund[148]	Sweden	1.6	(0.9–2.4)	Pesticide cohort
Hayes[75]	Unites States	1.2	(0.4–1.2)	Exposed to pesticides

* p < 0.05.
ALL = acute lymphocytic leukemia; AML = acute myelocytic leukemia; CLL = chronic lymphocytic leukemia; CML = chronic myelocytic leukemia; NHL = non-Hodgkin's lymphoma; NA = not available.

were small and relative risks (RRs) ranged from 1.1 to 1.4. There was no clear pattern by histologic type. In some studies,[16,17] histologic type was based on information from the death certificate, an approach with distinct limitations. The patterns by histologic type from incidence studies, however, were not entirely consistent either. In studies based on death certificates, farmers were at greater risk of chronic lymphatic leukemia (CLL) in Nebraska[17] and chronic myeloid leukemia (CML) in Wisconsin.[16] In the incidence studies, farmers from Sweden,[55] Tasmania,[63] and Iowa/Minnesota[21] experienced the greatest risk from CLL, whereas farmers in Missouri[24] had a deficit of CLL and the greatest excess for ALL. In Nebraska,[15] Iowa,[31] and Wisconsin[16] risks of leukemia were slightly higher among farmers born more recently than those born earlier, a pattern that suggests that the factors involved may have been those more recently introduced into the agricultural environment. These three studies evaluated leukemia risks by agricultural commodity, based on county of residence of the subject. Results were not highly consistent. Higher risks of leukemia occurred among farmers from heavy corn- and cattle-producing areas in Nebraska,[15] from corn, soybean, chicken, and herbicide areas in Iowa,[31] and corn, dairy products, fertilizer, and insecticide areas in Wisconsin.[16] Livestock farmers in New Zealand were at greater risk of leukemia (RR = 3.0) than other farmers,[111] but no association was observed between types of crops or animals raised in the study in Iowa and Minnesota.[21]

One of the earliest efforts to evaluate specific factors was by Donham et al.,[44] in which leukemia risks were evaluated among farmers who may have had contact with cattle carrying the bovine leukemia virus. Donham et al.[44] found that risk of acute lymphatic leukemia (ALL) was greater among men from heavy dairying counties in Iowa (RR = 1.5), particularly from counties where the herds were infected with bovine leukemia virus (RR = 1.7). On the other hand, the risk of leukemia and individual histologic types among dairy farmers in Wisconsin were similar to that among all farmers.[16] The bovine leukemia virus is readily transmitted among dairy cattle,[49,116] and to sheep and goats,[79] and in cell cultures,[66] but there is no serologic evidence to date that this virus can be transmitted to humans.[32,45] The epidemiologic and serologic data do not, therefore, provide strong evidence that cancer in humans is related to the bovine leukemia virus.

The viral hypothesis has recently been raised as an explanation for findings in New Zealand. Pearce and Reif[109] summarized information from a series of case-control studies in New Zealand that linked soft tissue sarcoma, non-Hodgkin's lymphoma, and acute myeloid leukemia with abattoir workers. Some abattoir workers may be exposed to chemicals in the treatment of pelts and plastics and their thermal decomposition products. Cancer risks among workers in these areas, however, were not different from other abattoir workers. Pearce and Reif[109] believe that these findings are consistent with a viral etiology.

Two studies have linked risk of leukemia with use of pesticides. Individuals reporting the use of DDT in Sweden[55] had elevated rates of CLL (RR = 1.8)), as did farmers in Iowa/Minnesota[21] (RR = 1.3), particularly for CLL (RR = 1.5). Among Iowa/Minnesota farmers,[21] leukemia was also associated with use of certain animal insecticides (crotoxyphos [RR = 11.1], dichlorvos [RR = 2.0], famphur [RR = 2.2], pyrethrins [RR = 3.7], and nicotine [RR = 1.6]). No significantly elevated risks, however, were associated with use of insecticides on crops. This difference in risk from use of pesticides on crops and animals may occur because animals are often treated in confined quarters where the farmer's potential for exposure could be greater. Leukemia has also been linked to pesticides in studies not specifically focusing on farmers.[27,85,90,91,129]

Hodgkin's Disease

Twelve of 15 comparisons of Hodgkin's disease in Table 2 found excesses of Hodgkin's disease among farmers, with two[8,86] being statistically significant. Analytic studies are inconsistent with regard to specific agents that might be involved. Hodgkin's disease has been linked with exposure to phenoxyacetic acids and chlorophenols[71,114] in Sweden, but not in the United States.[78] One difference between the Swedish and American studies is that in the U.S. all exposures occurred specifically among farmers, whereas in Sweden exposed persons may have included those in other occupations such as forestry and right-of-way workers who may have received higher exposures. Persson et al.[114] found Hodgkin's disease to be elevated among persons exposed to DDT (RR = 7.5), pesticides other than phenoxyacid herbicides or DDT (RR = 2.0), and creosote (RR = 10.7). Zahm et al.[155] found no association between insecticides, herbicides, or crops grown and Hodgkin's disease among Kansas farmers. In a study from Italy, the proportion of cases and controls exposed to herbicides did not indicate an association, although relative risks were not presented.[86] A cluster of Hodgkin's disease cases residing near a grain elevator has been linked to exposure to potential mitogenic factors.[127] The authors hypothesized a mechanism of chronic immune stimulation from grain dusts. This cancer was not excessive, however, among a large cohort of grain workers.[1] Another explanation might lie in the infectious model proposed by Gutensohn and Cole.[68] According to this hypothesis, delay in infection by the Epstein-Barr virus increases the risk of Hodgkin's disease. The relative isolation of farm families compared to urban dwellers might delay contact with the virus and thereby increase the risk of cancer. We are unaware of any studies that have tested this hypothesis in relation to farmers.

Multiple Myeloma

Fourteen of 19 comparisons in Table 2 found excesses of multiple myeloma among farmers, and 10 were statistically significant. In death certificate studies in Iowa[30] and Wisconsin,[34] the risk of multiple myeloma was greater among farmers residing in counties where insecticides were heavily used and in counties with large chicken inventories than among farmers residing in other counties. In Wisconsin,[34] the risk was greater among farmers residing in heavy insecticide-using counties if they were born after 1905 (RR = 2.8) than if born earlier (RR = 0.8). The farming experience of these younger farmers is more likely to encompass the chemical age of farming and suggests that factors recently introduced into the agricultural environment after the 1930s may be involved. Among participants in a prospective study conducted by the American Cancer Society,[20] multiple myeloma was associated with exposure to pesticides (RR = 2.1) and diesel exhausts (RR = 1.4). Farmers exposed to pesticides were at a particularly high risk. Compared to persons who were not farmers and unexposed to pesticides, the authors reported relative risks of 1.0 for multiple myeloma among nonfarmers exposed to pesticides, 1.7 among farmers unexposed to pesticides, and 4.3 among farmers exposed to pesticides. In another study in the U.S., exposure to pesticides, not exclusively among farmers, was associated with a significant risk (RR = 2.6).[100] Gallagher et al.[60] reported an interesting association between farmers exposed to processed grains and multiple myeloma (RR = 2.4), resembling reports of excesses from exposures to other organic dusts in the wood, leather, and textile industries,[122] which may point to a general effect of organic dusts.

Non-Hodgkin's Lymphoma

Eighteen of 29 comparisons in Table 2 showed excesses of non-Hodgkin's lymphoma among farmers. Although nine relative risks are statistically significant, none is greater than 2-fold. The agricultural factor most prominently linked with non-Hodgkin's lymphoma has been exposure to phenoxyacetic acid herbicides. This link was first noted in Sweden where a 6-fold risk was reported for those (farmers and others) exposed to phenoxyacetic acids or chlorophenols.[71] Studies of farmers in the U.S. and Canada generated similar findings. The risk of non-Hodgkin's lymphoma was significantly elevated among Kansas farmers using phenoxyacetic acid herbicides (RR = 2.2).[78] Risks rose with days per year of use of herbicides to over 7-fold among those reporting use of 21 or more days per year and who specifically reported they had used 2,4-D. This was a highly significant trend. This excess could not be accounted for by exposure to insecticides or other herbicides, or other risk factors for non-Hodgkin's lymphoma. A recent study of similar design in Nebraska also noted an increased risk of non-Hodgkin's lymphoma among farmers who mixed or applied the herbicide 2,4-D (RR = 1.5).[154] The relative risk rose to over 3-fold among farmers who reported using 2,4-D for 21 or more days per year, a pattern that could not be accounted for by other pesticide exposures. Farmers in Washington state with exposure to phenoxyacetic acid herbicides had a significantly elevated risk (RR = 1.3), but information on risk by days per year of use was not collected.[153] In a cohort mortality study of farmers in Saskatchewan, Canada, non-Hodgkin's lymphoma was also associated with use of herbicides.[147] Among farmers with operations of less than 1000 acres, relative risks rose with the number of acres sprayed with herbicides from 1.3 for < 100 acres, 1.9 for 100 to 249 acres, to 2.2 for 250 or more acres. No other cause of death showed this pattern. Although the association is with herbicides in general, the authors point out that in the 1960s 90% of herbicides used by weight in Saskatchewan was 2,4-D, and it still accounted for 75% of the use in the 1970s. It seems unlikely, therefore, that the association could be due to some herbicide other than 2,4-D. Persson et al.[114] reported nearly a 5-fold risk among persons exposed to phenoxyacetic acids, even though, as an occupation, farmers were not at excess risk. The proportion of non-Hodgkin's lymphoma cases in an Italian study reporting exposure with herbicides was approximately twice that reported among the controls, although relative risks were not presented.[86] Not all populations exposed to phenoxyacetic acid herbicides have had excess risks of non-Hodgkin's lymphoma. No excess was observed among all farmers in a case-control study from New Zealand.[112] Risks were not elevated among farmers most likely to have had contact with phenoxyacetic acid herbicides, nor did risks among exposed workers in New Zealand increase consistently with days per year of use,[108] as occurred in studies in Kansas[78] and Nebraska.[154] Among New Zealand farmers, relative risks were 0.9, 1.2, 2.2, and 1.1 for < 5, 5–9, 10–19, and 20 or more days per year of use, respectively.[108] Lymphoma was not excessive among Swedish pesticide applicators (RR = 1.01), among whom 72% reported they had used phenoxy acid herbicides.[149]

Factors in the agricultural environment other than phenoxyacetic acid herbicides have also been associated with non-Hodgkin's lymphoma. Although based on only three exposed cases, farmers in Kansas exposed to triazine herbicides experienced a relative risk of 2.2 (95% CI = 1.2–4.1) for non-Hodgkin's lymphoma that could not be accounted for by exposure to phenoxyacetic acid herbicides.[78] Few epidemiologic studies have evaluated the carcinogenic potential of triazine herbicides, but exposure to this chemical has been associated with ovarian cancer in a study in Italy.[46] Zahm et al.[154] reported that use of organophosphate insecticides by Nebraska farmers resulted in an increased risk of 2.4 that was independent of the effects of 2,4-D. Among Nebraska farmers, risk rose with days per year of organophosphate use, from 1.7 for 1–5 days, to 1.8 for 6–20 days, to 3.1 for 21 or more days. Fungicides were associated with non-Hodgkin's lymphoma among farmers from Kansas (RR = 2.1)[78] but not from Nebraska.[154] Among Saskatchewan farmers, risk was associated with fuel expenditures independently from risks from herbicide exposures.[147] The risk rose to 2.3 in the high expenditure category. The risk of non-Hodgkin's lymphoma among New Zealand farmers doing fencing work (RR = 1.4) could be due to their contact with pentachlorophenol used to preserve wooden posts.[112] In death certificate studies, non-Hodgkin's lymphoma was associated with hog, milk, and egg production and herbicide use in Iowa[30] and with hog, milk, chicken, and corn production and fertilizer, herbicide, and insecticide in Wisconsin.[33]

Lip Cancer

Nine of nine occupational surveys in Table 1 had excesses of lip cancer among farmers and five were significant excesses. These excesses are consistent with associations with many outdoor occupations and have been attributed to solar radiation. Case-control studies (see Table 2) in Sicily,[38] the United States,[82] and France,[69] with relative risks of 2.6, 3.2, and 5.3 among farmers, further indicate that farmers are at high risk of this rare cancer.

Skin Cancer

Among surveys of farmers, eight of 12 showed excesses of melanoma and seven of eight showed excesses of other skin cancer (Table 1). The excesses of both melanotic and nonmelanotic skin cancer among farmers is consistent with patterns by latitude of residence and likely related to heavy exposure to ultraviolet radiation because of the outdoor nature of their work.[88,128] Melanoma was elevated among New York farmers.[65] In a study in Great Britain farmers were found to be at particularly high risk for cancers on the arms and ears.[146] A few reports in the literature have associated skin cancer with various chemicals, including polychlorinated biphenyls, polycyclic aromatic hydrocarbons, arsenic, and pesticides,[87,128] and these are all substances with which farmers may have contact.

Brain Cancer

Fifteen of the 20 surveys in Table 1 found excesses of brain cancer among farmers, and five of seven studies in Table 2 noted excesses. The etiology of brain cancer is poorly understood, but a variety of chemical exposures, including solvents, lubricating oil, phenolic compounds, polycyclic aromatic hydrocarbons, electromagnetic radiation, and pesticides, have been postulated as risk factors.[138]

No association was observed between farming as an occupation and brain cancer in case-control studies in the United States[117,137] and Sweden.[94] The two studies in the U.S., however, were not located in major agricultural areas (one was in Los Angeles[117] and the other in New Jersey, Philadelphia, and New Orleans[137]).

Brain cancer was excessive among Missouri farmers, particularly for nonastrocytomas (RR = 5.3).[25] Elevated risks were observed among Italian[101,102] and New Zealand[121] farmers. The studies in Italy suggest that farmers who engaged in farming in more recent times had higher risks. Those engaged in farming only before 1960 had a relative risk of 0.9, those engaged both before and after 1960 had 2.5, and those engaged only after 1960 had 5.7.[101] The risk was also considerably greater among those employed as farmers for 10 or more years after 1960 (RR = 4.8) than among those who worked less than 10 years after 1960 (RR = 1.9). A later study by these investigators[102] found a slight excess of brain cancer among farmers who reported little use of agricultural chemicals (RR = 1.2), but a significant excess among those who relied on such chemicals (RR = 1.6). They observed relative risks of 2.0 among farmers who used insecticides and fungicides, 1.6 among those used herbicides, and 1.4 among those who used fertilizers. Use of herbicides and fertilizer in the absence of exposure to insecticides was not associated with brain cancer (RR = 0.9). In related investigations, brain cancer was more common among children who lived on farms than those who had not.[64,151] Higher levels of organochlorine compounds have been found in the adipose tissue of brain cancer patients than in noncancer patients.[140] Insecticides have well-known neurotoxic effects.[51] Some have been found in brain tissue,[76,118] so they are able to cross the blood-brain barrier. It should perhaps not be surprising if some insecticides prove to cause nervous system cancers in humans.

Soft-tissue Sarcoma (Connective Tissue)

Six of nine surveys in Table 1 showed excesses of cancer of the connective tissue among farmers, but none was statistically significant. Three of five studies in Table 2 had excesses among farmers. Several investigations in Sweden have linked soft-tissue sarcoma with exposure to phenoxyacetic acid herbicides and chlorophenols (not necessarily among farmers).[53,72,73] Relative risks were quite high among subjects exposed to phenoxyacetic acid herbicides from northern Sweden (RR = 5.3)[73] and southern Sweden (RR = 6.8).[53] A more recent study found an association with phenoxyacetic acids (RR = 3.3), but not with chlorophenols.[72] Women in Italy exposed to the phenoxyacetic acid, 2,4,5-T, during the weeding of rice fields had a significant excess of soft-tissue sarcoma (RR = 2.7).[144] No significant association between soft-tissue sarcoma and phenoxyacetic herbicides was seen in case-control studies in Kansas (RR = 1.4),[12] Washington (RR = 0.9),[153] and New Zealand (RR = 0.6).[131]

Contact with insecticides has been associated with soft-tissue sarcoma. Although Kansas farmers overall experienced no excess risk for soft-tissue sarcoma, there was a slight risk among those using insecticides (RR = 1.3) and a greater risk among those using insecticides on animals (RR = 1.6).[155] The risk rose with increasing time since first use to a relative risk of 4.9 among those first using insecticides on animals in 1945 or earlier.

Stomach Cancer

Twelve of 23 studies in Table 1 noted excesses for stomach cancer among farmers, with eight being statistically significant. Few analytic studies have focused on this association, but excesses were observed among farmers in six of six studies in Table 2. The case-control studies that have linked stomach cancer with farming in Iowa,[30] Kansas,[77] New York,[84] Iceland,[130] Chile,[4] and China[83] generally were not designed to identify specific factors in the agricultural environment that might be involved. The risk of stomach cancer, however, was particularly high among grain farmers in China.[83] A role for pesticides is suggested by the 5-fold risk observed among pesticide production workers in the study from China.[83] Stomach cancer has also occurred in excess among occupation cohorts exposed to herbicides and among laboratory animals in bioassays of certain pesticides (dichlorvos, alachlor, sufallate, chlorthalonil, dichlorobromopropane, and dichloropropene).[12] Nitrates have been associated with stomach cancer in epidemiologic and experimental investigations.[103] This is a particular concern regarding cancer risks among farmers because of the growing contamination of drinking water sources with nitrates in agricultural areas.[70]

Prostate Cancer

Seventeen of 24 comparisons in Table 1 showed excesses of prostate cancer among farmers. Ten of these excesses were statistically significant. Relative risks in the surveys and case-control studies were small (less than 2.0). Although no specific factors in the agricultural environment have been linked with this tumor, the excess among farmers is of special concern because prostate cancer is the most common tumor among men.

Testicular Cancer

Although only four of nine studies in Table 1 noted excesses of testicular cancer among farmers, the report of a 6-fold excess among farmers in the United States[99] generated several other evaluations. In Sweden, the incidence of testicular cancer increased more rapidly between 1961 and 1979 among agricultural workers than among other workers.[148] A small increase in risk occurred among farmers in England and Wales (RR = 1.57).[93] No excesses were observed, however, among American[22] or Danish farmers.[81] Despite the lack of an association with farmers in general,[22] self-reported exposure to pesticides by farmers in the study in the U.S.[75] was associated with relative risks of 1.2 (95% CI = 0.4–1.2) for all testicular cancers and 1.5 (95% CI = 0.9–2.7) for germinal cell tumors other than seminomas. A nonsignificant excess occurred among persons exposed to fertilizers (not necessarily farmers) in New York[74] and a nonsignificant excess (RR = 1.6) occurred among pesticide applicators.[148]

STUDIES OF RELATED OCCUPATIONS

Cancer risks have been assessed in relation to pesticide exposures in occupational groups other than farmers (see reviews by Axelson[6] and Blair[14]). Veterinarians who may share exposures to insecticides and zoonotic viruses and microbes with farmers experience elevated rates of cancer of the lymphatic and hematopoietic system, skin, and brain.[13] The leukemia excess among veterinarians was probably linked to x-ray exposure, because it was mostly confined to persons who practiced during the 1950s and 1960s when radiography was used without careful control. Skin cancer occurred among practitioners with large animal practices in accord with their greater exposure to sunlight. No specific agent was related to brain cancer, because this tumor was elevated in large and small animal veterinarians as well as nonpractitioners such as regulators and meat inspectors.

During handling of grains and livestock feeds, farmers may come into contact with grain dusts, aflatoxins, and fumigants. Studies of livestock feed processors in Denmark[107] and grain handlers in the United States[1] have noted excesses of lymphatic cancer (multiple myeloma in Denmark and non-Hodgkin's lymphoma in the U.S.). Cancers of the liver, gall bladder, and salivary glands were also elevated among Danish workers,[107] and pancreatic cancer was excessive among American grain workers.[1] The excess in the Danish workers may be due to aflatoxins because of their contact with peanut cakes, which are often heavily contaminated with fungi. Exposures to grain dusts and fumigants are the more likely explanations for the excesses among grain workers in the U.S., because aflatoxin is not as serious a problem in this industry as in the peanut industry.

Lymphatic and hematopoietic cancer has been associated with certain occupations in the United States Department of Agriculture (USDA). County extension agents experienced elevated mortality from Hodgkin's disease, non-Hodgkin's lymphoma, multiple myeloma, and leukemia and cancers of the colon, prostate, and brain.[2] The risk of leukemia rose with duration of employment as a county agent to nearly 3-fold among those employed for 15 or more years. Risks of multiple myeloma and non-Hodgkin's lymphoma were also greatest in the 15 or more year category, but the trends were not statistically significant. Forest and soil conservationists in the USDA experienced significant excesses of non-Hodgkin's lymphoma and cancers of the colon, prostate, and kidney.[3] A significant trend between non-Hodgkin's lymphoma and colon cancer was observed with duration of employment for both soil and forest conservationists.

CONCLUSIONS

Results from surveys in many countries indicate that farmers tend to have a lower mortality from all causes combined, heart disease, all cancer combined, and for specific tumors, particularly those of the esophagus, colon, bladder, and lung, than other occupational groups. Despite this favorable overall disease experience, studies often find that farmers have elevated risks for certain malignancies, including leukemia, Hodgkin's disease, non-Hodgkin's lymphoma, multiple myeloma, and cancers of the lip, stomach, skin (melanotic and nonmelanotic), prostate, brain, and connective tissue. The occurrence of these excesses in many investigations of different epidemiologic designs from a number of countries indicates that they are unlikely to be spurious findings. An intriguing point is that several of the cancers in excess among farmers (multiple myeloma, non-Hodgkin's lymphoma, melanoma, and cancer of the brain) are also tumors that are reportedly increasing in several countries around the world.[40] Understanding the reasons for the high rates among farmers may, therefore, provide leads to the causes for the rising rates in the general population.

The relative risks for most cancers among farmers are of small-to-moderate size (cancer of the lip is an exception), and considerable variability exists from study to study. Variation in estimates of risk is to be expected for several reasons. First, there may simply be chance variation. Even for clearly established causal factors for cancer, risk estimates vary by study. For example, prospective studies of cancer and smoking report relative risks of bladder cancer from 1.4 to 3.0.[136] Second, any exposure classification scheme that groups all farmers together is likely to be inaccurate and cause variation in estimates, because all farmers do not have the same exposures. Third, even in investigations where attempts are made to assess specific agricultural exposures, the method employed may influence risk estimates.[18] In case-control studies of non-Hodgkin's lymphoma and herbicide use, risks rose significantly with increasing frequency of use, but not with years of use or acres treated.[78,154] Misclassification of exposures must certainly exist in studies of farmers and, in general, it has been well-established that misclassification of exposure in epidemiologic studies typically reduces relative risks and dilutes exposure-response gradients. Given the difficulty of making accurate quantitative assessments of agricultural exposures and the tendency for misclassification to bias risk estimates toward the null value, it is not surprising that relative risks are small and vary from study to study.

Attempts to identify the specific agents in the agricultural environment that might account for these excesses among farmers have only recently begun, and additional studies with this goal are needed. Some factors have already been linked to cancer risks among farmers. The excesses of cancer of the lip and skin among farmers are likely due to exposure to solar radiation. Exposure to pesticides has been associated with cancers of the lymphatic and hematopoietic system and brain. Associations between phenoxyacetic acid herbicides and non-Hodgkin's lymphoma in several countries from case-control and cohort designs and the existence of sharp exposure-response gradients build a strong case for a role for these herbicides in the development of non-Hodgkin's lymphoma among farmers. Organophosphate insecticides and fungicides may contribute to farmers' risk of non-Hodgkin's lymphoma, leukemia, soft-tissue sarcoma, and brain cancer, but the evidence is not as strong for phenoxyacetic herbicides and non-Hodgkin's lymphoma. There are few data to indicate which factors might account for the reported excesses of cancer of the stomach and prostate. Stomach cancer has been linked with ingestion of nitrates, and, given the growing contamination of the drinking water from fertilizer runoff, this deserves a more thorough evaluation.

In the United States, government attention to issues of exposure and chronic disease in agriculture has not been as focused as for other industries,[52] because work on the farm typically is performed by family members and is not affected by state or federal labor regulations.[141] This appears to be changing somewhat, because the Occupational Safety and Health Administration has announced a series of meetings around the country to discuss the development of Permissible Exposure Levels for agriculture. In the meantime, health care providers in rural areas can help fill this void by being aware of potential chronic disease risks associated with agricultural practices and reinforcing the need for prudent use of agricultural chemicals by providing advice regarding potential hazards. Training programs to enhance physicians' skills in diagnosis and treatment of chronic disease arising from agricultural exposures would be timely.

Additional support is needed for research on cancer risks in the agricultural community. The major limitation in studies of cancer among farmers is the difficulty in accurately estimating relevant exposures. Farmers have contact with a variety of chemicals, and these exposures change over time. This creates uncertainty in relating cancer to specific chemicals, particularly in studies where exposure is based on subject recall. Undoubtedly current assessment techniques result in considerable misclassification by exposure. Nondirectional misclassification, the type most likely to occur in this situation, tends to reduce risk estimates and to dilute exposure-response gradients.[18] Although this problem does not tend to create false positive findings, it is not reassuring that hazards may be missed because of inaccurate evaluation of exposures. The problem of accurate assessment of exposure is not unique to studies of farmers but must be faced in most epidemiologic investigations of diseases with long latencies. Studies of dietary factors associated with cancer are equally difficult. In contrast with diet, however, relatively little methodologic research has been conducted with respect to the reliability and validity of the techniques employed to estimate agricultural exposures, and such work is urgently needed. Two approaches could be employed to address this problem. Methodologic investigations are needed to identify the best techniques for characterizing exposures in retrospective studies. For example, methodologic studies should be undertaken to evaluate the comparability of information obtained from farmers themselves versus their next-of-kin, from interviews and reinterviews, from records of farm activities versus interviews, from different air and biologic monitoring techniques, and from monitoring versus interviews and records.[18] Prospective studies offer another approach for dealing with uncertainties associated with exposure assessment. This design requires large numbers of subjects when the focus is on relatively rare diseases such as cancer.

REFERENCES

1. Alavanja MCR, Blair A, Masters MN: Cancer mortality in the U.S. flour industry. JNCI 82:840–848, 1990.
2. Alavanja MCR, Blair A, Merkle S, et al: Mortality among agricultural extension agents. Am J Ind Med 14:167–176, 1988.
3. Alavanja MCR, Blair A, Merkle S, et al: Mortality among forest and soil conservationists. Arch Environ Health 44:94–101, 1989.
4. Armijo R, Orellana M, Medina E, et al: Epidemiology of gastric cancer in Chile: I. Case-control study. Int J Epidemiol 10:53–56, 1981.
5. Albanes D, Blair A, Taylor PR: Physical activity and risk of cancer in the NHANES I population. Am J Public Health 79:744–750, 1989.
6. Axelson O: Pesticides and cancer risks in agriculture. Med Oncol Tumor Pharmacother 4:207–217, 1987.
7. Axelson O, Steenland K: Indirect methods of assessing the effects of tobacco use in occupational studies. Am J Ind Med 13:105–118, 1988.
8. Balarajan R: Malignant lymphomas in agricultural and forestry workers in England and Wales. Public Health 102:585–592, 1988.
9. Balarajan R, Acheson ED: Soft tissue sarcomas in agriculture and forestry workers. J Epid Comm Health 38:113–116, 1984.
10. Band PR, Spinelli JJ, Gallagher RP, et al: Identification of occupational cancer risks using a population-based cancer registry. In Band P: Occupational Cancer Epidemiology. Recent Results in Cancer Research 120. Berlin, Springer-Verlag, 1990, pp 106, 182–189.
11. Bernard SM, Cartwright RA, Darwin CM, et al: Hodgkin's disease: Case control epidemiological study in Yorkshire. Br J Cancer 55:85–90, 1987.
12. Blair A, Axelson O, Franklin C, et al: Carcinogenic effects of pesticides. In Baker SR, Wilkinson CF: The Effects of Pesticides on Human Health. Princeton, NJ, Princeton Sci Publ Co, Adv Mod Environ Toxicol XVIII:201–260, 1990.
13. Blair A, Hayes HM Jr: Mortality patterns among US veterinarians, 1947–1977: An expanded study. Int J Epidemiol 11:391–397, 1982.
14. Blair A, Malker H, Cantor KP, et al: Cancer among farmers—A review. Scand J Work Environ Health 11:397–407, 1985.
15. Blair A, Thomas TL: Leukemia among Nebraska farmers: A death certificate study. Am J Epidemiol 110:264–273, 1979.
16. Blair A, White DW: Death certificate study of leukemia among farmers from Wisconsin. JNCI 66:1027–1030, 1981.
17. Blair A, White DW: Leukemia cell types and agricultural practices in Nebraska. Arch Environ Health 40:211–214, 1985.
18. Blair A, Zahm SH: Methodologic issues in exposure assessment for case-control studies of cancer and herbicides. Am J Ind Med 18:285–293, 1990.
19. Blair SN, Kohl HW, Paffenbarger RS Jr, et al: Physical fitness and all-cause mortality—A prospective study of healthy men and women. J Am Med Assoc 262:2395–2401, 1989.
20. Boffetta P, Stellman SD, Garfinkel L: A case-control study of multiple myeloma nested in the American Cancer Society prospective study. Int J Cancer 43:554–559, 1989.
21. Brown LM, Blair A, Gibson R, et al: Pesticide exposures and other agricultural risk factors for leukemia among men in Iowa and Minnesota. Can Res 50:6585–6591, 1990.
22. Brown LM, Pottern LM: Testicular cancer and farming. Lancet i:1356, 1984.

23. Brownson RC, Reif JS, Chang JC, Chang JC: Cancer risks among Missouri farmers. Cancer 64:2381–2386, 1989.
24. Brownson RC, Reif JS: A cancer registry-based study of occupational risk for lymphoma, multiple myeloma, and leukemia. Int J Epidemiol 17:27–32, 1988.
25. Brownson RC, Reif JS, Chang J, Davis JR: An analysis of occupational risks for brain cancer. Am J Public Health 80:169–172, 1990.
26. Brownson RC, Zahm SH, Chang JC, Blair A: Occupational risk of colon cancer—An analysis by anatomic subsite. Am J Epidemiol 130:675–687, 1989.
27. Buckley JD, Robison LL, Swotinksy R, et al: Occupational exposures of parents of children with acute nonlymphocytic leukemia: A report from the Childrens Cancer Study Group. Cancer Res 49:4030–4037, 1989.
28. Buesching DP, Wollstadt L: Cancer mortality among farmers. JNCI 72:503, 1984.
29. Burmeister LF: Cancer mortality in Iowa farmers, 1971–1978. JNCI 66:461–464, 1981.
30. Burmeister LF, Everett GD, Van Lier SF, Isacson P: Selected cancer mortality and farm practices in Iowa. Am J Epidemiol 118:72–77, 1983.
31. Burmeister LF, Van Lier Sf, Isacson P: Leukemia and farm practices in Iowa. Am J Epidemiol 115:720–728, 1982.
32. Caldwell GG, Baumgartener L, Carter C: Seroepidemiologic testing in man for evidence of antibodies to feline leukemia virus and bovine leukemia virus. Bibl Haematol 43:238–241, 1976.
33. Cantor KP: Farming and mortality from non-Hodgkin's lymphoma: A case-control study. Int J Cancer 29:239–247, 1982.
34. Cantor KP, Blair A: Farming and mortality from multiple myeloma: A case-control study with the use of death certificates. JNCI 72:251–255, 1984.
35. Cassel J, Bartel AG, Kaplan BH, et al: Occupational and physical activity and coronary heart disease. Arch Intern Med 128:920–928, 1971.
36. Central Bureau of Statistics. Smoking habits n Sweden: A mail survey—Spring, 1963. Stockholm, 1965.
37. Cuzick J, De Stavola B: Multiple myeloma—a case-control study. Br J Cancer 57:516–520, 1988.
38. Dardanoni L, Gafa L, Paterno R, Pavone G: A case-control study on lip cancer risk factors in Ragusa (Sicily). Int J Cancer 34:335–337, 1984.
39. Danmarks Statistik. Dodelighed og erhverv, 1970–75. Statistiske undersogelser nr 37. Kobenhavn, 1979.
40. Davis DL, Hoel D, Fox J, Lopez A: International trends in cancer mortality in France, West Germany, Italy, Japan, England and Wales, and the USA. Lancet 336:474–481, 1990.
41. Decoufle P, Stanislawizyk K, Houten L, et al: A retrospective survey of cancer in relation to occupation. National Institute for Occupational Safety and Health. DHEW (NIOSH) Publ. No. 77–178. Cincinnati, OH, 1977.
42. Delzell E, Grufferman S: Mortality among white and nonwhite farmers in North Carolina, 1976–1978. Am J Epidemiol 121:391–402, 1985.
43. Donham KJ: Hazardous agents in agricultural dusts and methods of evaluation. Am J Ind Med 10:205–220, 1986.
44. Donham KJ, Berg JW, Sawin RS: Epidemiologic relationships of the bovine population and human leukemia in Iowa. Am J Epidemiol 112:80–92, 1980.
45. Donham KJ, Van DerMaaten MJ, Miller JM, et al: Seroepidemiologic studies on the possible relationships of human and bovine leukemia: Brief communication. JNCI 59:851–853, 1977.
46. Donna A, Crosignani P, Robutti F, et al: Triazine herbicides and ovarian epithelial neoplasms. Scand J Work Environ Health 15:47–53, 1989.
47. Dubrow R, Wegman DH: Occupational characteristics of cancer victims in Massachusetts 1971–1973. National Institute for Occupational Safety and Health. DHEW (NIOSH) Publ. No. 84–109. Cincinnatti, OH, 1984.
48. Dubrow R, Paulson JO, Indian RW: Farming and malignant lymphoma in Hancock County, Ohio. Br J Ind Med 45:25–28, 1988.
49. Dutcher RM, Larkin EP, Marshak RR: Virus-like particles in cow's milk from a herd with high incidence of lymphosarcoma. JNCI 33:1055–1064, 1964.
50. Dutkiewicz J, Jablonski L, Olenchock SA: Occupational biohazards: A review. Am J Ind Med 14:605–623, 1988.
51. Echobichon DJ, Davies JE, Doull J, et al: Neurotoxic effects of pesticides. In Baker SR, Wilkinson CF: The Effects of Pesticides on Human Health. Princeton, NJ, Princeton Sci Pub Co, Adv Mod Environ Toxicol XVIII:131–199, 1990.
52. Emanuel DA, Draves DL, Nycz CR: Occupational health services for farmers. Am J Ind Med 18:149–162, 1990.

53. Eriksson M, Hardell L, Berg NO, et al: Soft-tissue sarcomas and exposure to chemical substances: A case-referent study. Br J Ind Med 38:27–33, 1981.

54. Fasal E, Jackson EW, Klauber MR: Leukemia and lymphoma mortality and farm residence. Am J Epidemiol 87:267–274, 1968.

55. Flodin U, Fredriksson M, Persson B, Axelson O: Chronic lymphatic leukaemia and engine exhausts, fresh wood, and DDT: A case-referent study. Br J Ind Med 45:33–38, 1988.

56. Flodin U, Fredriksson M, Persson B: Multiple myeloma and engine exhausts, freshwood, and creosote: A case-control study. Am J Ind Med 12:519–529, 1987.

57. Franceschi S, Serraino D, Bidoli E, et al: The epidemiology of non-Hodgkin's lymphoma in the northwest of Italy: A hospital-based case-control study. Leuk Res 13:465–472, 1989.

58. Fredriksson M, Bengtsson N, Hardell L, Axelson O: Colon cancer, physical activity, and occupational exposures—A case-control study. Cancer 9:1838–1842, 1989.

59. Fox AJ, Goldblatt PO: Longitudinal study of sociodemographic mortality differentials, 1971–1975. Office of Population Censuses and Surveys. Her Majesty's Stationery Office, Series LS No. 1, London, 1980.

60. Gallagher RP, Spinelli JJ, Elwood JM, Skippen DH: Allergies and agricultural exposures as risk factors for multiple myeloma. Br J Cancer 48:853–857, 1983.

61. Gallagher RP, Threlfall WJ, Jeffries E, et al: Cancer and aplastic anemia in British Columbia farmers. JNCI 72:1311–1315, 1984.

62. Garabrant DH, Peters JM, Mack TM, Bernstein L: Job activity and colon cancer risk. Am J Epidemiol 119:1005–1014, 1984.

63. Giles GG, Lickiss JN, Baikle MJ, et al: Myeloproliferative and lymphoproliferative disorders in Tasmania, 1972–80: Occupational and familial aspects. JNCI 72:1233–1240, 1984.

64. Gold E, Gordis L, Tonascia J, Szklo M: Risk factors for brain tumors in children. Am J Epidemiol 109:309–319, 1979.

65. Graham S, Marshall J, Haughey B, et al: An inquiry into the epidemiology of melanoma. Am J Epidemiol 122:606–619, 1985.

66. Graves DC, Ferrer JF: In vitro transmission and propagation of bovine leukemia virus in monolayer cell cultures. Cancer Res 36:4152–4159, 1976.

67. Guralnick L: Mortality by occupation and cause of death. DHEW (Vital Statistics Special Rep. No. 53(3)), Washington, DC, 1963.

68. Gutensohn N, Cole P: Epidemiology of Hodgkin's disease in the young. N Engl J Med 300:1006–1011, 1979.

69. Haguenoer JM, Cordier S, Morel C, et al: Occupational risk factors for upper respiratory and upper digestive tract cancers. Br J Ind Med 47:380–383, 1990.

70. Hallenberg GR: Nitrates in Iowa groundwater. In D'Itri FM, Wolfson LL: Rural Groundwater Contamination. Chelsea, MI, Lewis Publ., pp 23–68.

71. Hardell L, Eriksson M, Lenner P, Lundgren E: Malignant lymphoma and exposure to chemicals, especially organic solvents, chlorophenols and phenoxy acids: A case-control study. Br J Cancer 43:169–176, 1981.

72. Hardell L, Eriksson M: The association between soft-tissue sarcomas and exposure to phenoxyacetic acids: A new case-referent study. Cancer 62:652–656, 1988.

73. Hardell L, Sandstrom A: Case-control study: Soft-tissue sarcomas. Br J Cancer 39:711–717, 1979.

74. Haughey BP, Graham S, Brasure J, et al: The epidemiology of testicular cancer in upstate New York. Am J Epidemiol 130:25–36, 1989.

75. Hayes RB, Brown LM, Pottern LM, et al: Occupation and risk for testicular cancer: A case-control study. Int J Epidemiol 19:825–831, 1990.

76. Hayes WJ Jr: Toxicology of Pesticides. Baltimore, Williams & Wilkins, 1975.

77. Higginson J: Etiologic factors in gastrointestinal cancer in men. JNCI 37:537–549, 1966.

78. Hoar SK, Blair A, Holmes FF, et al: Agricultural herbicide use and risk of lymphoma and soft-tissue sarcoma. J Am Med Assoc 256:1141–1147, 1986.

79. Hoss HH, Olsen C: Infectivity of bovine C-type virus for sheep and goats. Am J Vet Res 35:633–637, 1974.

80. Howe GR, Lindsay JP: A follow-up study of a ten-percent sample of the Canadian labor force: I. Cancer mortality in males, 1965–1973. JNCI 70:37–44, 1983.

81. Jensen OM, Olsen JH, Osterlind A: Testis cancer risk among farmers in Denmark. Lancet i:794, 1984.

82. Keller AZ: Cellular types, survival, race, nativity, occupations, habits and associated diseases in the pathogenesis of lip cancers. Am J Epidemiol 91:486–499, 1970.

83. Kneller RW, Gao Y, McLaughlin JK, et al: Occupational risk factors for gastric cancer in Shanghai, China. Am J Ind Med 18:69–78, 1990.

84. Kraus AS, Levin ML, Gerhardt PR: A study of occupational associations with gastric cancer. Am J Public Health 47:961-970, 1957.
85. Laval G, Tuyns AJ: Environmental factors in childhood leukemia. Br J Ind Med 45:843-844, 1988.
86. LaVecchia C, Negri E, D'Avanzo B, Franceschi S: Occupation and lymphoid neoplasms. Br J Cancer 60:385-388, 1989.
87. Lee JAH: Melanoma. In Schottenfeld D, Fraumeni JF Jr: Cancer Epidemiology and Prevention. Philadelphia, W.B. Saunders, 1982, pp 984-995.
88. Lee JAH, Strickland D: Malignant melanoma: Social status and outdoor work. Br J Cancer 41:757-763, 1980.
89. Linos A, Kyle RA, O'Fallon WM, Kurland LT: A case-control study of occupational exposures and leukemia. Int J Epidemiol 9:131-135, 1980.
90. Lowengart RA, Peters JM, Cicioni C, et al: Childhood leukemia and parents' occupational and home exposures. JNCI 79:39-46, 1987.
91. Malone KE, Koepsell TD, Daling JR, et al: Chronic lymphocytic leukemia in relation to chemical exposures. Am J Epidemiol 130:1152-1158, 1989.
92. Matthews MLV, Dougan LE, Thomas DC, Armstrong BK: Interpersonal linkage among Hodgkin's disease patients and controls in Western Australia. Cancer 54:2571-2579, 1984.
93. McDowall M, Balarajan R: Testicular cancer and employment in agriculture. Lancet i:510-511, 1984.
94. McLaughlin JK, Malker HSR, Blot WJ, et al: Occupational risks for intracranial gliomas in Sweden. JNCI 78:253-257, 1987.
95. McLaughlin JK, Linet M, Stone BJ, et al: Multiple myeloma and occupation in Sweden. Arch Environ Health 43:7-10, 1988.
96. McMichael AJ, Hartshorne JM: Mortality risks in Australian men by occupational groups, 1968-1978. Med J Austr 1:253-256, 1982.
97. Milham S Jr: Leukemia and multiple myeloma in farmers. Am J Epidemiol 94:307-310, 1971.
98. Milham S Jr: Occupational mortality in Washington state, 1950-1979. National Institute for Occupational Safety and Health. DHHS (NIOSH) Publ. No. 83-116, Cincinnati, OH, 1983.
99. Mills PK, Newell GR, Johnson DE: Testicular cancer associated with employment in agriculture and oil and natural gas extraction. Lancet i:207-210, 1984.
100. Morris PD, Koepsell TD, Daling JR, et al: Toxic substance exposure and multiple myeloma: A case-control study. JNCI 76:987-994, 1986.
101. Musicco M, Filippini G, Bordo BM, et al: Gliomas and occupational exposure to carcinogens: Case-control study. Am J Epidemiol 116:782-790, 1982.
102. Musicco M, Sant M, Molinari S, et al: A case-control study of brain gliomas and occupational exposure to chemical carcinogens: The risk to farmers. Am J Epidemiol 128:778-785, 1988.
103. Nomura A: Stomach. In Schottenfeld D, Fraumeni JF Jr: Cancer Epidemiology and Prevention. Philadelphia, W.B. Saunders, 1982, pp 624-637.
104. Notkola VJ, Husman KRH, Laukkanen VJ: Mortality among male farmers in Finland during 1979-1983. Scand J Work Environ Health 13:124-128, 1987.
105. Nandakumar A, Armstrong BK, DeKlerk NH: Multiple myeloma in Western Australia: A case-control study in relation to occupation, father's occupation, socioeconomic status and country of birth. Int J Cancer 37:223-226, 1986.
106. Oleske D, Golomb HM, Farber MD, Levy PS: A case-control inquiry into the etiology of hairy cell leukemia. Am J Epidemiol 121:675-683, 1985.
107. Olsen JH, Dragsted L, Autrup H: Cancer risk and occupational exposure to aflatoxins in Denmark. Br J Cancer 58:392-396, 1988.
108. Pearce N: Phenoxy herbicides and non-Hodgkin's lymphoma in New Zealand: Frequency and duration of herbicide use. Br J Ind Med 46:143-144, 1989.
109. Pearce N, Reif JS: Epidemiologic studies of cancer in agricultural workers. Am J Ind Med 18:133-142, 1990.
110. Pearce NE, Sheppard RA, Fraser J: Case-control study of occupation and cancer of the prostate in New Zealand. J Epid Comm Health 41:130-132, 1987.
111. Pearce NE, Sheppard RA, Howard JK, et al: Leukemia among New Zealand agricultural workers—A cancer registry-based study. Am J Epidemiol 124:402-409, 1986.
112. Pearce NE, Sheppard RA, Smith AH, Teague CA: Non-Hodgkin's lymphoma and farming: An expanded case-control study. Int J Cancer 39:155-161, 1987.
113. Pearce NE, Smith AH, Fisher DO: Malignant lymphoma and multiple myeloma linked with agricultural occupations in New Zealand cancer registry-based study. Am J Epidemiol 121:225-237, 1985.

114. Persson B, Dahlander A, Fredriksson M, et al: Malignant lymphomas and occupational exposures. Br J Ind Med 46:516–520, 1989.
115. Petersen GR, Milham S Jr: Occupational mortality in the state of California, 1959–1961. National Institute for Occupational Safety and Health. DHEW (NIOSH, NIH) Publ. No. 80-104, Rockville, MD, 1980.
116. Piper CE, Abt DA, Ferrer JF, Marshall RR: Seroepidemiologic evidence for horizontal transmission of bovine C-type virus. Cancer Res 35:2714–2716, 1975.
117. Preston-Martin S, Mack W, Henderson BE: Risk factors for gliomas and meningiomas in males in Los Angeles County. Cancer Res 49:6137–6143, 1989.
118. Radomiski JL, Deichman WB, Clizer EE: Pesticide concentrations in the liver, brain, and adipose tissue of terminal hospital patients. Food Cosmet Toxicol 6:209–220, 1968.
119. Rafnsson V, Gunnarsdottir H: Mortality among farmers in Iceland. Int J Epidemiol 18:146–151, 1989.
120. Reif J, Pearce N, Fraser J: Cancer risks in New Zealand farmers. Int J Epidemiol 18:768–774, 1989.
121. Reif J, Pearce N, Fraser J: Occupational risks for brain cancer: A New Zealand cancer registry-based study. J Occup Med 31:863–867, 1989.
122. Riedel DA, Pottern LM, Blattner WA: Epidemiology of multiple myeloma. In Wiernik BA, Canellos CP, Kyle RA, Schiffer CA: Neoplastic Diseases of the Blood, 2nd ed. New York, Churchill Livingstone, 1990 (in press).
123. Saftlas AF, Blair A, Cantor KP, et al: Cancer and other causes of death among Wisconsin farmers. Am J Ind Med 11:119–129, 1987.
124. Schumacher MC: Farming occupations and mortality from non-Hodgkin's lymphoma in Utah. J Occup Med 27:580–584, 1985.
125. Schumacher MC, Delzell E: A death-certificate case-control study of non-Hodgkin's lymphoma and occupation in men in North Carolina. Am J Ind Med 13:317–330, 1988.
126. Schuman LM, Mandel J, Blackard C, et al: Epidemiologic study of prostatic cancer: Preliminary report. Can Treat Rep 61:181–186, 1977.
127. Schwartz RS, Callen JP, Silva J Jr: A cluster of Hodgkin's disease in a small community. Am J Epidemiol 108:19–26, 1978.
128. Scotto J, Fraumeni JF Jr: Skin (other than melanoma). In Schottenfeld D, Fraumeni JF Jr: Cancer Epidemiology and Prevention. Philadelphia, W.B. Saunders, 1982, pp 996–1011.
129. Shu XO, Gao YT, Brinton LA, et al: A population-based case-control study of childhood leukemia in Shanghai. Cancer 62:635–644, 1988.
130. Sigurjonsson J: Occupational variations in mortality from gastric cancer in relation to dietary differences. Br J Cancer 21:651–656, 1967.
131. Smith AH, Pearce NE, Fisher DO, et al: Soft tissue sarcoma and exposure to phenoxyherbicides and chlorophenols in New Zealand. JNCI 73:1111–1117, 1984.
132. Stark AD, Chang H, Fitzgerald EF, et al: A retrospective cohort study of mortality among New York state farm bureau members. Arch Environ Health 42:204–212, 1987.
133. Steineck G, Wiklund K: Multiple myeloma in Swedish agricultural workers. Int J Epidemiol 15:321–325, 1986.
134. Statistics Sweden. Dodsfalls registret 1961–1970. Stockholm, 1981.
135. Stubbs HA, Harris J, Spear RC: A proportionate mortality analysis of California's agricultural workers, 1978–1979. Am J Ind Med 6:305–320, 1984.
136. Surgeon General. Smoking and Health—A report of the Surgeon General. Department of Health, Education, and Welfare (DHEW publication no. (PHS) 79-50066, USGPO). Washington, DC, 1979.
137. Thomas TL, Fontham ETH, Norman SA, et al: Occupational risk factors for brain tumors. Scand J Work Environ Health 12:121–127, 1986.
138. Thomas TL, Waxweiler RJ: Brain tumors and occupational risk factors—A review. Scand J Work Environ Health 12:1–15, 1986.
139. Tollerud DJ, Brinton LA, Stone BJ, et al: Mortality from multiple myeloma among North Carolina furniture workers. JNCI 74:799–801, 1985.
140. Unger M, Olsen J: Organochlorine compounds in the adipose tissue of deceased patients with and without cancer. Environ Res 23:257–263, 1980.
141. U.S. Department of Labor. Child Labor Requirements for Agriculture, United States, 1984, Fair Labor Standards Act. Child Labor Bulletin No. 102, WH Publication No. 1295, 1984.
142. Vena JE, Graham S, Zielezny M: Lifetime occupational exercise and colon cancer. Am J Epidemiol 123:775–780, 1986.
143. Verluys JJ: Cancer and occupation in the Netherlands. Br J Cancer 3:162–185, 1949.

144. Vineis P, Terracini B, Ciccone G, et al: Phenoxy herbicides and soft-tissue sarcomas in female rice weeders. Scand J Work Environ Health 13:9–17, 1987.
145. Walrath J, Rogot E, Murray J, Blair A: Mortality patterns among US veterans by occupation and smoking status. US Government Printing Office (NIH Publ. No. 85-2756), Washington, DC, 1985.
146. Whitaker CJ, Lee WR, Downes JE: Squamous cell skin cancer in the northwest of England, 1967–69, and its relation to occupations. Br J Ind Med 36:43–51, 1979.
147. Wigle DT, Semenciw RM, Wilkins K, et al: Mortality study of Canadian male farm operators: Non-Hodgkin's lymphoma mortality and agricultural practices in Saskatchewan. JNCI 82:575–582, 1990.
148. Wiklund K, Dich J, Holm LE: Testicular cancer among agricultural workers and licensed pesticide applicators in Sweden. Scand J Work Environ Health 12:630–631, 1986.
149. Wiklund K, Dich J, Holm LE: Risk of malignant lymphoma in Swedish pesticide applicators. Br J Cancer 56:505–508, 1987.
150. Wiklund K, Einhorn J, Wennstrom S, Rapaport E: A Swedish cancer-environment register available for research. Scand J Work Environ Health 7:64–67, 1981.
151. Wilkins JR, Sinks T: Parental occupation and intracranial neoplasms of childhood: Results of a case-control interview study. Am J Epidemiol 132:275–292, 1990.
152. Williams RR, Stegens NL, Goldsmith JR: Associations of cancer site and type with occupation and industry from the Third National Cancer Survey Interview. JNCI 59:1147–1185, 1977.
153. Woods JS, Polissar L, Severson RK, et al: Soft tissue sarcoma and non-Hodgkin's lymphoma in relation to phenoxyherbicide and chlorinated phenol exposure in western Washington. JNCI 78:899–910, 1987.
154. Zahm SH, Weisenburger DD, Babbitt PA, et al: A case-control study of non-Hodgkin's lymphoma and the herbicide 2,4-dichlorophenoxyacetic acid (2,4-D) in eastern Nebraska. Epidemiology 1:349–356, 1990.
155. Zahm SH, Blair A, Holmes FF, et al: A case-referent study of soft-tissue sarcoma and Hodgkin's disease—Farming and insecticide use. Scand J Work Environ Health 14:224–230, 1988.

CLIFTON D. CRUTCHFIELD, PhD, CIH
STEVEN T. SPARKS, MD

EFFECTS OF NOISE AND VIBRATION ON FARM WORKERS

Clifton D. Crutchfield, PhD, CIH
Director, Industrial Hygiene
Division of Community and
    Environmental Health
University of Arizona
Tucson, Arizona

Steven T. Sparks, MD
Section of Preventive and
    Occupational Medicine
Department of Family and
    Community Medicine
University of Arizona College
    of Medicine
Tucson, Arizona

Reprint requests to:
Clifton D. Crutchfield, PhD, CIH
Director, Industrial Hygiene
Division of Community and
    Environmental Health
University of Arizona
1435 N. Fremont Ave.
Tucson, AZ 85719

Many farmers still function as small independent businessmen and as such are not bound by Occupational Safety and Health Administration (OSHA) regulations.[29] As a result, the information and inspection functions that form an important part of health and safety programs in other occupational sectors are generally missing in the agricultural arena. The diffuse nature of farming operations, in contrast to most industrial operations, also makes the widespread dissemination and implementation of health and safety practices for farmers much more challenging.

The lack of specific health and safety programs in many farming operations resulted in an estimated 1,300 agricultural deaths and 120,000 farm-related injuries in 1989.[32] An incidence rate of 48.8 occupational illnesses per 10,000 full-time agricultural workers was reported for 1988 by the Bureau of Labor Statistics (BLS).[32] This illness figure is conservative in that the BLS survey did not include farms with fewer than 11 employees. Therefore, the magnitude of health and safety hazards confronted by agricultural workers on the numerous small farming operations that are characteristic of rural America is not precisely known. This chapter focuses on the hazards of noise and vibration, which are common to most farming operations.

NOISE

Definition of Noise Problem
Data from the Public Health Service's Health Promotion and Disease Prevention Questionnaire indicate that farm operators head the

list of persons concerned about exposure to occupational risks.[35] More than 50% of the farm operators surveyed recognized a health risk associated with their work conditions. Exposure to noise was the condition reported most frequently. Of all workers who reported exposure to health-endangering work conditions, 32% were concerned about possible hearing loss.

Noise-induced hearing loss is a major public health problem. Its occurrence among farm personnel has long been recognized.[26,36] However, the distribution and severity of hearing loss have proven more difficult to study among farm populations than in more concentrated occupational settings, such as factories.

Noise is commonly described as unwanted sound. The physical nature of sound is defined as a variation in ambient pressure in a medium that can be detected by the human ear. It is usually generated by either a vibrating surface or by turbulence in a flowing fluid or gas. The pressure variation propagates through the medium by wave motion. The characteristic components of a sound wave are its frequency and amplitude. Sound frequency, which we perceive as pitch, is measured in Hertz (Hz). The frequency response range of a healthy young ear extends from about 20 Hz up to 20,000 Hz.

Sound amplitude, which we perceive as loudness, is measured in decibels (dB). The range of sound pressure variations to which the ear can respond is extremely large, covering approximately six orders of magnitude. A decibel (log) scale is conventionally used to compress the range into a more manageable form. The relationship between sound pressure, measured in micropascals (μPa), and sound pressure level measured in dB is given in equation 1.

$$L_p \text{ (dB)} = 20 \log_{10} (P/P_o)$$

where L_p = sound pressure level, dB
 P = sound pressure, μPa
 P_o = reference sound pressure (20 μPa)

The threshold of hearing is considered to be 0 dB, which is equivalent to a pressure variation of 20 μPa. This means that the ear is capable of responding to a sound pressure that is more than a billion times lower than atmospheric pressure. The upper limit of the ear's effective response to pressure is generally considered to be the threshold of pain, which occurs at a pressure of about 200 million μPa or 140 dB.

The human ear's response to frequency and intensity is not uniform throughout its response range. At sound pressure levels below 90 dB, the ear is not as responsive to low frequencies ($<$ 700 Hz) as it is to frequencies of 1,000 Hz and greater. Consequently, an electronic weighting network is built into sound-measuring equipment to more closely align its response to that of the ear. An "A" weighting network has been adopted by OSHA, whose standards are referenced to sound pressure levels measured on the "A" scale, or dBA.[10]

Physiology and Effects of Noise

The basic physiology of the ear can be broken down into three sections. The outer ear, which consists of the pinna and the auditory canal, is separated from the middle ear by the tympanic membrane (eardrum). Sound pressure variations detected by the eardrum are transmitted through the middle ear by the three small bones of the ossicular chain. These bones are arranged to provide some lever amplification to the stapes, which terminates the chain by oscillating in and out of

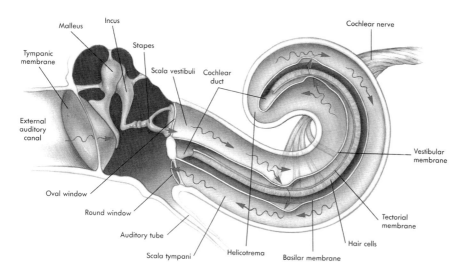

FIGURE 1. Effect of sound waves on cochlear structures. Sound waves strike the tympanic membrane and cause it to vibrate. This vibration causes the three bones of the middle ear to vibrate, which causes the membrane of the oval window to vibrate. This vibration causes the perilymph in the scala vestibuli to vibrate, which causes the fluid in the cochlear duct and basilar membrane to vibrate. Short sound waves (high pitch) cause the basilar membrane near the oval window to vibrate, and longer sound waves (low pitch) cause the basilar membrane some distance from the oval window to vibrate. Sound is detected in the hair cells of the organ of Corti, which is attached to the basilar membrane. Vibrations are transferred to the perilymph of the scala tympani and to the round window where they are dampened. (From Seeley RR, Stephens TD, Tate P: Anatomy and Physiology. St. Louis, C.V. Mosby, 1989, p 485, with permission.)

the oval window of the inner ear. The areal ratio of the tiny stapes compared to the eardrum also generates a significant amount of amplification to help overcome the signal losses associated with transmitting sound waves from air into the fluid-filled inner ear (Fig. 1).

The inner ear consists of a three-chambered organ called the cochlea which is shaped like a snail's shell (Fig. 2). Sound wave propagation through the cochlea is wavelength (reciprocal of frequency)-dependent. The waves travel down the scala vestibuli, across the organ of Corti, and back through the scala tympani to the round window where the sound energy exits the inner ear. Sound wave propagation across the organ of Corti stimulates hair cells located there and produces the nerve impulses which are interpreted as sound in the brain. The location of a hair cell and its displacement amplitude are directly related to the frequency and intensity of the initiating sound wave.

Noise-induced Hearing Loss. Excessive noise exposure over a period of years can lead to permanent damage to the hair cells of the cochlea. If the noise exposure occurs over a broad range of frequencies (white noise), a characteristic hearing loss at around 4,000 Hz is often seen on audiograms. This loss is associated with the permanent loss of hair cells in the region of the cochlea responsible for detecting 4,000 Hz wavelengths. As the noise insult continues, the hearing loss will spread to adjacent areas of the cochlea, and both lower and

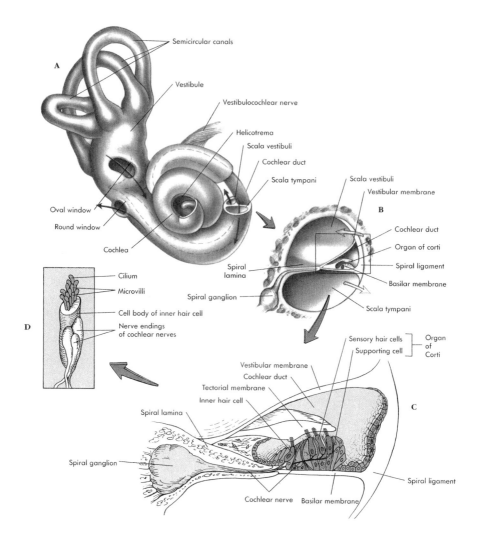

FIGURE 2. Elements of the inner ear. *A,* Location of the cochlear duct and organ of Corti. Insets show, *B,* an enlarged section of the cochlea and, *C,* an even greater enlargement of the organ of Corti. *D,* A greatly enlarged individual sensory hair cell. (From Seeley RR, Stephens TD, Tate P: Anatomy and Physiology. St. Louis, C.V. Mosby, 1989, p 483, with permission.)

higher frequency losses will occur. When the loss extends into the frequency range of 500 to 2,000 Hz, a person begins to experience difficulty understanding human speech. Although the speech patterns continue to be loud enough to be heard, differentiation of consonant sounds becomes increasingly difficult as the hearing loss spreads down through the primary speech frequencies.

   Other Causes of Hearing Loss. It is important to differentiate noise-induced hearing loss from other causes of hearing impairment. **Presbycusis** results from the spontaneous degeneration of the hearing system that accompanies aging. Like noise-induced hearing loss, presbycusis also tends to affect the higher frequencies to a greater extent. In many cases, some portion of hearing losses is attributable to noise sources outside the workplace. **Sociacusis** is a term that has been used to define hearing loss that has its origins in the loud noises encountered in many of our society's recreational activities, such as listening to amplified music and hobbies such as shooting. **Nosoacusis** refers to hearing damage caused by other factors, such as hereditary defects, certain ototoxic drugs, and barotrauma.[2]

Noise Sources and Standards

The current OSHA permissible exposure limit for continuous noise is 90 dBA as a time-weighted average over an 8-hour shift.[10] The Hearing Conservation Amendment to the OSHA noise standard, which became effective in 1985, established an action level of 85 dBA.[11] When the time-weighted average noise exposure exceeds 85 dBA, specific actions must be taken to reduce the exposure level or time. The OSHA standard is based upon a 5 dB exchange rate, which means that the allowable exposure time is cut in half for each 5 dB increase in average noise exposure above the action level. For example, exposure to a noise source that averaged 100 dBA would only be allowed under the standard for a period of 2 hours per day.

Agricultural practices involve a number of operations with noise sources that exceed 90 dBA when they operate. Noise from farm tractors in particular poses a serious threat of hearing loss to operators.[26,36] Although tractor cabs that were originally designed for weather protection and safety were found to actually increase the noise exposures of their drivers, a great deal has been accomplished by manufacturers in recent years to reduce in-cab noise levels. Since 1976, British legislation has specified a maximum operator noise exposure of 90 dBA for new tractors.[28]

Several other types of machinery used in agriculture also produce high noise levels. In addition to tractors and various types of harvesters, equipment such as grain dryers, brush hogs, and chain saws generate significant noise exposures. Many farmers also listen to the radio at a high volume setting in order to hear above the noise of operating machinery. It has been suggested that many farmers also participate in noisy sports such as hunting and snowmobiling.[39]

Studies that report specific sound levels generated by the wide variety of farm machinery are limited. However, Broste et al. did report sound level measurements from a small pilot study of farm operations.[6] Of 31 tractors surveyed, only one was found to operate below the current OSHA action level of 85 dBA at full throttle. Noise measurements were made at ear level in the driver's seat with the cab window open if so equipped.

A farm worker's exposure to noise is generally more variable both in terms of intensity and duration than the noise patterns experienced in other types of industry. However, research has shown that the variability does not offer any significant advantage in protecting the hearing of the farm worker.[28]

An important study by Thelin et al. compared hearing loss among male farmers in Missouri to nonfarmers and office workers.[39] It was found that the rate of failure to hear 1,000 and 2,000 Hz tones at 20 dB and a 4,000 Hz tone at 25 dB was lowest for office workers and highest for farmers. The finding was significant at the 2,000 and 4,000 Hz frequencies. Of special interest was the finding that the farmers had a higher failure rate at those two frequencies in every age group from

25 to 64 years. Of the farmers aged 25 to 64 years old, 16.8% had a hearing loss sufficient to interfere with speech communication, compared to 6.2% of the office workers. This finding points to a greater need for active measures directed towards protecting the hearing of agricultural workers in the younger age groups.

In the study by Broste et al., hearing loss was studied among high school farm students.[6] Students were grouped into four categories depending on their degree of participation in farm work. Broste found a higher rate of hearing loss at each tested frequency for the two student groups with the greatest noise exposure. The difference between the groups was greatest at higher frequencies, which is consistent with a pattern of early noise-induced hearing loss. Considering the results of previous studies in adult farmers, this finding suggests that adult hearing loss may begin in childhood.

Data used to establish the current OSHA standard were derived primarily from studies involving adults. It is unclear whether such a standard will provide sufficient protection for children (assuming full compliance). In Broste's study,[6] only 9% of the farm students tested reported use of hearing protection when working in noisy areas. This indicates a great need for preventive measures directed at this age group.

Farriers are a specialized group of workers in animal husbandry. In the shoeing of horses, farriers are exposed to dangerously high levels of noise. When horseshoes are hammered on an anvil for final fitting, sound levels may range from 98 to 120 dBA, with most readings above 108 dBA.[27] The ring of an anvil is essentially continuous noise because the impacts are normally spaced less than 1 second apart. Time spent shoeing horses may amount to 2 or more hours per day, resulting in a noise exposure with definite potential for hearing damage. According to Holler, the use of hearing protectors among farriers is not a common practice.[18]

Modern pig breeding facilities represent yet another source of possible noise exposure for workers engaged in animal husbandry. Kristensen and Gimsing reported acoustical measurements in a facility housing 1,100 pigs.[25] During the feeding process, noise levels ranged from 95 to 104 dBA in the feed alleys. The time period during which these sound levels were maintained was not stated. However, in similar situations, noise from the squealing and shrieking of the pigs usually lasted about 45 minutes for two periods during each day. Workers were also exposed to noise from high-pressure sprayers used for cleaning the pig sties. Noise levels were reported to range from 98 to 105 dBA when the sprayers were being used. Measurements were made at 50 cm to the side of the worker's ear. The machinery used for grinding and mixing the feed produced a noise-induced hearing loss in a 45-year-old pig breeder, which was felt with reasonable certainty to be due to his work exposures. Use of hearing protectors is recommended in this type of animal facility during noisy periods.

Control of Noise Exposures

Classic approaches to controlling excessive noise exposures involve attacking the problem at the noise source, along the noise propagation path, or at the point of the exposed receiver. Noise control at the source includes strategies such as reducing the driving force that creates the noise, isolating the driving force from vibrating surfaces, or surrounding the source in a sound-dampening enclosure. Improved designs of tractor engine compartments and exhaust mufflers are examples of the application of noise control at the noise source.

The variable nature of farm tasks makes noise control along the path of sound propagation more difficult to achieve on the farm relative to industrial operations. Many farm operations are conducted outdoors, where sound propagation tends to follow the inverse square law. Consequently, distance can be used to good advantage in reducing noise exposures by separating as much as possible the majority of farm workers from significant noise sources such as tractors or harvesters. In an outdoor location without significant reflective surfaces, a doubling of the distance between source and receiver will yield a four-fold decrease in noise exposure intensity.

Hearing-protection devices represent the most commonly applied noise control at the point of the receiver. The level of noise reduction that can be achieved with earplugs and earmuffs depends upon the frequency spectrum of the noise exposure. Figure 3 gives an indication of the reductions that can be achieved if the hearing protective devices are properly and consistently used. Ensuring that such devices are readily available and maintained in a sanitary condition, and that farm workers are properly trained in their use, represent significant challenges in the setting of the typical small farm.

Data describing the extent of hearing protection use among adult farm workers are not readily available. It is common knowledge that many industrial

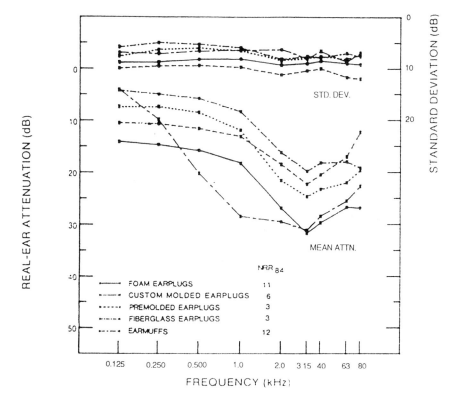

FIGURE 3. Real world attenuation for five types of hearing protectors. (Reproduced from Berger,[1] with permission.)

workers are reluctant to comply with noise regulations, even when motivated by their supervisors and safety officers. Among factory workers in New Zealand, for example, 55% of those exposed to noise levels greater than 85 dBA had been issued hearing protection devices.[9] Only 43% were actually using them. It is likely that a much lower percentage of farm workers are actually using hearing protection devices with regularity.

Concern has also been expressed over the resistance of some farm equipment operators to the introduction and use of quiet cabs. Drivers must be able to detect problems that develop with their equipment, such as changes in load. Quieter and safer ways of monitoring equipment operation have been suggested.[13]

What can be done to prevent the development of noise-induced hearing loss among farm workers? Farm workers as a group are more geographically spread than workers in other industries and are often fiercely independent. To make matters worse, a large portion of the farm labor force is excluded from the hearing conservation programs mandated by the Occupational Safety and Health Administration for the rest of American industry.

It has been pointed out that information can best be disseminated to farm workers through agencies and associations with which they commonly deal.[39] Migrant farm workers are most difficult to reach. Because of the prevalence of noise in farm operations, information on prevention of noise-induced hearing loss should be given a prominent place in materials that farmers read. Use of hearing protectors should be actively promoted, and these devices should be made readily available. It may be necessary for local health departments to take the lead in this area. Special efforts need to be directed toward protecting children who are involved in farm work.

Programs such as the one developed by the University of Minnesota Agricultural Extension Service could do much to fill the need for educating farmers to better protect their health.[29] Packaged instructional units were designed for use by county agents, vocational teachers, and chemical distributors. Workshops were then held throughout the state to train people in the use of these materials. Such a program could be of tremendous value if fully implemented in every state.

VIBRATION

Sources and Types

The machines operated by modern farmers not only produce excessive noise but also may produce hazardous levels of vibration. Apparently there is some synergism between the effects of overexposure to noise and the effects of overexposure to vibration. Miyakita et al. in their study of forestry workers in Japan found a relationship between noise-induced hearing loss and vibration-induced white finger (VWF).[30] A greater hearing loss was observed in chain-saw operators with VWF than in those operators who did not exhibit any signs of VWF. The presence of VWF suggests greater vibration amplitude, which would also generate higher noise levels.

The differences observed in the Miyakita study were statistically significant for workers with 5 to 9 years of exposure but not for the groups with 10 to 14 years of exposure. The reason for such an effect remains obscure, but it was suggested that inter-individual differences in susceptibility to noise and vibration may be involved. It has been hypothesized that vibration may induce a reflex vasoconstriction of the inner ear that is mediated through the sympathetic nervous system.[33] The Miyakita study confirmed the results of previous studies.[20,21]

There are two principal types of vibration exposure. Whole-body vibration is transmitted either through the feet when standing on a vibrating platform or through the buttocks when seated in a vehicle. Localized vibration is generally transmitted from vibrating tools through the hands into the upper extremities.

Studies on prevalence of vibration exposure in the United States showed that 8 million workers were exposed to occupational vibration.[3] Over 1.2 million of those workers were exposed to hand and arm vibration.

Effects of Whole-body Vibration

There is a lack of solid evidence on the long-term effects of exposure to whole-body vibration.[19] Much more research has been done on the acute effects of intense vibration, which causes discomfort and thereby leads to poor performance. The extent to which the acute effects of vibration are relevant to farming operations is unknown. Acute effect data from both laboratory experiments and practical experience form the basis for the regulations and guidelines that have been established concerning vibration exposure.

The most commonly reported long-term sequelae of exposure to whole-body vibration are low back pain, early degeneration of the spinal system, and herniation of the lumbar disc.[19] Studies of the effects of whole-body vibration on parts of the body other than the low back have not produced conclusive results. A number of epidemiologic studies have shown evidence of an increased risk of low back pain among drivers of tractors as well as other types of machinery.[42] Low back pain from various causes appears to occur at an earlier age among those exposed to whole-body vibration.

A literature review by Seidel and Heide included 18 studies on tractor drivers or drivers of other agricultural machinery.[34] They concluded that there is an increased risk of spinal column damage and damage to the peripheral nervous system due to intense long-term whole body vibration. Effects on other systems including the digestive system, peripheral veins, female reproductive organs, and the vestibular system were stated to have a lower probability of occurrence.

Another review by Hulshof and van Zanten analyzed 19 studies conducted prior to 1987.[19] Their focus was restricted to effects on the thoracic and lumbar spines. After rating each reviewed study according to an objective set of exposure, health effects, and methodologic criteria, most scores were found to be relatively low. Even though there was limited information in many of the studies reviewed, a "strong tendency in a similar direction was found" which led the reviewers to conclude that whole body vibration is harmful to the spinal system. Among the four studies of agricultural tractor drivers that were reviewed, only one was rated as moderately informative.

A study by Gruber and Zippermann found that experienced motor coach operators had a greater prevalence of spinal disorders and vertebrogenic pain.[16] In another cohort study by Gruber, truck drivers exhibited a higher incidence of degenerative changes of the spinal column and displacement of the intervertebral disc.[17] A recently reported study of New York City Transit Authority subway operators found that the high prevalence of back problems in the population does appear to be related to high whole-body vibration exposure, as well as to other ergonomic factors, including poor seat design.[22a]

A case-control study by Kelsey and Hardy compared the risk of acute herniated lumbar disc among different occupations.[24] For those spending greater than half of their work time driving, an increased risk of disc herniation was noted. A relative risk of 4.67 (p < 0.02) was calculated for truck drivers. An even higher risk would be expected for operators of farm machinery because of the greater prevalence of vibrating sources.

Hulshof reviewed a study of helicopter pilots by Fisher that found a higher prevalence of low back pain as well as degenerative changes of the spine compared to a control group of other pilots.[19] Vibrational forces in the vertical axis from agricultural tractors without suspension systems are on the same order of magnitude as those encountered in helicopters. Weighted root mean square (RMS) accelerations ranged from 0.4 to 1.25 m/s^2 for tractors, compared with 0.1 to 1.5 m/s^2 for helicopters. Comparisons of this nature have some inherent difficulties, but the evidence in helicopter pilots does suggest a need for caution concerning whole-body vibration exposures among farmers.

In the cross-sectional study by Dupuis and Zerlett, a group of earth-mover operators was compared with a control group not exposed to vibration.[12] Subjective reporting of spinal discomfort was much higher among the exposed workers. Lumbar syndrome was reported by 68.7% of the workers, followed by 18.2% reporting problems with the cervical spine. Only 6.8% of the surveyed workers reported trouble in the thoracic region. Both mechanical overloading of the spine and metabolic disturbances of the disc were proposed as possible mechanisms for the premature degenerative changes of the spine.

Whole-body vibration was also studied in crane operators.[12] Operators of farm tractors are expected to experience similar exposure to vibration, although again there are no good comparative data. Vibration measurements in overhead traveling cranes ranged from 0.1 to 0.8 m/s^2. Bongers et al. attributed a significant excess in extended sickness absences among crane operators with greater than 5 years of work exposure to intervertebral disc disease.[4] Furthermore, absences related to disc disease lasted longer among those workers exposed to vibration.

In their study of 3,920 family practice patients, Frymoyer et al. found a significant correlation between truck driving and low back pain.[14] It was also found that low back pain was associated with cigarette smoking, particularly when smoking was accompanied by a chronic cough.

Vibration is considered a significant factor in the etiology of back pain, along with other mechanical stresses related to acceleration and deceleration. Possible reasons for the identification of driving as a risk factor for low back pain were considered by Kelsey and Hardy.[24] More pressure is exerted on the lumbar discs while sitting than while either standing or lying down. There is also evidence that most motor vehicle seats do not provide adequate support for the lower back.[23]

Even more rare effects have been reported from exposure to vibration. A case of pneumomediastinum in an 18-year-old male was apparently due to the use of a pneumatic drill for 7 hours during his first day on a new job.[43]

The production of such effects is not without biologic plausibility. A number of studies have demonstrated physiologic abnormalities related to whole-body vibration exposure. For example, nutrition of the intervertebral disc is compromised in the presence of excessive vibration. Such a compromise could lead to earlier than expected disc and vertebral degeneration.[32] Neuropharmacologic abnormalities such as altered concentrations of substances in the dorsal root ganglion cell bodies have been shown to result from low frequency whole-body vibration.[32] Such altered physiology may well contribute to early degenerative changes of the spine.

A problem common to all of these studies was a general lack of data describing exposure magnitudes and time histories. It should be pointed out that disorders of the spinal column associated with whole-body vibration are multifactorial. There is no specific disease caused by whole-body vibration alone, as there is when the extremities are exposed to segmental vibration.[15,19] The reviews also pointed out that whole-body vibration may exacerbate other pre-existing conditions.[34] Of interest to farmers is the caution raised by several authors regarding a potential greater risk for musculoskeletal damage in juveniles exposed to excessive whole-body vibration. Farm children need to be protected from excessive exposure until their skeletons have developed full mechanical loading capacity.

Vibration Standards

There is currently no national standard covering vibration exposures. The American Conference of Governmental Industrial Hygienists (ACGIH) has recommended a threshold limit value for hand-arm vibration, which is summarized in Table 1. A guideline for whole-body vibration is currently under study by the ACGIH.

It is important for the practicing physician to have a strategy for determining the work-relatedness of degenerative changes in the spinal column that may be related to whole-body vibration exposure. Differentiation is difficult because such changes are commonly associated with advancing age, even in the unexposed population.[12] However, when workers exposed to excessive vibration have degenerative changes beyond what is expected for their age, vibration as a potential causative agent should be explored. Work patterns associated with the vibration should be examined and altered where necessary to prevent further disease progression. More effective isolation of the worker from the vibration source by incorporating items such as vibration mounts, shocks, and additional padding should be considered. Work schedules and tasks can also be administratively rotated to decrease the duration of exposures.

TABLE 1.   Threshold Limit Values for Exposure of the Hand to Vibration in Either X, Y, Z Directions*

	Values of the Dominant,[b] Frequency-Weighted, rms, Component Acceleration Which Shall Not Be Exceeded $a_K,(a_{K_{eq}})$	
Total Daily Exposure Duration[a]	m/s²	g[c]
4 hours and less than 8	4	0.40
2 hours and less than 4	6	0.61
1 hour and less than 2	8	0.81
Less than 1 hour	12	1.22

[a] The total time vibration enters the hand per day, whether continuously or intermittently.
[b] Usually one axis of vibration is dominant over the remaining two axes. If one or more vibration axis exceeds the Total Daily Exposure, then the TLV has been exceeded.
[c] g = 9.81 m/s².
* (Reproduced from ACGIH,[41] with permission.)

Effects of Hand-Arm Vibration

One other recognized sequela of exposure to vibration is vibration-induced white finger (VWF) disease. VWF has been identified as a major occupational hazard resulting from the use of vibratory tools. Although statistics for the occurrence of the syndrome among farm workers are lacking, it is likely that farmers who frequently use chain saws are at increased risk. Forestry workers who use chain saws are known to have a high prevalence of this disorder.[38]

Vibration-induced white finger is a multisystem disorder of the peripheral circulatory system, nerves, muscles, and joints.[40] It is characterized by episodic blanching of the fingers. In the early stages of the disease, a tingling of the fingers becomes noticeable, which later progresses to numbness. With further exposure, episodes of blanching may occur when touching cold objects. In severe cases, blanching of the fingers can occur whenever the body is exposed to a cold environment. Both hands are usually affected more or less equally. The thumbs are seldom involved except in the most severe cases.

Exposure to cold is always involved in cases of VWF, although other factors are thought to be contributing.[40] Exposure to high humidity, driving of motor vehicles, and even stress are among these other factors. Smoking increases the risk of VWF rather dramatically. Blanching may sometimes occur at rest. Such periodic attacks typically last from 10 to 40 minutes. Sensation is lost in the involved finger during the attack, but acute pain usually accompanies the restoration of circulation.

Along with circulatory disturbances, direct injury to the peripheral nerves, muscles, bones, and joints is also involved with exposures to hand-arm vibration.[7] Abnormalities of the skin are also observed. In the end, the fingers become stiff, painful, swollen, and clumsy due to the lack of tactile sensation.[8] Workers with VWF experience difficulty in performing job tasks because of discomfort, clumsiness, and loss of sensation in the fingers and hands. Hobbies and other outdoor activities are also adversely affected.[15]

It is important to differentiate VWF from idiopathic Raynaud's phenomenon and from secondary Raynaud's syndrome associated with autoimmune diseases. Carpal tunnel syndrome must also be excluded. It has been reported that, among nonvibration-exposed agricultural workers in France, the underlying incidence of Raynaud's phenomenon is about 2%.[15] In Great Britain, a prevalence of 5.3% has been reported.[38]

Chain-saw users are particularly vulnerable to VWF. Among forestry workers in Quebec, a prevalence of 30.5% was observed among users compared to a rate of 8.7% among nonusers.[40] The latter figure probably includes workers with idiopathic Raynaud's syndrome plus those with the syndrome secondary to other causes. For those who had used chain saws for 20 or more years, the prevalence rate was over 50%. Interestingly, for those using the chain saw for more than 10 years, the relative risk was 3.60 for nonsmokers and 6.55 for smokers. In this study, 5.4% of cases had only blanching of the fingers (grade 1), 57.6% had to use some relief measures (grade 2) or methods of prevention (grade 3), and 37% received medical treatment (grade 4) or considered looking for other work (grade 5). Other factors found to predispose workers to VWF were a family history of idiopathic Raynaud's phenomenon, previous injuries to the arms, climate, and type of residence occupied during the wood-cutting season.

Bovenzi et al. found osteoarthritis of the wrist joints to be significantly greater among their vibration-exposed study population.[5] The prevalence of radiographic abnormalities of the elbow was also significantly higher in the vibration group than in the control group. Contrary to some previous studies, no evidence of increased prevalence of bone cysts in the hands was found for the vibration-exposed subjects. The development of such abnormalities was felt to depend on the characteristics of the vibration exposure (frequency, amplitude, direction, and exposure time), on ergonomic factors such as posture of the hands and arms and handgrip force, and on individual susceptibility to vibration. As the interval between vibration exposures decreases, recovery time for the hand is reduced, resulting in a more hazardous work process with greater potential for producing VWF.[38]

Use of impact power tools may also lead to pain, stiffness, and weakness in the arms and shoulders.[31] Although contested, there is evidence that vibration also causes bone cysts and early osteoarthritis.[5] Resonance in other organs from severe vibration may also cause pain or dysfunction. According to Futatsuka and Ueno, chronic low back pain and even stomach trouble occur regularly as a result of exposure to vibration.[11]

A questionnaire study by Musson et al. of percussive tool users in the Netherlands provided evidence that vibration is a risk factor for pain or stiffness of the back, neck, and upper extremities.[31] There appears to be only limited evidence for segmental vibration having a role in other reported symptoms, such as headache, fatigue, insomnia, and stress. This same study indicated that only 25% of the workers with complaints of VWF were receiving medical care.

A number of abnormalities have been found in VWF patients, including: (1) proliferation of the arterial intima and hypertrophy of the media, leading to segmental hypertrophy of the peripheral digital arteries, (2) degeneration and demyelination of peripheral nerves, with sensitivity to autonomic stimuli, and (3) collagenization of the dermis.[7] Such a combination of factors leads to an alteration in blood flow both before and after an episode of vibration exposure. Brown et al. reported a seeming paradox among workers with severe VWF when an episode of vibration exposure "resulted in decreased blood flow resistance in the distal vascular bed of the fingers."[7]

Currently, there is no established treatment for VWF other than terminating the patient's exposure to vibration. If this is done early enough in the course of the disease, the symptoms will resolve spontaneously, in most cases within a few months to a year.[8] If, on the other hand, the worker is not removed from the vibration exposure, the syndrome may progress to a point of severe impairment.

SUMMARY

A variety of significant health effects are associated with occupational exposures to noise and vibration, which are an integral part of many agricultural operations. Since vibrating surfaces represent one of the primary sources of noise, exposures to both types of physical stressors are commonly encountered. The effects of noise and vibration exposures may be exacerbated among farm workers because they tend to be more isolated than workers in other types of industry. As a consequence, access to health and safety information, medical care, and hazard control technology may be more restricted.

Medical practitioners who serve the agricultural community must be aware of the consequences of exposures to noise and vibration. A primary duty involves conducting baseline and periodic examinations to catch diseases associated with such exposures at an early stage, when the condition is still reversible. In addition, the practitioner's role also includes prevention of disease through education of workers regarding the effects of noise and vibration and through helping specify procedures and strategies that will result in exposure reductions.

REFERENCES

1. Berger E: Using the NRR to estimate the real world performance of hearing protectors. Sound and Vibration 17:12–18, 1983.
2. Berger E, Morrill J, Ward W, Royster L: Noise and Hearing Conservation Manual. Akron, American Industrial Hygiene Association, 1986.
3. Blair S, Allard K: Prevention of trauma: A cooperative effort. J Hand Surg 8:649–654, 1983.
4. Bongers P, Boshuizen H, Hulshof C, Koemeester A: Long-term sickness absence due to back disorderes in crane operators exposed to whole-body vibration. Int Arch Occup Environ Health 61:59–64, 1988.
5. Bovenzi M, Fiorito A, Volpe C: Bone and joint disorders in the upper extremities of chipping and grinding operators. Int Arch Occup Environ Health 59:189–198, 1987.
6. Broste S, Hansen D, Strand R, et al: Hearing loss among high school farm students. Am J Public Health 79:619–622, 1989.
7. Brown T, Blair W, Gabel R, et al: Effects of episodic air hammer usage on digital artery hemodynamics of foundry workers with vibration white finger disease. J Occup Med 30:853–862, 1988.
8. Cohen S, Bilinski D, McNutt NS: Vibration syndrome: Cutaneous and systemic manifestations in a jackhammer operator. Arch Dermatol 121:1544–1547, 1985.
9. Department of Health, Wellington: Noise-induced hearing loss. New Zealand Med J 98:815, 1985.
10. Department of Labor, Occupational Safety and Health Administration: 29 CFR Part 1910.95: Occupational Noise Exposure. Federal Register 36:10518, No. 105, May 29, 1971.
11. Department of Labor, Occupational Safety and Health Administration: 29 CFR Part 1910: Occupational Noise Exposure; Hearing Conservation Amendment. Federal Register 46:42622–42639, No. 162, Aug. 21, 1981.
12. Dupuis H, Zerlett G: Whole-body vibration and disorders of the spine. Int Arch Occup Environ Health 59:323–336, 1987.
13. Futatsuka M, Ueno T: Vibration exposure and vibration-induced white finger due to chain saw operation. J Occup Med 27:257–264, 1985.
14. Frymoyer J, Pope M, Costanza M, et al: Epidemiologic studies of low-back pain. Spine 5:419–423, 1980.
15. Gemne G: Pathophysiology and multifactorial etiology of acquired vasospastic disease (Raynaud syndrome) in vibration-exposed workers. Scand J Work Environ Health 8:243–249, 1982.
16. Gruber G, Zippermann H: Relationship between whole body vibration and morbidity patterns among motor coach operators. DHEW/NIOSH Report No. 75-104, Cincinnati, Ohio, 1975.
17. Gruber G: Relationship between whole body vibration and morbidity patterns among interstate truck drivers. DHEW/NIOSH Report No. 77-167, Cincinnati, Ohio, 1977.
18. Holler A: Occupational hazard of farriers. Am Ind Hyg Assoc J 45:34–38, 1984.
19. Hulshof C, van Zanten B: Whole-body vibration and low-back pain. A review of epidemiologic studies. Int Arch Occup Environ Health 59:205–220, 1987.
20. Iki M, Kurumatani N, Hirata K, et al: Association between vibration-induced white finger and hearing loss in forestry workers. Scand J Work Environ Health 12:365–370, 1986.
21. Iki M, Kurumatani N, Hirata K, et al: An association between Raynaud's phenomenon and hearing loss in forestry workers. Am Ind Hyg Assoc J 46:509–513, 1985.
22. James C, Aw T, Harrington J, et al: A review of 132 consecutive patients referred for assessment of vibration white finger. J Soc Occup Med 39:61–64, 1989.
22a. Johanning E, Wilder DG, Landrigan PJ, Pope MH: Whole-body vibration exposure in subway cars and review of adverse health effects. J Occup Med 33:605–612, 1991.
23. Keegan J: Alterations of the lumbar curve related to posture and seating. J Bone Joint Surg 35:589–603, 1953.
24. Kelsey J, Hardy R: Driving of motor vehicles as a risk factor for acute herniated lumbar intervertebral disc. Am J Epidemiol 102:63–73, 1975.
25. Kristensen S, Gimsing S: Occupational hearing impairment in pig breeders. Scand Audiol 17:191–192, 1988.
26. Lierle D, Reger S: The effect of tractor noise on the auditory sensitivity of tractor operators. Ann Otol Rhinol Laryngol 67:372–388, 1958.
27. MacKenzie S: Beware the anvil's ring. Equus 17:57–58, 1978.

28. Matthews J: Ergonomics and farm machinery. J Soc Occup Med 33:126–136, 1983.
29. McJilton C, Aherin R: Getting the message to the farmer. Am Ind Hyg Assoc J 43:467–471, 1982.
30. Miyakita T, Miura H, Futatsuka M: Noise-induced hearing loss in relation to vibration-induced white finger in chain saw workers. Scand J Work Environ Health 13:32–36, 1987.
31. Musson Y, Budorf A, Van Drimmelen D: Exposure to shock and vibration and symptoms in workers using impact power tools. Ann Occup Hyg 33:85–96, 1989.
32. National Safety Council: Accident Facts, 1990 Edition. Chicago, National Safety Council, 1990.
33. Pyykko I, Starck J, Farkkila M, et al: Hand-arm vibration in the aetiology of hearing loss in lumberjacks. Br J Ind Med 38:281–289, 1981.
34. Seidel H, Heide R: Long-term effects of whole-body vibration: A critical survey of the literature. Int Arch Occup Environ Health 58:1–26, 1986.
35. Shilling S, Brackbill R: Occupational health and safety risks and potential health consequences perceived by U.S. workers, 1985. Public Health Reports 102(1):36–46, 1987.
36. Stone E: Report on a survey of farm workers' hearing. Proc Agricultural Engineering Symposium. Silsoe, 1967 (quoted in #9).
37. Talamo J: The perception of machinery indicator sounds. Ergonomics 25:41–51, 1982.
38. Taylor W: Vibration white finger in the workplace. J Soc Occup Med 32:159–166, 1982.
39. Thelin J, Joseph D, Davis W, et al: High-frequency hearing loss in male farmers in Missouri. Public Health Reports 98(3):268–273, 1983.
40. Theriault G, DeGuire L, Gingras S, et al: Raynaud's phenomenon in forestry workers in Quebec. Can Med Assoc J 126:1404–1408, 1982.
41. Threshold Limit Values for Chemical Substances and Physical Agents. Cincinnati, American Conference of Governmental Industrial Hygienists, 1990.
42. Weinstein J, Pope M, Schmidt R, et al: Neuropharmacologic effects of vibration on the dorsal root ganglion. Spine 13:521–525, 1988.
43. Zoltie N, Walker D: Spontaneous pneumomediastinum associated with vibration injury. J Royal Coll Surg (Edinb) 29:189, 1984.

W. DANNY BROWN, PhD, MD

HEAT AND COLD IN FARM WORKERS

From Federal Employee
  Occupational Health
U.S. Public Health Service,
  Region X
Seattle, Washington

The opinions and assertions contained herein are the private views of the author and are not to be construed as official or reflecting the views of the Department of Health and Human Services, the U.S. Public Health Service, or the Division of Federal Employee Occupational Health.

Correspondence to:
W. Danny Brown, PhD, MD
Regional Occupational Physician
Federal Employee Occupational
  Health
U.S. Public Health Service,
  Region X
2201 Sixth Avenue, Mail
  Stop RX-21
Seattle, WA 98121-2500

Humans, like other mammals, have the ability to maintain a body temperature within narrow limits. This characteristic is known as homeothermy and allows humans to carry out a wide range of activities without substantial influence by the environment. A protected human may tolerate environmental temperature variation of $-30°C$ to $+80°C$, but a variation in deep body temperature of only $4°C$ can be tolerated. Maximal limits for a living cell are about $-1°C$ and $+45°C$, but temperatures $> 45°C$ can only be tolerated for a short period of time. The consequences of exceeding the normal range of body temperature include mere loss of comfort, impairment of physical and mental performance, and, under extreme conditions, thermal injuries and illnesses. Because it is easier to protect from overcooling than from overheating, physiologic mechanisms have developed to aid in compensating for overheating.

A person who works outdoors, as farm workers must, face definite environmental hazards from heat and cold. Most farm workers have little, if any, training in the evaluation of thermal stress. Instrumentation for the assessment of thermal conditions is not readily available to most farm workers, aside from the standard dry-bulb thermometer. Farm workers often work long hours, perform jobs with heavy workloads, and encounter thermal conditions of both extreme cold and extreme heat. Clothing appropriate to the thermal conditions may not be available. Inadequate rest, poor nutrition, and low aerobic conditioning may add to the difficulties of tolerating thermal stress. When thermal injuries or illnesses do occur, medical care may be geographically distant and the time to treatment delayed for several hours. In addition to providing an overview of the assessment of heat and cold stress and the physiological responses to heat and cold, this chapter is intended to provide practical advice for health practitioners with farm worker patients on avoiding thermal injuries and illnesses.

The incidence of thermal injuries and illnesses among farm workers is unknown. There is no national surveillance system for monitoring these disorders. In 1955 to 1963, 15 deaths were attributed to heat stroke among farm workers in California.[11] Case histories of death due to heat stroke have been reported in a field worker and a laborer.[32] A study in tractor drivers found a level of heat stress sufficient to be a work performance or health hazard.[22] As would be expected, the number of deaths attributable to heat stroke increases during periods of particularly hot weather.[12] The National Safety Council estimates 338 heat-related deaths occurred in the U.S. during 1987, the latest year for which such figures are available.[25]

THERMOREGULATION

Heat Exchange

To prevent and appropriately manage heat-related illnesses, an understanding of heat stress and the pathophysiology of thermoregulation is necessary. Thermoregulation represents the summation of the processes controlling heat production, heat loss, and/or heat gain. Body temperature is determined by the balance between heat accumulation, whether generated by physical activity or gained from the environment, and heat dissipation. Heat storage is the result of either excessive heat accumulation or a reduced ability to dissipate body heat, illustrated in Figure 1. Thermoregulation can be expressed in the form of a simple equation:

$$M \pm C \pm D \pm R = E$$

where M = metabolism
C = convection
D = conduction
R = radiation
E = evaporative cooling from sweating

For body temperature to remain stable, the two sides of the equation must remain equal.

Metabolism is a sequence of chemical reactions that occur as muscles perform work. These chemical reactions consume fuel, generate energy, and produce by-products that must be eliminated. All of these reactions are exothermic and combine to produce the basal metabolic rate. This basal metabolism produces approximately 50–60 kcal/m^2/hour or about 100 kcal/hour for a 70 kg "average" man.

Strenuous physical exertion can produce a marked elevation in the amount of heat produced due to metabolism, on the order of 10- to 20-fold. Certain metabolic conditions such as hyperthyroidism and drugs such as sympathomimetic amines may increase body heat production. Physical tasks that might be performed by farm workers and the associated metabolic heat production are listed in Table 1.

Conduction is the transfer of heat from warmer to cooler objects through direct contact. Only a small fraction—about 20%—of the body's heat is lost through conduction, because air is a good insulator. Temperature loss during

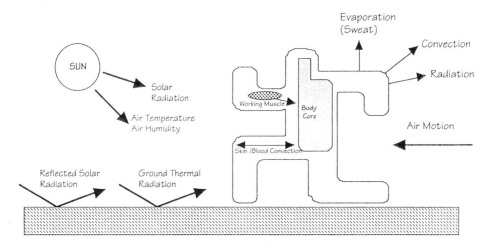

FIGURE 1. "Solar Man" illustrates sources of heat gain and loss in an outdoor farm worker.

immersion in cold water will be much greater, however, due to the significant greater thermal conductivity of water.

Convection represents heat transfer from the air and is due to air and water vapor molecules circulating around the body. Three factors determine how much heat is transferred. One factor is the insulating effect of clothing. Clothing adds insulation in such a manner that the more skin that is covered and/or the thicker the cover, the lower the rate of heat transfer. The second factor is air velocity. The higher the air velocity, the greater the rate of heat transfer. The third factor is the temperature difference between the air and the skin. The larger the difference, the greater the heat transfer will be. When the air temperature exceeds the skin temperature (about 36°C), heat is gained by the body. When the air temperature is less than the skin temperature, the body is cooled by convection.

Radiation is heat transfer by electromagnetic waves (infrared). Radiant heat exchange occurs between two solid bodies. The warmth felt when standing near a hot stove is an example. Two factors affect the amount of radiant heat transfer. First, the more the skin is covered or the thicker the clothing, the less the transfer of heat. In addition, if the clothing has a shiny surface, the infrared radiation is

TABLE 1. Metabolic Heat Production During Various Agricultural Activities

Activity	Kcal/hour
Mowing	360–600
Tractor Plowing	250
Thrashing	300
Weeding	180–480
Brush cleaning	360
Log carrying	200
Milking by hand	200–370
Tree felling with a saw	510–750
Stacking firewood	330–400

Modified from Astrand and Rodahl.[3]

reflected. Second, the average temperature difference between the skin and the surrounding objects determines radiant heat transfer. Radiant heat transfer can contribute significantly to the heat load of individuals working outside; heat gain from the sun can be up to 300 kcal/hour.

Evaporation represents the cooling of the skin by the evaporation of sweat. This is the primary mechanism for cooling the body, especially as the ambient temperature rises. Since the heat necessary to evaporate the sweat is taken from the skin, the skin temperature is reduced. In this manner, heat brought to the skin from the muscles by the blood as well as the heat gained from the environment is removed from the body. The required rate of sweat evaporation is adjusted to balance heat gain from the sum of M, C, and R. The sweat rate does reach a maximum, however, which is determined by the physiologic limit to the amount of sweat a given individual can produce and to the evaporative cooling limitation of the environment. The physiologic limit to sweating in a given individual is generally about 1–2 liters per hour in the untrained individual, but it can exceed 3–4 liters per hour in selected individuals. The environmental limitation on evaporative cooling is determined by clothing insulation, air velocity, and humidity. As clothing insulation increases, the maximum loss due to sweat decreases. As air velocity increases, the maximum evaporation rate increases. Finally, air humidity relates to the amount of water in the air. Most of the time, air humidity is much less than the humidity of sweat at the skin surface, but as air humidity increases, evaporative cooling decreases.

Physiologic Responses to Heat

The hypothalamus serves as the neural control point for thermoregulation. It utilizes sensory information from the body's core and periphery to control the sweating mechanism, cardiovascular system, and muscular function. In general terms, the hypothalamus acts as a "thermostat" to detect changes in body temperature and initiates physiologic responses to maintain the body temperature at a set point. The brain is well perfused and responds rapidly to changes in blood temperature. When heat strain occurs, the body must increase blood flow to take heat away from the muscles to the skin and to increase the sweat rate to dissipate heat by evaporative cooling. Heat loss from the skin by convection and radiation is maximized by increased skin blood flow, which also carries heat convectively from the core to the surface. The main role of elevated skin blood flow in a warm environment, however, is to deliver the heat necessary to evaporate sweat.

During work in the heat, the heart cannot provide enough cardiac output to meet both the peak needs of all the body's organ systems and the need for dissipation of body heat. The autonomic nervous system and the endocrine system control the allocation of blood flow among organ systems. The increase in blood supply to active working muscles is balanced by a progressive vasoconstriction of inactive vascular beds, especially in the digestive system. If continuous work in the heat is required, the heart rate gradually rises as the heart is unable to maintain the stroke volume due to the fall in central venous volume from hypohydration; water is lost in sweat and the circulatory system tries to maintain flow to exercising muscles as well as to the skin.

Sweat glands are present in abundance in the skin. Under cholinergic stimulation, they secrete a hypotonic solution composed of 99.5% water by weight. Each liter of sweat evaporated from the skin surface represents a loss of approximately 560 kcal of heat to the environment; sweat that drips from the skin does not cool the body.

Two hormones are important in thermoregulation, the antidiuretic hormone (ADH) and aldosterone. ADH is released by the pituitary and reduces water loss through the kidney, but it has no effect on the water loss through the sweat glands. Aldosterone is released from the adrenal glands and reduces sodium loss through the kidney and the sweat glands.

Acclimatization

On repeated exposure to hot environments, a process of adaptation occurs in which physiologic processes respond to heat in a more efficient fashion, resulting in a better individual tolerance to heat stress. Once acclimatized, an individual may work safely in conditions that previously would have resulted in heat-related illness or even death. Daily exposure to work and heat causes acclimatization over a period of 10 to 14 days. Acclimatization only occurs if the intensity of work is sufficient to increase the body temperature. Work that does not elevate the body temperature does not produce this adaptive phenomenon. The level of acclimatization is relative to the initial level of the farm worker's physical fitness and the total heat stress experienced by the farm worker. A farm worker who does only light work indoors in a hot environment will not achieve the level of acclimatization needed to work outdoors with the additional heat load from the sun or to do harder physical work in the same hot environment indoors. Similarly, an unacclimatized farm worker in excellent physical condition can withstand considerably more heat stress than an unconditioned farm worker.

It is generally agreed that 2 to 4 hours per day of work in the hot environment offers a good practical approach to acclimatization. Work levels can start at about 50% of the full level and progress by about 10% per day, using either an adjustment in the amount of time or work. Acclimatization to work in hot, humid environments provides adaptive benefits that also apply in hot, desert environments; the critical factor appears to be the total heat load experienced by the farm worker. Prolonged absence from the work environment results in some loss of acclimatization, although some effects of acclimatization persist for several weeks. Some reduction in work level is recommended on a return to work.

The physiologic changes during acclimatization include a lower body temperature, a reduced heart rate, increased sweat production, and the production of a more hypotonic sweat response to work in the heat, as shown in Figure 2. A classic feature of the heat acclimatized state is a smaller increment in rectal temperature at a given work level. Failure to replace the water lost in sweat will retard or prevent the development of acclimatization.

Farm workers, although acclimatized to a certain set of conditions of heat and work load, may experience difficulties during sudden seasonal shifts in environmental temperature. At such times, cases of heat-related illness may occur.

HEAT-INDUCED ILLNESS

Several disorders are related to exposure to heat stress. Some, such as heat rash ("prickly heat"), are relatively minor. The important heat-related illnesses are heat cramps, heat edema, heat syncope, heat exhaustion, and heat stroke.

Heat cramps are painful spasms of muscles used during work (arms, legs, or abdominal muscles). Heat cramps tend to occur when the farm worker has ceased activity and is resting, in contrast to athlete's cramps, which tend to occur during exercise and are relieved by muscle massage. Individuals who are at risk for heat cramps are those who produce large quantities of sweat and receive adequate

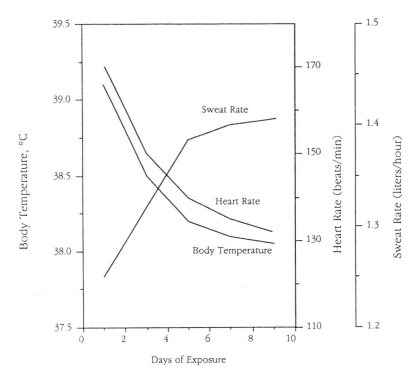

FIGURE 2.   Typical physiologic changes occurring during acclimatization to hot working conditions.

replenishment of water but inadequate NaCl replacement. The most likely cause is hyponatremia. Prevention can usually be assured by providing copious amounts of water and increasing the daily intake of salt. Severe cases can be treated with intravenous saline (0.9% NaCl).

Heat edema refers to slight dependent edema of the ankles and feet in unacclimatized individuals, who usually offer a history of prolonged standing or sitting. There is no significant functional impairment and the disorder is self-limited. Therapy should be limited to elevation of the lower limb.

Heat syncope is dizziness or fainting that occurs in a person who has been exposed to a hot environment and for which no other apparent cause can be found. The cause appears to be pooling of blood in dilated vessels of the skin and lower parts of the body, with subsequent cerebral ischemia. The disorder is self-limiting, because falling to a horizontal position increases cerebral perfusion; the fall, however, may result in serious injury. Individuals at risk, e.g., cardiac patients or patients taking diuretics, should be warned to avoid prolonged standing in the heat and to assume a sitting or horizontal position whenever presyncopal symptoms develop. Acclimatization will reduce the likelihood of heat syncope.

Heat exhaustion, also known as heat prostration, is the most common heat-related illness. It is characterized by a constellation of constitutional symptoms (weakness, fatigue, frontal headache, nausea, vomiting, anorexia, impaired judgment) and may be accompanied by cramps, dizziness, and syncope. Heat exhaustion lies somewhere in a continuum between mild heat illness and heat stroke. Heat exhaustion should be differentiated from heat stroke by the modest elevation of core temperature (37.5°C to 38.5°C), lack of severe central nervous system dysfunction, and the lack of elevated transaminases in the peripheral blood.

Two types of heat exhaustion have been described, either that due to water depletion or due to salt depletion. Water depletion heat exhaustion results from insufficient fluid replacement and has been noted to occur in various types of laborers, including hay balers.[17] Inadequate fluid replacement results in progressive dehydration and hypernatremia. There is a steady increase in body temperature and pulse rate, declining sweat rate, fatigue, weakness, vertigo, intense thirst, and impaired judgment. Left untreated, water depletion heat exhaustion may progress to heat stroke. Farm workers will not replace all water lost while working in the heat through voluntary drinking, usually replenishing about two-thirds of water loss.

Salt depletion heat exhaustion occurs when large volumes of sweat are replaced with adequate water but inadequate salt. Thirst is not a predominant symptom of this type, and urine flow and sweat rate remain normal. Unlike heat cramps, which are also associated with hyponatremia, symptoms are systemic. Symptoms and signs resemble those of water depletion heat exhaustion, but body temperature may be normal or even low.[17]

Most cases of heat exhaustion are of a mixed type; treatment involves fluid replacement, with the type and amount of fluid guided by the clinical and laboratory (electrolytes, blood urea nitrogen, hematocrit, serum, and urine osmolality) assessment. The body water deficit can be estimated by assuming that the water loss is universally proportional to the increase in the concentration of sodium. For example, the "ideal" 70 kg patient has 42 liters of estimated total body water (total body water [TBW] = 70 kg × 60% total body water). If the serum Na^+ is 160 mEq/liter, the water deficit is estimated as follows:

$$\text{Water deficit (L)} = TBW - (TBW \times \text{desired } [Na^+]/\text{observed } [Na^+])$$
$$= 42\ L - (42\ L \times 140\ \text{mEqL}^{-1}/160\ \text{mEqL}^{-1})$$
$$= 42\ L - 36.7\ L = 5.3\ L$$

The rate of fluid administration should be controlled, because overly rapid correction may result in cerebral edema, seizures, and death. The water deficit should be replaced over 36 to 48 hours once the patient is hemodynamically stable. If the patient is conscious and not vomiting, oral replacement is the preferred route. Treatment can be less vigorous in cases of salt depletion heat exhaustion, which generally require only 1 to 2 liters of fluid intravenously as normal saline before symptomatic improvement is observed.[17]

Heat stroke is a medical emergency. Heat stroke occurs when the body's homeostatic mechanisms are unable to meet the demands of heat stress. Body temperature increases to extreme levels, producing multisystem dysfunction and tissue damage. The classic description of heat stroke includes (1) a major disruption of central nervous system function (delirium, seizures, coma), (2) a lack of sweating, and (3) a rectal temperature in excess of 41°C.[34] Observations on the clinical progression of heat stroke have been made only after the admission of patients to hospitals, which may vary in time from about 30 minutes to several hours after onset. It is clear that in some cases of heat stroke sweating may be present.[8] In cases of exertional heat stroke, sweating may continue in up to 50% of cases.[17] The presence of sweating does not rule out the diagnosis of heat stroke, and a failure of the sweat glands is not the cause of heat stroke. Due to the time interval between the onset of the disorder and the presentation to emergency medical facilities, some cooling may occur; the initial rectal temperature may not be elevated above 41°C and may not represent a maximum.[31] A high index of suspicion must be maintained, and a diagnosis of heat stroke considered when environmental conditions conducive to heat illness are present.

Heat stroke has been subdivided into two forms based upon the presentation, treatment, and prevention: classic and exertional.[18] Classic heat stroke will be only briefly reviewed here. Exertional heat stroke is the more likely entity to occur in farm workers who are performing physical tasks in a hot environment. The major features of classic heat stroke and exertional heat stroke are listed in Table 2.

Classic heat stroke occurs during periods of sustained high temperatures and humidity, such as summer heat waves; usually temperatures and humidity remain high both day and night.[14] Active sweating continues constantly but eventually fails. The elderly and debilitated are at greatest risk for classic heat stroke, often having inadequate access to effective household cooling or ready access to water. Farm workers may be included in this category, because they may continue to work until late in life and not leave the work force as in other occupations. Additional risk factors include chronic disease, alcoholism, certain medications (diuretics, anticholinergics, neuroleptics, and antihypertensives), and mental disorders.[16]

Of more concern in farm workers is the threat of **exertional heat stroke**. Farm workers, by necessity, are physically active and may be working vigorously in the open during periods of high temperature and humidity. For example, during the late summer months, average daily temperatures and humidity may reach their

TABLE 2.   Comparison of Classic and Exertional Heat Stroke*

Feature	Classic	Exertional
Age group	Very young, very old	Men 15–45 years old
Health status	Chronic illness common	Usually healthy
History of febrile illness or immunization	Unusual	Common
Activity	Sedentary	Common in football players, military recruits, competitive runners
Drug use	Sweat depressants, diuretics, haloperidol, phenothiazines	Amphetamines, cocaine
Sweating	Usually absent	Often present
Respiratory alkalosis	Dominant	Mild
Lactic acidosis	Absent or mild	Often marked
Acute renal failure	<5% of patients	30% of patients
Rhabdomyolysis	Seldom severe	Severe
Hyperuricemia	Modest	Severe
Creatinine:BUN[†] ration	1:10	Elevated
CPK[†], aldolase	Mildly elevated	Markedly elevated
Hypocalcemia	Uncommon	Common
DIC[†]	Mild	Marked
Hypoglycemia	Uncommon	Common

* Some features are common to both types: lack of heat acclimatization, dehydration, salt depletion, hyperthermia (> 106°F), cutaneous flushing and mottling, coma, psychotic behavior, convulsions while cooling, shock, adult respiratory distress syndrome, hypokalemia, hypernatremia, hypophosphatemia or hyperphosphatemia, and poikilothermia during recovery.
† BUN = blood urea nitrogen; DIC = disseminated intravascular coagulopathy; CPK = creatine kinase.
Reproduced from Knochel,[17] with permission.

peaks; this period may be an active time for the harvesting of some crops. The basic mechanism of exertional heat stroke involves a failure of the body's ability to dissipate excess endogenous heat. Exertional heat stroke has been reported in military personnel,[15] marathon runners,[40] other athletes,[23] miners and other industrial workers who perform strenuous jobs in a hot environment,[35] and field workers.[32]

The pathophysiology of exertional heat stroke is uncertain, but an "energy depletion" model has been proposed.[13] This model suggests that an exercise-induced thermal imbalance leads to an energy imbalance within the cells and subsequent changes in sodium permeability. This model is also able to account for the beneficial effects of cooling, which alters the sodium influx in the favor of cellular stabilization.

In addition to the symptoms previously described for classic heat stroke, exertional heat stroke is associated with elevated levels of serum enzymes (aspartate transaminase, alanine transaminase, lactic dehydrogenase, creatine kinase) and hypotension. Treatment of heat stroke must include basic airway management and circulatory support. The cornerstone of treatment is cooling. Mortality rates from heat stroke have been shown to increase when cooling is delayed.[36] Delays in cooling are usually attributable to a failure to make the diagnosis or a lack of proper cooling facilities. In areas where heat stroke is likely to occur, prior consideration should be given to the problem and a management plan developed. The modalities of cooling include total body immersion and rubbing the body surface with ice.[18] A specific unit for total body cooling, the Makkah body cooling unit, has been described.[39] During treatment, attention must be given to the potential complications of heat stroke: rhabdomyolysis, disseminated intravascular coagulation, and acute renal failure.[18]

Heat Stress Tolerance Limits

The Occupational Safety and Health Administration defined heat stress as the aggregate of environmental and physical factors that constitute the total heat load imposed on the body.[27] Based upon the material presented thus far, it can be concluded that many factors determine the physiologic strain imposed by heat. These factors include individual variations in body size and fat content, the state of physical fitness, acclimatization, and external factors such as convective air currents, radiant heat gain, intensity of work, amount, type, and color of clothing, and most important, the relative humidity. All these factors may play a role on the total heat burden to farm workers.

In addition to the risks on health presented by heat stress, thermal stress can be linked to an increase in unsafe work behavior. The accumulation of heat in the body during longer and more intense exposures gradually builds up fatigue and a corresponding decrease in endurance. The relationship between unsafe work behavior and thermal stress seems to follow a U-shaped curve, with increases in unsafe behavior occurring at high heat levels (WBGT over 23°C).[28] There have not been enough studies, however, to establish heat stress limits for accident prevention.

The most effective way to control heat-related illnesses and injuries is to prevent their occurrence. Considerable attention has been given to the evaluation of an environment in terms of its potential heat challenge. Numerous attempts have been made to generate standards, rules, or guidelines concerning work in the heat. The Heat Stress Index (HSI) developed by Belding and Hatch[24] is widely accepted as a method of providing a quantitative description of the heat components of an environment. The HSI is complex and difficult to use, however.

The need for a measure of occupational heat stress that is easy to use and understand has led to the support of the Wet Bulb Globe Temperature (WBGT). To use the WBGT as a basis for occupational heat decisions requires that estimates or measurements be made of the metabolic workload and the thermal components of the environment. The WBGT has been adopted by the American Conference of Governmental Industrial Hygienists (ACGIH) with the concurrent establishment of Threshold Limit Values (TLV) for heat stress. The National Institute for Occupational Safety and Health (NIOSH) revised its WBGT-based recommendations in 1986. NIOSH recommends two standards, one for acclimatized workers (the Recommended Exposure Limit, or REL) and one for unacclimatized workers (Recommended Alert Limit, or RAL).[24] Both NIOSH recommendations represent 8-hour time-weighted averages that are not to be exceeded for a given level of metabolic heat, as shown in Figures 3 and 4. Both recommendations are

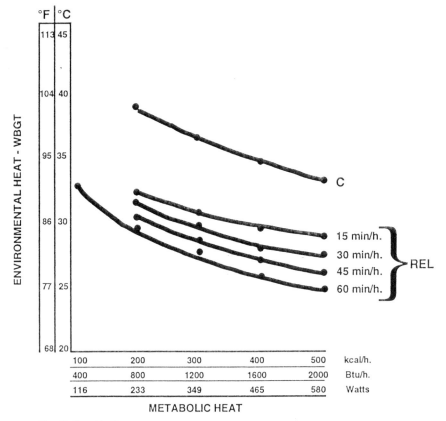

C = Ceiling Limit

REL = Recommended Exposure Limit

*For "standard worker" of 70 kg (154 lbs) body weight and

1.8 sq. meters (19.4 sq. feet) body surface

FIGURE 3. NIOSH Recommended Exposure Limit for heat-acclimatized workers.

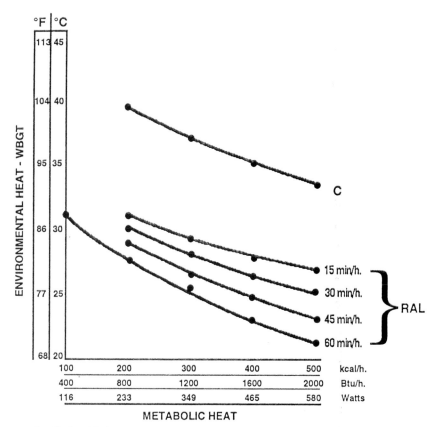

C = Ceiling Limit

RAL = Recommended Alert Limit

*For "standard worker" of 70 kg (154 lbs) body weight and

1.8 sq. meters (19.4 sq. feet) body surface

FIGURE 4.   NIOSH Recommended Alert Limit for heat-unacclimatized workers.

based on the assumption that almost all healthy farm workers should be able to tolerate the recommended total heat load without substantially increasing their risk of incurring acute adverse health effects. The ACGIH has adopted NIOSH's REL for acclimatized workers as its current TLV recommendation.[1] Because both the TLV and the REL are based on metabolic heat in addition to environmental heat load, an estimation (using examples such as in Table 1) or an actual measurement of metabolic heat is required.

Outdoor farm work usually involves a solar load. In these cases, the WBGT is calculated as follows: WBGT = 0.7 NWB + 0.2 GT + 0.1 DB, where NWB is the natural wet bulb temperature, DB is the dry bulb temperature, and GT is the globe temperature. Indoor or outdoor work with no solar load is calculated as follows: WBGT = 0.7 NWB + 0.3 GT. Instruments that measure each component and even perform a WBGT calculation are available commercially.

TABLE 3. Categorization of Heat Stress Using the Apparent Temperature

Category	Apparent Temperature (°F)	Heat Syndrome
Caution	80° to 90°	Fatigue possible with prolonged exposure and physical activity.
Extreme Caution	90° to 106°	Heat cramps, and heat exhaustion *possible* with prolonged exposure and physical activity.
Danger	106° to 130°	Heat cramps, and heat exhaustion *likely*. Heat stroke *possible* with prolonged exposure and physical activity.
Extreme Danger	> 130°	Heat stroke *very likely*.

Source: U.S. Weather Service

In 1984, the National Weather Service adopted the Apparent Temperature (AT) Index[37] for its heat wave advisories. The AT value can be calculated as follows: $AT = -2.65 + 0.994 \, Ta + 0.015 \, Td^2$, where Ta = dry bulb temperature and Td = dew point temperature. The Ta and Td values are obtainable through local weather reports. A range of AT values is used to categorize the potential for heat-related illness, as shown in Table 3. The AT index may be one of the easiest for farm workers to use due to the ready availability of the temperature indices. It is not intended, however, for the assessment of occupational heat stress and does not include a contribution for metabolism.

Personal Monitoring

Personal monitoring is a method to assess the farm worker's response to a heat exposure while working. Two physiologic responses to heat stress that are generally recognized as important candidates for assessment are body temperature and heart rate. Body temperature measurements are usually impractical for the agricultural environment. Obtaining rectal temperatures is usually unacceptable. Oral temperatures are unreliable. Heart rate, however, can be measured directly by palpation or by surface electrodes. With the increase in popularity of physical fitness, numerous electronic devices for measuring heart rate are available. If it is suspected that an exposure to heat stress may be excessive, the recovery heart rate pattern can be examined using a method developed by Fuller and Smith.[10] To use this technique, the farm worker must stop working for 4 minutes. From 30 to 60 seconds after the work, the heart beats should be counted and multiplied by 2 (rate P1). From 150 to 180 seconds (2.5 to 3 minutes), the heart beats should be counted and multiplied by 2 (rate P3). The decision logic is as follows:

P3 < 90: no excessive strain
P3 > 90 and P1–P3 > 10: marginal stress
P3 > 90 and P1–P3 < 10: high stress

If marginal stress is indicated, work should proceed with caution (reduced workload and further checks). If high stress is indicated, work should be terminated. Although this method has not been completely validated, it may provide a reasonable field estimate of heat strain.

Work Practices

There are other work practices that may help farm workers avoid heat-related illness and injury. Physicians who are involved in the care of farm workers should instruct them to:

- Schedule heavy work during cooler parts of the day or postpone to later days, when a heat stress index indicates that heat-related illness is a possibility.
- Where possible, take measures to reduce the physical workload, such as increased mechanization, changing the job, or distributing tasks across more farm workers.
- Dress appropriately for the job and the hot environment. Loose, lightweight clothing will aid evaporative cooling. A wide-brimmed hat should be worn when working in the sunshine.
- Perform work in a cool, shaded area if the job permits.
- Establish a schedule for work and rest, based upon the heat stress index and the level of work to be done.
- Learn to recognize the signs and symptoms of heat disorders and to give first aid when needed.
- Establish an acclimatization program, which will benefit new farm workers and any unacclimatized ones.
- Improve overall physical fitness, which will improve heat tolerance.
- Be well rested at the start of work periods. Fatigue lowers the body's resistance to heat stress.
- Provide adequate water supplies during hot working conditions. It is best to plan to have as many liters of replacement fluid (water or electrolyte replenishing solution) available as there are person-hours of heat exposure. Water breaks may need to be mandatory, since satisfying thirst alone will not provide the needed replacement.
- Alcoholic beverages should be prohibited.

COLD-ASSOCIATED ILLNESS

Cold presents another environmental hazard to farm workers. Harvesting crops, feeding livestock, and repairing machinery in the field are just some of the activities that may require farm workers to work in temperatures that are near to or below freezing.

The same mechanisms (conduction, convection, radiation) that function in gain of heat by the body from the hot environment, also serve as the routes of loss of heat from the body to the cold environment. Heat loss by **conduction** is usually minimal, since there is a reflex withdrawal from cold objects. Under certain conditions, such as being buried in snow or immersed in cold water, conduction may assume an important role. Heat loss by conduction is also many times more rapid in wet clothes than with dry clothing. Perspiration or rain reduce the insulating properties of clothing.

Body heat loss may also occur through **convection.** The body maintains a warm microclimate of air adjacent to the skin. If this thin layer is removed by wind or air currents, cooling will result. As air movement increases, the effect of "wind chill" becomes more important. Wind chill causes heat to be lost from the body faster than would be the case in still air. Wind chill tables (Table 4) quantitate the risk. For example, a wind at a speed of 10 MPH reduces an ambient temperature of 0°F to the equivalent of –24°F, greatly increasing the risk of cold-related injuries.

Radiation of heat occurs from uncovered surfaces, especially hands, face, head, and neck, and is the usual predominant source of heat loss. Additional heat loss occurs through the evaporation of sweat and through respiration.

Ambient Temperature, °F														
40	35	30	25	20	15	10	5	0	-5	-10	-15	-20	-25	-30
Equivalent Temperature, °F														
40	35	30	25	20	15	10	5	0	-5	-10	-15	-20	-25	-30
37	33	27	21	16	12	6	1	-5	-11	-15	-20	-26	-31	-36
28	21	16	9	4	-2	-9	-15	-21	-27	-33	-38	-46	-52	-58
22	16	11	1	-5	-11	-18	-25	-36	-40	-45	-51	-58	-65	-72
18	12	3	-4	-10	-17	-25	-32	-39	-46	-53	-60	-67	-76	-82
16	7	0	-7	-15	-22	-29	-37	-44	-52	-59	-67	-74	-83	-88
13	5	-2	-11	-18	-26	-33	-41	-48	-56	-63	-70	-79	-87	-94
11	3	-4	-13	-20	-27	-35	-43	-49	-60	-67	-72	-82	-90	-98
10	1	-6	-15	-21	-29	-37	-45	-53	-62	-69	-76	-85	-94	-100

Wind Speed MPH: Calm, 5, 10, 15, 20, 25, 30, 35, 40

Exposed Flesh Can Freeze in 60 Seconds

Exposed Flesh Can Freeze in 30 Seconds

TABLE 4. Wind Chill Table.

Source: National Weather Service

When the body is exposed to a cold environment, it has two types of normal physiologic reactions. First, constriction of superficial blood vessels in the skin and subcutaneous tissue shunts blood away from the body surface where it will lose heat to a cooler environment. Second, there is an increase in metabolic heat production through voluntary movement and shivering. Cold-induced shivering increases oxygen consumption about four times, involves a specific frequency range (8–11 Hertz), and invokes a remarkable synchronization of different muscle groups.[26] Different physiologic mechanisms predominate at different body temperatures. Between 35°C and 32.2°C, heat production is primarily from shivering and endocrinologic mechanisms that are coupled with vasoconstriction. From 32.2°C to 24°C, vasoconstriction but not shivering is present, and metabolic heat production decreases. Below 24°C, heat conservation fails.[19]

Cold-Induced Injuries

Cold injuries involve the extremities and/or the body's core. Cold injuries may involve freezing or may be nonfreezing. Several factors may predispose a farm worker to cold injury (Table 5). All outdoor workers, including farm workers, are at risk for cold injuries.

Cold injuries of the extremities are most likely in the cheeks, nose, external ear, fingers, toes, hands, and feet. **Frost nip** is the least severe cold injury and represents reversible ice crystal formation in the skin surface. It is associated with intense vasoconstriction and usually develops slowly and painlessly. The symptoms usually resolve spontaneously with warming, and no tissue is lost. The involved area should be warmed by rubbing or blowing warm air.

Chilblains result from repeated exposure of bare skin to cold water or from wet cooling of an extremity over hours or days at temperatures slightly above freezing. Chilblains usually refer to lesions of the hands and feet. Trench foot (immersion foot) represents a more severe form of the injury occurring in the lower extremities, which is most often seen in the military and in seamen and fishermen. The skin is erythematous at first but turns pale. Paresthesia and anesthesia are characteristic. Two to three days following rewarming, hyperemia develops with intense pain, additional swelling, redness, heat, blistering, hemorrhage, ecchymoses, and sometimes cellulitis, gangrene, or thrombophlebitis. Chronic cold sensitivity, hyperhidrosis, and hyperpigmentation are potential long-term sequelae. Management consists of elevation, gradual rewarming, and protection from pressure sores.

Frostbite is caused by the actual freezing of soft tissue. It is usually seen with extremely cold temperatures in conjunction with the wind. Given long enough exposure, bare skin will begin to freeze at –2°C (28°F). Exposed areas of skin are most commonly involved. Unlike thermal burns, frostbite has not been given a classification system. A staging system has been suggested, however, based upon symptoms and signs.[9] Frostbite begins with local swelling and redness, and

TABLE 5.   Risk Factors for Cold Injury

Age (very young or very old)
Poor nutrition
Fatigue
Alcohol
Smoking
Any condition affecting peripheral circulation (arterial disease, tight clothing)
Inadequate insulating clothing

paresthesia or anesthesia. The skin is white with a "waxy" appearance and may feel hard if the frostbite is deep. A comprehensive protocol for the treatment of frostbite has been recommended.[21] Treatment is directed toward blocking direct cellular injury and toward prevention of progressive microvascular thrombosis and tissue loss. All but the most minor frostbite cases should be hospitalized.

Hypothermia represents systemic cold injury and is arbitrarily defined as a core temperature of less than 35°C (95°F). Accidental hypothermia is the major cause of death in people engaged in outdoor recreation and a significant public health problem in the elderly and debilitated, although the exact incidence in the United States is not clear.

Hypothermia can be easily overlooked. Standard clinical thermometers only extend to 34.4°C (94°F), and the signs and symptoms of hypothermia are nonspecific. Its onset is so gradual that frequently the victim and those around him or her fail to notice the onset. Initial clinical findings include drowsiness, slurred speech, irritability, impaired coordination, general weakness and lethargy, combativeness, and a cool skin and face. Figure 5 outlines the various levels of hypothermia and the corresponding signs and symptoms. Comprehensive reviews of the pathophysiology, presentation, and treatment of hypothermia are available.[7,9]

Work Practices

There are also some work practices that may help farm workers avoid cold-related illness and injury. Primary prevention of hypothermia is desirable due to the difficulties of treatment in the field. Physicians may instruct farm workers to take the following preventive measures for cold-related injury:

- Learn to recognize the signs and symptoms of cold disorders and how to give first aid when needed.
- Improve general physical conditioning.
- Maintain good nutrition and have adequate rest prior to beginning to work in the cold.
- Avoid dehydration.
- Wear layers of clothing to allow adjustment for overheating or overcooling. Wool offers the best natural fabric.
- Cover areas of the body with a high surface to volume ratio (hands, ears, and head) to reduce heat loss.
- Wear clothing that allows water vapor to escape.
- Use rain gear if necessary to keep clothing dry.
- Avoid alcohol since it may impair the thermoregulatory response to cold.
- Remember that acclimatization to cold offers less benefit than in the case of heat, because humans possess little capacity for adaptation to prolonged cold exposure.

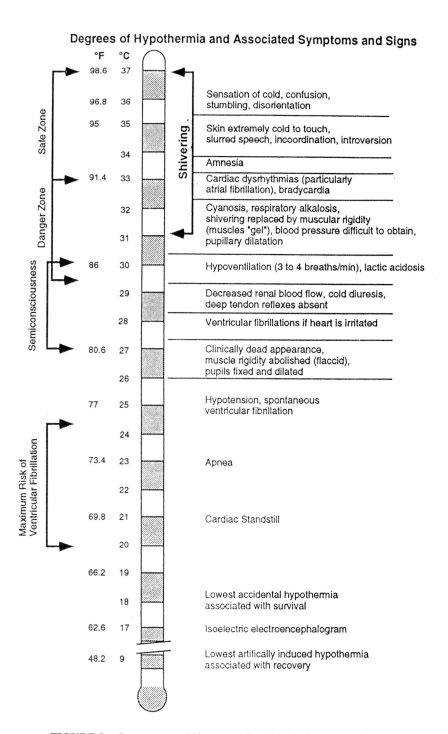

FIGURE 5. Symptoms and signs at various levels of hypothermia.

REFERENCES

1. American Conference of Governmental Industrial Hygienists: Threshold Limit Values and Biological Indices. Cincinnati, ACGIH, 1990.
2. Armstrong LE, Hubbard RW, Jones BH, Daniels JT: Preparing Alberto Salazar for the heat of the 1984 Olympic marathon. Phys Sportsmed 14:73–81, 1986.
3. Astrand PO, Rodahl K: Textbook of Work Physiology: Physiological Basis of Exercise, 2nd ed. New York, McGraw-Hill, 1986.
4. Avellini BA, Shapiro Y, Fortney SM, et al: Effects on heat tolerance of physical training in water and on land. J Appl Physiol 53:1291–1298, 1982.
5. Bean WB, Eichna LW: Performance in relation to environmental temperature: Reactions of normal young men to simulated desert environment. Fed Proc 2:144–158, 1943.
6. Collins KJ: The action of exogenous aldosterone on the secretion and composition of drug-induced sweat. Clin Sci 30:207–221, 1966.
7. Danzl DF, Pozos RS, Hamlet MP: Accidental hypothermia. In Auerbach PS, Geehr EC (eds): Management of Wilderness and Environmental Emergencies. St. Louis, C.V. Mosby, 1989, pp 35–76.
8. Dukes-Dobos FN: Hazards of heat exposure. A review. Scand J Work Environ Health 7:73–83, 1981.
9. Fritz RL, Perrin DH: Cold exposure injuries: Prevention and treatment. Clin Sports Med 8:111–128, 1989.
10. Fuller FH, Smith PE: The effectiveness of preventive work practices in a hot work shop. In Proceedings of a NIOSH Workshop on Recommended Heat Stress Standards, DHHS Publication No. 81-108, Washington, DC, 1980, pp 32–42.
11. Gilbert A, O'Rourke PF: Effects of rural poverty on the health of California's farmworkers. Public Health Rep 83:827–839, 1968.
12. Heat related deaths—Missouri 1979–1988. MMWR 38:437–439, 1989.
13. Hubbard RW, Armstrong LE: Hyperthermia: New thoughts on an old problem. Phys Sportsmed 17:97–113, 1989.
14. Jones TS, Liang AP, Kilbourne EM, et al: Morbidity and mortality associated with the July 1980 heat wave in St. Louis and Kansas City, MO. JAMA 247:3327–3331, 1982.
15. Kerstein MD, Wright D, Connelly J, Hubbard R: Heat illness in hot/humid environments. Milit Med 151:308–311, 1986.
16. Kilbourne EM: Illness due to thermal extremes. In Last JM (ed): Maxcy-Rosenau's Public Health and Preventive Medicine, 12th ed. New York, Appleton-Century-Crofts, 1986, pp 703–714.
17. Knochel JP: Heat stroke and related heat stress disorders. Dis Mon 35:301–377, 1989.
18. Knochel JP: Environmental heat illness. An eclectic review. Arch Intern Med 133:841–864, 1974.
19. Maclean D, Emslie-Smith D: Accidental Hypothermia. Philadelphia, J.B. Lippincott, 1977.
20. McArdle WD, Katch FI, Katch VL: Exercise Physiology: Energy, Nutrition, and Human Performance, 2nd ed. Philadelphia, Lea & Febiger, 1986.
21. McCauley RL, Hing DN, Robson MC, Heggers JP: Frostbite injuries: A rational approach based on the pathophysiology. J Trauma 23:143–147, 1983.
22. Miller CW: Heat exhaustion in tractor drivers. Occup Health (Lond) 34(8):361–365, 1982.
23. Murphy RJ: Heat illness in the athlete. Am J Sports Med 12:258–261, 1984.
24. National Institute for Occupational Safety and Health: Criteria for a Recommended Standard: Occupational Exposure to Hot Environments. DHHS Publication No. 86-113, Washington, DC, 1986.
25. National Safety Council: Accident Facts. 1990 Edition, Chicago, National Safety Council, 1990.
26. Pozos RS, Israel D, McCutcheon R, et al: Human studies concerning thermal-induced shivering, postoperative "shivering," and cold-induced vasodilation. Ann Emerg Med 16:1037–1041, 1987.
27. Ramsey JD: Stress standard: OSHA's advisory committee recommendations. Nat Saf News 89–95, 1975.
28. Ramsey JD, Burford CL, Beshir MY, Jensen RC: Effects of workplace thermal conditions on safe work behavior. J Saf Res 14:105–114, 1983.
29. Reuler JB: Hypothermia: Pathophysiology, clinical settings, and management. Ann Intern Med 89:519–527, 1978.
30. Rowell LB: Cardiovascular aspects of human thermoregulation. Circ Res 52:367–379, 1983.
31. Shapiro Y, Seidman DS: Field and clinical observations of exertional heat stroke patients. Med Sci Sports Exerc 22:6–14, 1990.
32. Sherman R, Copes R, Stewart RK, et al: Occupational death due to heat stroke: Report of two cases. Can Med Assoc J 140:1057–1058, 1989.

33. Shibolet S, Coll R, Gilat T, Sohar E: Heatstroke: Its clinical picture and mechanism in 36 cases. Q J Med 36:525–548, 1967.
34. Shibolet S, Lancaster MC, Danon Y: Heat stroke: A review. Aviat Space Environ Med 47:280–301, 1976.
35. Spain WH, Ewing WM, Clay EM: Knowledge of causes, controls aids prevention of heat stress. Occup Health Saf 54:27–33, 1985.
36. Spring CL: Heat stroke: Modern approaches to an ancient disease. Chest 77:461–472, 1980.
37. Steadman RG: A universal scale of apparent temperature. J Climate Applied Metereol 23:1674–1687, 1984.
38. Talbott JH: Heat cramps. Medicine (Baltimore) 14:232–241, 1935.
39. Weiner JS, Khogali M: A physiological body-cooling unit for treatment of heat stroke. Lancet i:507–509, 1980.
40. Whitworth JA, Wolfman MJ: Fatal heat stroke in a long distance runner. Br Med J (Clin Res) 287:948–951, 1983.
41. Wyndham CH, Strydom NB, Morrison JF, et al: Responses of unacclimatized men under stress of heat and work. J Appl Physiol 6:681–690, 1954.
42. Yarborough BE, Hubbard RW: Heat-related illness. In Auerbach PS, Geehr EC (eds): Management of Wilderness and Environmental Emergencies. St. Louis, C.V. Mosby, 1989, pp 119–143.

CARYL S. SHAVER, MD
THEODORE TONG, PharmD

CHEMICAL HAZARDS TO AGRICULTURAL WORKERS

Caryl S. Shaver, MD
Section of Preventive and
  Occupational Medicine
Department of Family and
  Community Medicine
The University of Arizona College
  of Medicine
Tucson, Arizona

Theodore Tong, PharmD
Director, Arizona Poison
  Information Center
College of Pharmacy
The University of Arizona
Tucson, Arizona

Reprint requests to:
Theodore Tong, PharmD
The University of Arizona College
  of Pharmacy
Room 344D
Tucson, AZ 85721

CHEMICAL HAZARDS IN AGRICULTURE

Agriculture is an extremely diverse industry. The hazards on a Midwestern dairy farm may be very different from the hazards existing on a California produce farm. Even for a single type of farm, the risks may vary widely through the seasons, with hazards of the summer growing season being quite different from the hazards in winter, when stored crops are opened for use. Farmers also tend to be "do it yourself" types.[17] It is routine to repair one's own equipment, and financial constraints make it common to get by with less than optimal equipment. This leads to inexperienced workers using potentially dangerous equipment and chemicals in rushed circumstances—clearly a risky affair.

The agriculture industry is also quite complex. It is difficult for individual farmers to be uniformly knowledgeable about all potential dangers from chemical hazards on a farm. Farmers do not have safety personnel on staff as do other industries where hazardous chemicals are used. Some chemicals may be in the form of consumer products and therefore may have product information available. However, many chemical hazards, such as manure gas and silo gas, are produced on the farm itself, and the farmer may not be aware that a danger exists. In many situations the only resources a farmer may have available are the County Agricultural Service, state or local pesticide office, Poison Control Center, and the community physician, if one exists.[17] It is, therefore, very important that any physician practicing in an agricultural area be aware of potential agricultural chemical hazards, because in many cases he or she will be the primary contact person for health and safety information.

This discussion will survey potential hazards to farmers' health from chemicals. Certainly, the most dramatic health risks from agricultural chemicals involve pesticides of various sorts, particularly the organophosphates. For that reason, discussions of agricultural chemical hazards are usually overshadowed by these pesticides. However, in this paper the focus will be on the acute toxicity of chemical hazards, other than pesticides, likely to be present in an agricultural setting. The focus will be process-oriented wherever possible. Processes covered here include: (1) fertilizer use, (2) equipment use and repair, (3) sterilization and fumigation operations, (4) animal confinement hazards, and (5) the use of stored products (such as silo-opening hazards). Because pesticides are covered extensively in other reference sources, their toxicity will be summarized at the conclusion of this article and will not be discussed in depth.

In this discussion it is also important to remember the littlest farmers, i.e., children. Children constitute a large portion of the labor force on many family farms. Exposure to farm chemicals at an early age may have far-reaching effects that are, as yet, undiscovered. Very little is known about the health effects of most farm chemicals on infants and children. In addition, even when not acting in the labor force directly, some chemical hazards (such as nitrates from fertilizer or pesticide residues brought home on clothing) can adversely affect the health of farm infants and children.

FERTILIZER APPLICATION HAZARDS

Anhydrous Ammonia

Fertilizer is usually a combination of nitrogen, phosphates, potassium, and other plant nutrient materials of a variety of types. Most commonly, it is in the form of a granular material that is spread on the soil. Other forms include slurry or sludge from animal wastes and anhydrous ammonia.

One-third of emergency department visits caused by agricultural chemical exposures in a 21 county area in Nebraska in 1985 were due to anhydrous ammonia exposure from its use as a fertilizer.[72] Anhydrous ammonia, a source of nitrogen, is stored in liquid form in pressurized tanks. These tanks are pulled behind a tractor and the ammonia is sprayed directly onto fields. Exposure can occur during application or during connection of a tank to spraying equipment. Freezing burns of the skin and eyes due to heat loss caused by the vaporization of anhydrous ammonia can occur if contact is made with the liquid as it escapes from the container. The most severe burns result from direct contact with ammonia in the liquid form. Anhydrous ammonia is very water-soluble and forms a strongly alkaline solution that can produce severe burns of the skin, eyes, and mucous membranes.[72] Liquefacient necrosis of tissues results and, as with any strongly alkaline chemical, penetration to deep tissues can occur. First and second degree burns and blistering of the skin can result.[64] Ocular exposure to anhydrous ammonia can be serious and in some cases requires referral to an ophthalmologist due to the severity of corneal burns. Mild keratitis and conjunctivitis can be treated with supportive measures.[11]

The most severe health risk is due to inhalation. Anhydrous ammonia can cause adult respiratory distress syndrome (ARDS), bronchiolitis obliterans, and chronic bronchiectasis if inhaled in its gaseous form. Fatalities have occurred as a result.[8,39,77] Pulmonary fibrosis may also result, even if the initial insult is survived.[86]

Differing exposure times and concentrations lead to differing pulmonary syndromes. High concentrations (2500–6500 ppm or greater)[70] for short periods of time can result in partial- to full-thickness burns of the face, neck, exposed extremities and cornea. These patients are likely to have serious burns of the upper airway and may require intubation to avert upper airway obstruction. Fortunately, these patients can expect to recover with few sequelae.

In patients exposed to lower concentrations (~ 100–2500 ppm or greater)[70] of anhydrous vapor for longer periods of time, devastating burns of the entire tracheobronchial tree, rather than upper airway obstruction, will result. This is because the anhydrous ammonia in vapor form can be inhaled throughout the pulmonary system. At lower levels, the upper respiratory irritation effects can be tolerated somewhat longer, leading to an increased dose in the lower respiratory tract. Once deep in the lungs, it can combine with water present on the mucosal surfaces to cause alkali burns of the small airways, which leads to acute pulmonary edema. In these cases, initial presenting symptoms may not represent the actual severity of the injury. Early pulmonary function tests may be abnormal and provide the only clue of impending pulmonary failure. It is crucial to the success of medical management to realize that even with severe pulmonary damage, the initial chest x-ray films may be normal and initial arterial blood gas studies may be normal or show only mild hypoxemia. While no clear recommendations for medical management exist, successful early management has included steroids, mechanical ventilation, and antibiotics.[8]

After the initial injury, an exacerbation is not uncommon 2 to 3 weeks after exposure. Gradual deterioration of pulmonary function can continue for 2 to 6 months, followed by a slight improvement. In some cases, pulmonary impairment may result from ventilation-perfusion deficits and moderate obstructive airway function.[8]

Other Fertilizer Hazards

There are numerous fertilizer preparations available, many in granular form. The use of granular fertilizers has not been associated with systemic health problems. A more insidious threat from the use of fertilizers results from the nitrate contamination of ground water. High levels of nitrates in the soil and nitrates and nitrites in the ground water can also have profound health effects, both on adult farmers and their children. This contamination is due to application of chemical fertilizer, but feedlot and barnyard run-off and sewage disposal systems also contribute to the problem (from nitrates and ammonia in excrement). Ground-water contamination of well water can cause infant death due to methemoglobin (well water methemoglobinemia syndrome).[9,16,23,43,44] Methemoglobinemia is generally not a problem for adults because they have adequate amounts of methemoglobin reductase. Methemoglobinemia in adults is a consideration in animal confinement units, however, and this will be discussed below.

The long-term effects of nitrates in the water supply on many farms are of great concern. Nitrosamines are formed through the combination of nitrates with secondary amines in the body. Nitrosamines are potent carcinogens.[48,59] Nitrates can also be converted to nitrites by bacteria in the mouth to increase the nitrite pool, facilitating the formation of nitroso- compounds.[44,60] There is a possible relationship between nitrate in the drinking water and the incidence of stomach and esophageal cancer.[12,14,26,46] Non-Hodgkin's lymphoma has also been associated with elevated levels of nitrates in the drinking water in farming communities.[81]

EQUIPMENT USE AND REPAIR

Gasoline

A variety of organic solvents, gasoline, and diesel fuel may be present on a farm. Often farmers will maintain their own gasoline and diesel supply tanks. In addition to using gasoline as a fuel, they may also use it as a solvent. Risks of exposure to solvents and fuels include skin contact (and possible systemic absorption), ingestion with resulting pulmonary aspiration, and inhalation of vapors.[80] Of these potential exposures, inhalation is the most common occupational exposure. Gasoline vapors are pulmonary tract irritants and may cause headache, dizziness, flushed face, dysphagia, slurred speech, nausea, anorexia, dullness, and mental confusion. At higher concentrations, central nervous system depression predominates. Vomiting, delirium, cyanosis, coma, seizures, and respiratory depression may result. Inhalation of concentrations greater than 5000 ppm can be rapidly fatal. Microhemorrhages in organs may also occur.[15,24] Sudden death may occur due to cardiac sensitization, with resultant arrhythmia in gasoline inhalation as well as from inhalation of other volatile organic compounds.[51]

Dermal effects of gasoline and other volatile organic solvents usually are limited to dermatitis secondary to defatting of the skin. Severe chemical burns can result from immersion accidents if the skin is in prolonged contact with gasoline.[34]

By far the greatest potential risk from the use of gasoline and organic solvents is due to the flammability of the compounds.[67] This is particularly true in agricultural applications, where appropriate safety precautions may not be followed due to failure to recognize risk or the prohibitive cost of safety devices. A fire or injury on a farm can be quite serious due to the distance from municipal emergency equipment. The presence of storage tanks may present confined-space hazards that may not be appreciated by the farmer.

Siphoning of gasoline from one vehicle to another can be a common agricultural practice, particularly in times of short supply and during periods of isolation due to inclement weather. An outbreak of aspiration of siphoned gasoline occurred during a blizzard in 1978 because gasoline was being transferred to snowblowers and snowmobiles.[49] The gastrointestinal effects of gasoline are minimal, but aspiration of even small amounts of petroleum products can result in severe pulmonary damage.[53]

Other Organic Solvents

Other solvents used in agricultural settings include degreasers such as toluene, paint thinners and strippers, mineral spirits, and various petroleum solvents. Kerosene is often used in small indoor heaters.[13] Even though industrial uses of solvents account for the largest quantities of solvents used, often the workers exposed to the highest levels are occasional users, because they may not have protective equipment available and may not appreciate the risks.[73]

Many solvent toxicities are similar to gasoline toxicity. Major routes of exposure are through inhalation of vapors and through skin contact.[73] Ingestion is usually rare in the occupational use of solvents. Many pesticides also use short-chain organic solvents as a carrier.[13] Therefore, it may be important to consider the toxicity of the solvent carrier in addition to the toxicity of the pesticide itself. Most nonhalogenated solvents are flammable and, just as with gasoline, pose fire and explosion hazards.

Organic solvents are mild respiratory irritants; most are anesthetic at high concentrations. Many of them have been associated with hepatotoxicity and some are associated with renal toxicity. Again, serious pulmonary sequelae may result from aspiration into the lungs following ingestion, but this is uncommon with the occupational use of these solvents. One must consider the children on a farm, as the risk of accidental poisoning is significant when these solvents are accessible by children.

Equipment Repair

Farm workers can be exposed to metals by a variety of routes. It is common for a farmer to repair his own equipment and occasionally to repair equipment using a welding process. There are innumerable types of welding processes. The most common health effects from welding are due primarily to inhalation of metal fumes and the production of ozone, nitrogen dioxide, and carbon monoxide.[76] The metal fume produced depends on the type of welding and the materials being welded. The main component of welding fume is iron oxide (Fe_3O_4), and the majority of these particles can be of respirable size.[78] Other components can include fluorides and hexavalent chromium (particularly when welding on stainless steel), manganese, zinc oxide, cadmium oxide, aluminum oxide, and nickel.[50]

Health effects can include acute lung injury, pulmonary edema, and pneumonitis, particularly from ozone[52] and nitrogen dioxide[65] production. Metal fume fever can occur in the agricultural setting.[37] Metal fume fever is commonly associated with welding of galvanized steel.[75] Occupational asthma can result from welding procedures.[47] Ocular damage and keratitis may also result from inadequate eye protection. There are other types of chronic health effects associated with welding, but these are unlikely to be associated with the sporadic use of welding procedures in an agricultural setting.

STERILIZATION AND FUMIGATION PRACTICES

Fumigants

The type of agricultural product produced dictates the procedures used to maintain cleanliness and inhibit spoilage of products. Fumigation is a common method of sterilizing farm products such as grains. Fumigants are materials in a vapor, gas, or smoke form. They are used to fill the atmosphere in a container enclosing the product. The container (usually a rail car or grain elevator) is closed up and the chemical has the desired effect. The most danger is during initial application of the chemical and especially upon opening the container, because the person opening the container does not always appreciate the danger involved.

Grain producers may use fumigation to retard insect infestation and mold growth. Other common uses of fumigants include the use of gases or vapors to destroy bacteria or rodents.[56] The major exposure to many fumigants may be in large grain terminals and not directly on the farm. Today, however, many farmers are storing grain products for longer periods of time themselves.[1] This introduces new risks to farm workers unfamiliar with fumigant toxicities.

Common fumigants include a number of compounds with significant toxicity. Health hazard evaluations of several grain elevators revealed "80/20" (the

TABLE 1.   Common Fumigants

Halocarbons	
Carbon tetrachloride	Ethylene dibromide
Chloroform	1,3-Dichloropropene
Chloropicrin	Dibromochloropropane
Methyl bromide	Ethylene dichloride
Oxides and Aldehydes	
Ethylene oxide	Propylene oxide
Formaldehyde	Paraformaldehyde
Acrolein	
Sulfur and Phosphorus Compounds	
Sulfur dioxide	Carbon disulfide
Phosphine (from aluminum phosphide)	Sulfuryl fluoride
Cyanide	
Hydrogen cyanide	Acrylonitrile
Primary Insecticides	
Methoxychlor	Malathion

1. Morgan DP: Recognition and Management of Pesticide Poisonings, 3rd ed. Washington, D.C., U.S. Environmental Protection Agency, U.S. Government Printing Office, 1983.
2. Zaebst D, Morelli-Schroth P, Blake L: Summary of recent environmental assessments of exposure to grain fumigants at export, inland, and country elevators. In Dosman JA, Cockcroft DW (eds): Principles of Health and Safety in Agriculture. Boca Raton, FL, CRC Press, 1989.

name for a mixture of carbon tetrachloride [80%] and carbon disulfide [20%]), ethylene dibromide, phosphine, malathion/methoxychlor mixtures, chloroform, and methyl bromide.[87] Chloroform, chloropicrin, ethylene dichloride, dichlorpropene and -ane, sulfuryl fluoride, and dibromochloropropane (DBCP) are also common fumigants (Table 1). Ethylene dibromide has recently been banned for use as a fumigant because it has been shown to be carcinogenic, mutagenic, and a reproductive hazard.[63] DBCP is restricted as well. DBCP is a reproductive hazard, causing testicular failure in men.[79] Other fumigants include ethylene oxide, propylene oxide, formaldehyde, propanil, hydrogen cyanide, and acrylonitrile.[79]

Fumigants in general are extremely penetrating agents and most personal protective devices are of minimal effectiveness. Respiratory tract injury is the most common sequela of fumigants. Sulfur dioxide, chloropicrin, formaldehyde, and acrolein are so irritating that it is unlikely a sufficient dose can be inhaled to damage the lung; however, laryngeal edema or bronchospasm can result. Methyl bromide, phosphine, and ethylene oxide on the other hand are not as irritating to the upper respiratory tract but can cause severe deep pulmonary injury and pulmonary edema.

Dermal injury can also result with some fumigants, ranging from mild chemical burns to vesiculation and ulceration. Fumigants are also irritating to the eyes, and liquid fumigants can cause corneal ulceration. Most fumigants are central nervous system depressants to varying degrees. Hepatotoxicity and renal damage can also occur.[79]

Chloropicrin is a severe skin, eye, and pulmonary irritant similar to tear gas. Most persons cannot tolerate even concentrations of < 1 ppm for more than 30 seconds.[3] Because of its severe irritant effects, it is commonly used in low concentrations as a warning agent in other fumigant preparations that do not have warning properties.

Carbon disulfide has been associated with neuropsychiatric changes, a parkinsonian syndrome associated with pyramidal tract damage, and peripheral neurotoxicity in grain storage workers.[68] It also is associated with decreased sperm counts in workers in a variety of occupations.[82] Carbon tetrachloride is predominantly a hepatotoxin and may be a carcinogen.

Phosphine (aluminum phosphide) can cause chest tightness, vomiting, diarrhea, and CNS effects.[45] Acute inhalation can result in pulmonary edema, CNS and myocardial depression, and death.[84] It also can self-ignite, posing a fire and explosion hazard. Phosphine is increasingly used as other agents such as ethylene dibromide are being phased out.[78] Phosphine can also be generated by the ignition of zinc phosphide pellets, which are dropped into animal burrows as a rodenticide and caninicide, and poisoning has resulted.[74] If the initial insult is survived, hepatic necrosis and acute tubular necrosis can follow.[79]

Methyl bromide is used as a soil fumigant and nematocide. When used in this manner, it is injected into the soil, which is then covered with plastic sheets. A neurologic syndrome has been reported in persons removing these sheets.[38] Methyl bromide use as a fumigant has caused 60 fatalities from 1953–1981.[53] Methyl bromide use is increasing due to concerns about the carcinogenicity of two other fumigants, ethylene dibromide and 1,2 dichloropropane.

Other fumigants are used in other applications. Formaldehyde is used as a sterilant in mushroom growing[71] and other operations. In addition to respiratory and skin irritation, it is a potential sensitizing agent and can cause an asthma-like response in sensitive workers.[2,38]

Hydrogen cyanide use is restricted due to its severe toxicity, but it is important to note here because a specific antidote is available. Hydrogen cyanide's major toxicity is due to its binding to cytochrome oxidase. This essentially halts all cellular respiration. The toxic effects can be blocked by the administration of thiosulfate. The thiocyanate complex produced by administration of thiosulfate is much more readily detoxified by the liver.

Cyanide poisoning is rapidly fatal in adequate doses, often with death following seizure activity. In the instance of exposure, after resuscitation and decontamination, amyl nitrate ampules should be broken and inhaled for 15 to 30 seconds of each minute until sodium nitrite solution is administered. Cyanide antidote kits are available from Eli Lilly Company. They contain amyl nitrate ampules, sodium nitrite solution, and sodium thiosulfate solutions, with complete instructions and adequate supplies for administration of the antidote.[70] Kits should be available where cyanide is used and workers instructed on the use of the kit. Intravenous medications supplied in the kit can be administered by emergency response personnel at the scene to minimize delay in treatment. Of note, acrylonitrile is metabolized to hydrogen cyanide and similar toxicity can result.

Chlorine and hydrochloric acid as well as bleach (sodium hypochlorite) are commonly used as cleaning and disinfecting agents in dairy or other agricultural facilities. Hypochlorite solutions used for dairy sanitizers may contain up to 50% hypochlorite and can be more damaging than household bleach solutions, which contain from 5% to 15% hypochlorite.[28] All of these agents can cause pulmonary damage if inhaled in the gaseous form. They can also cause skin burns and blistering, which may be severe.

Rodenticides

Control of larger pests such as rats, mice, and prairie dogs often is a concern in agricultural situations. Rodenticides are the most common method of control. Many agents have been used, but many are severely toxic and their use is restricted

TABLE 2.   Rodenticides

Coumarins	
Dicoumarol	Warfarin
Culmachlor	Coumatetralyl
Indandiones	
Chlorophacinone	Pival
Diphacinone	
Organochlorines	
DDT	Endrin
Botanicals	
Red Squill	Strychnine
Organophosphates	
Gophacide	
Pyrinimilureas	
RH-787 (Vacor no longer available)	
Miscellaneous	
ANTU	Phosphorus
Sodium fluoroacetate	Fluoroacetamide
Thallium sulfate	Zine phosphide
Yellow phosphorus	Crimidine
Norbormide	

1. Morgan DP: Recognition and Management of Pesticide Poisonings, 3rd ed. Washington, D.C., U.S. Environmental Protection Agency, U.S. Government Printing Office, 1983.
2. Meister RT (ed): Farm Chemicals Handbook, 75th ed. Willoughby, OH, Meister Publishing Company, 1989.

to licensed applicators (Table 2). Anticoagulants are the most commonly available rodenticides, namely, warfarin and diphacinone. Little toxicity has been encountered from the agricultural application of these agents. In rare cases, coumarin-type anticoagulants have caused skin ecchymoses and necrosis in users, not associated with ingestion.[79] Significant toxicity has occurred through accidental ingestion by children and pets, however.

Strychnine, sodium fluoroacetate, and fluoroacetamide are also used and have severe toxicities.[71] Strychnine is a natural poison that acts directly on central nervous system tissues to cause seizures and muscular tightness. It causes death, probably as a result of impaired respiration during seizures.[29] Sodium fluoroacetate (Compound 1080) and fluoroacetamide (Compound 1081) are extremely toxic agents that block the metabolism of citrate in the tricarboxylic acid cycle, inhibiting oxidative energy metabolism. This leads to apprehension, nausea, vomiting, and cyanosis, which can progress to seizures, ventricular fibrillation, and death.[35,60] The use of sodium fluoroacetate and fluoroacetamide is restricted to licensed applicators due to their toxicity.[27]

Alpha napththylthiourea (ANTU) is used as a rodenticide, but many rat strains have a variable resistance to it. It is, therefore, now not as useful as it once was. It is a selective rodent toxin that acts by causing pulmonary edema in the animal. It is felt that humans are resistant to ANTU toxicity.[62]

Phosphine is also used as a rodenticide and was discussed above. Thallium was used as an animal control agent, but due to its severe neurotoxicity and fatality rate, its use is severely restricted in the U.S.[30]

Arsenic-containing compounds were at one time commonly used as insecticides, herbicides, and fungicides. The use of arsenicals as insecticides has been banned, but organoarsenicals (ammonium and monoammonium methane arsonate, cacodylic acid, disodium, and monosodium methane arsonate) are still used as herbicides. They still are used in some wood preservatives.[37] Arsenic-containing compounds may in some instances still be used as rodenticides.[56]

Fungicides

Fungicides are used on crops as a protective treatment, both on seeds to be used for planting and on trees, shrubs, and vegetable crops. They are usually applied as suspensions or dusts to seeds or soil.[56] Major categories are included in Table 3. Some agents have been discussed already under fumigants. Many fungicides have significant toxicity; others are associated with mild occupational toxicity, usually only mild skin irritation. Those associated only with skin irritation or mild toxicity include: hexachlorobenzene, pentachloronitrobenzene, terrazole, chlorothalonil, and the dicarboximides.[79] The metallo-dithiocarbamates and ethylene dithiocarbamates are moderately irritating to skin and mucous membranes. Thiram is a bis dithiocarbamate. It inhibits aldehyde dehydrogenase and is associated with a disulfuram-type reaction to alcohol.[79] It is a carcinogen and teratogen in animals, although this has not been reported in humans.[70] Benomyl is a carbamate, but it does not cause inhibition of acetyl cholinesterase. It, too, is a mild irritant.[79]

Cyclohexamide is highly toxic but not well absorbed dermally.[79] Organomercury compounds are common fungicides. Alkyl and phenyl mercuric salts are associated with a neurologic syndrome typified by ataxia, weakness, visual impairment, and delirium.[79] Numbness and tingling, paresthesias, seizures, muscle spasms, salivation, lacrimation, gastrointestinal disturbance, and kidney damage can also result. Alkyl mercury compounds are also respiratory and skin irritants.[6,42,70]

Dinitrophenols and pentachlorophenols are highly toxic; some are used as fungicides. Dinitrophenols can be well-absorbed through skin and lung. Severe

TABLE 3.   Fungicides

Inorganic	
Sulfur	
Mercury (alkyl and phenyl)	Copper
Organic	
Dithiocarbamates	Thiazoles
Aromatics	Terrazole
Hexachlorobenzene	Anilazine
Pentachlorophenol	Systemics
Chlorothalonil	Oxathiins
Dicarboximides	Oxycarboxin
Captan Folpet	Fumigants
Captafol	Chloropicrin
Antibiotics	Methyl bromide
Cyclohexamide	Methylisothiocyanate
Streptomycin	Dinitrophenols
Organotins	Dinocap (Karathane)
Fentin	Aliphatic nitrogens
Hydroxide	Dodine

1. Morgan DP: Recognition and Management of Pesticide Poisonings, 3rd ed. Washington, D.C., U.S. Environmental Protection Agency, U.S. Government Printing Office, 1983.
2. Meister RT (ed): Farm Chemicals Handbook, 75th ed. Willoughby, OH, Meister Publishing Company, 1989.

occupational toxicity can result. The toxicity of the nitrophenols is similar to that of the nitrocresols, although they exhibit less toxicity systemically.[33] Their toxicity is manifested by a stimulation of oxidative phosphorylation in cell mitochondria by uncoupling of carbohydrate oxidation with phosphorylation. This causes pyrexia, tachycardia, and dehydration and can lead to cerebral edema and toxic psychosis. Hepatotoxicity and renal toxicity may occur; agranulocytosis has been reported with dinitrophenol.[79] Pentachlorophenol is a potent skin, eye, and upper respiratory tract irritant. Its toxicity also includes the uncoupling of oxidative phosphorylation and resultant hypermetabolic state, similar to the dinitrophenols and dinitro-ortho cresols.[5,31,33,85]

ANIMAL CONFINEMENT HAZARDS

Modern intensive agricultural methods have also changed the way animals are reared. Animals are often housed in densely populated confinement facilities. Here the animals, usually cattle, pigs, or fowl, live out their lives preparing for market. These large enclosures often have a holding tank for excrement below the facility. The wastes drain through floor grates into a containment area. These wastes also can be swept out and stored in a separate containment vessel outside the building. Both storage methods, above ground and below the building, can be dangerous.

It is estimated that one-half million people are involved in swine confinement work and another one-half million are exposed to the confinement rearing of poultry, beef, veal, and dairy animals.[21] Toxic gases are commonly produced from the degradation of animal wastes by anaerobic degradation by facultative microbes. Although 150 different gases may be formed, the fixed gases of methane, ammonia, carbon dioxide, carbon monoxide, and hydrogen sulfide are the most important.[19] Toxic dusts resulting from animal dander, fecal material, and animal feeds may also be present. Many of these dusts are of respirable size. Also included in these dusts are pollens and mold spores, which grow readily in the warm humid atmosphere in these buildings.[18]

Ammonia levels in swine confinement units can exceed the threshold limit value (TLV). Ammonia can absorb onto respirable particles in humid environments.[57] High levels of hydrogen sulfide (H_2S) can occur, particularly during agitation of the manure material, which takes place when pumping the material out into the storage container.[19,21] Hydrogen sulfide may give an odor warning at low levels, but at concentrations over 150 ppm, the olfactory system may be paralyzed and danger may go undetected. Exposure has resulted in fatalities on numerous occasions.[19] Carbon dioxide (CO_2) levels may result in asphyxiation but do not seem to cause any acute pulmonary toxicity.[21] Carbon monoxide is often present but seems more related to the use of propane heaters in the confinement buildings than to the decomposition of wastes.[21] Methane may also accumulate and can be an explosion hazard at levels below the asphyxiation level.[57]

Acute toxicity resulting from work in an animal confinement unit can manifest itself by one or more of several mechanisms. Oxygen depletion may occur in a high methane atmosphere or due to carbon dioxide production by animals, particularly if there is a failure of the ventilation system. Acutely lethal levels of hydrogen sulfide, carbon dioxide, ammonia, and other gases may result during initial agitation of the manure below the animal confinement building in the course of cleaning or removal. Animals have also succumbed to the gases produced. Entering an enclosed waste-containing area below ground level may be acutely hazardous, because CO_2 and H_2S are heavier than air and will be in high concentration in this enclosed space.[20]

Waste-storage structures separate from the animal confinement areas are often in the form of manure pits. Similar toxicities to the aforementioned have resulted from entering the manure pit.[32,58,66] The toxicity in these circumstances is thought primarily due to hydrogen sulfide gas. High levels of hydrogen sulfide have caused immediate death in freestanding manure pits.[19] Drowning can also occur when a worker is overcome by the gases present in the pit and falls into the waste material.

Hydrogen sulfide gas can inhibit cytochrome oxidase activity, blocking cellular respiration similar to cyanide poisoning. There is controversy regarding treatment of hydrogen sulfide gas poisoning with nitrites, as is commonly done with cyanide poisoning. Nitrite treatment may increase methemoglobin concentrations and may have a detrimental effect.[7,32]

The most prominent health effect of working in animal confinement buildings is a pattern of acute and chronic pulmonary complaints. Pulmonary edema, asthma, bronchitis, bronchiolitis, airway obstruction, and organic dust toxic syndrome have all been reported by animal confinement workers.[57] Airway obstruction is the most common complaint.[22] Changes in pulmonary function have been loosely associated with levels of ammonia, carbon dioxide, hydrogen sulfide, and total particles.[19]

ACUTE FEED-ASSOCIATED ILLNESS

Feeds are often stored in silos at the time of harvest. Silos come in several forms, but in most cases the feed is preserved by the relative oxygen-limited anaerobic environment deep in the feed. An upper portion of feed forms a fermented layer that protects the deeper layers. This upper layer often contains extremely high levels of microorganisms such as molds.[55] A syndrome is related to the opening of silos that contain stored grains, commonly corn or hay. It is termed silo-filler's syndrome (SFS). SFS is caused by nitrogen oxides (NO, NO_2, and N_2O_4) produced by the fermentation of nitrates contained in the silage. These nitrogen oxides react with enzymes to form nitrites and oxygen. These nitrites combine with organic acids forming nitrous acid, which further decomposes into nitrogen oxides.[61] It is not uncommon to observe a heavy red-brown layer above the silage that represents the nitrogen dioxide gas. This visible layer should serve as a warning of dangerous conditions and entrance should be avoided.

Concentrations of NO has been recorded at > 500 ppm, NO_2 at > 300 ppm and CO_2 concentrations at 78% in the air at a height of 1 foot above the silage in an unventilated, newly opened silo. Levels of NO_2 of 150–1900 ppm are probably common, but levels up to 4000 have been reported.[10] For comparison, the current short-term exposure limit (STEL) recommended for NO_2 by the American Conference of Governmental and Industrial Hygienists is 5 ppm.[4] In addition to the high levels of nitrogen oxides, the relative hypoxia may lead to hyperventilation, compounding deep lung exposure.[61] NO_2 is an irritant, but only a comparably mild to moderate one, allowing serious damage to deep lung tissue to occur before being forced out of a silo contaminated with dangerous levels of NO_2.[41] Refer to Appendix I for safe silo opening practices.

Nitrogen dioxide, when inhaled, reacts with airway water to form acids that burn airways and alveolar surfaces. This has led to pulmonary edema and bronchiolitis obliterans, which is, in some reported case series, fatal up to 29% of the time.[61,69]

The clinical presentation is related to the degree of injury, which is closely related to exposure. Upper respiratory irritation may be noted immediately, but usually there is a delay of symptoms for several hours. Minimal exposure can cause only mild tracheobronchitis and a dry, nonproductive cough that resolves spontaneously. With more severe exposure, bronchiolitis and focal bronchopneumonia occur. The initial presentation then is characterized by cough, dyspnea, cyanosis, chest pain, nausea, and vomiting. Often with a more severe exposure, the symptoms will resolve, but there will be a relapse 2 to 3 weeks later with dyspnea, cough, and fever. Death has been reported both in the initial exposure and the relapse. With severe exposure, pulmonary edema rapidly develops. If the initial episode is survived, a relapse can occur, just as with lesser episodes.[61] The relapse is felt due to bronchiolitis obliterans, which represents the destruction of deep bronchiolar cells and subsequent sloughing of necrotic cells.[41] Sudden death upon initial exposure is due to acute laryngospasm reflex, respiratory arrest, or simple asphyxiation.[41,61] Numerous case reports support the use of corticosteroids for respiratory distress or pulmonary edema.[41] While most who survive pulmonary edema or bronchiolitis obliterans do not develop significant respiratory impairment, an occasional individual will develop persistent pulmonary dysfunction.

The chronic effects of low-level exposure to NO_2 are unclear. It is felt by some that long-term exposure does not lead to emphysema or chronic bronchitis,[41] but reports of reactive airways disease and chronic shortness of breath in 8 out of 19 survivors of SFS have been reported. Animal studies have also demonstrated a form of chronic pulmonary disease similar to emphysema associated with chronic NO_2 exposure. Brief exposures also result in transient airflow restriction.[69]

SFS is to be contrasted with hypersensitivity pneumonitis and silo unloader's syndrome (SUS). Farmer's lung disease (FLD) is a hypersensitivity pneumonitis reaction to inhaled thermophilic actinomycete elements. It occurs in the winter, when hay and moldy crops are fed to animals by the farmer, whereas SFS occurs in the late summer and early fall harvesting months. FLD usually presents a delayed (6 to 8 hours from exposure), reversible, acute, restrictive disorder. It will be discussed in greater detail elsewhere.

SUS has been reported to occur as a distinct entity from SFS. SUS is associated with a massive exposure to the moldy elements at the top of a silo, generally occurring during the removal of the topmost layer of silage from a newly opened silo. SUS is typified by a syndrome of fever, malaise, chills, and cough without significant pulmonary function changes or positive serological assays as in FLD. Mild respiratory alkalosis may be present. Severe pulmonary failure and death have not been reported in SUS. The chest x-ray is normal in SUS but shows hazy infiltrates in FLD. SUS often occurs in clusters, particularly when several people are exposed to the same moldy silage. SUS is thought to be a relatively common occurrence, but one that frequently goes unreported.[69]

PESTICIDE USAGE

The term **pesticides**, as used in this section, refers to insecticides, herbicides, defoliants, molluscicides, nematocides, algicides, and acaracides. Pesticide exposure can occur under many circumstances. These are:

1. While diluting and mixing the commercial material with water or other substance.

2. While loading the prepared pesticides into the apparatus used for application, such as tanks, ground rigs, backpack applicators, or hand-held sprayers.

3. During application, spray can be blown in the wrong direction and hit workers or bystanders, causing inhalation exposure or dermal contact.

4. During cropdusting, workers serve as flaggers. This job requires standing at the end of fields to mark the rows for crop-dusting planes.

5. During field and orchard work, such as harvesting, picking, or pruning, workers come into contact with pesticide residues on crops, leaves, and fruit.

6. Migrant lifestyle sometimes forces these workers to live temporarily in the fields or orchards where they work. If spraying has occurred, the ground, food, clothing, and water for drinking and washing can all be contaminated.

7. Accidents and spills are always a possibility, especially during mixing, loading, and spraying. Accidental ingestion by a child should not be overlooked.

8. Homes and gardens also have uses for many of these chemicals, for pest control, for example.

9. Contamination of food, water, and air can occur in the work or home environment, especially due to spills or from accidental spraying.

Pesticide exposures carry multiple risks, ranging from dermatitis, various types of cancer, neurologic and behavioral abnormalities, reproductive disorders, liver damage, and inhibition of cholinesterase activity. Table 4 lists reported associations between pesticides and health risks to farmers. Table 5 lists pesticide categories, selected compounds in each category, acute health effects, signs and symptoms of exposure, and laboratory diagnostic tests to order.

It is important to remember that a pesticide also consists of the technical grade chemical formulated with diluents, many of which are organic solvents, additives, or other inert ingredients. These inert ingredients can be toxic as well; many are organic solvents.

Certain pesticides are of concern for their reproductive toxicity, but there are few studies of reproductive toxicity for men or women. However, recent studies have produced evidence of reproductive toxicity in animals for certain pesticides. Table 6 lists those pesticides.

Another large problem causing exposure is misuse of the chemical compound in a manner inconsistent with its labeling.[26a] The correct type of respirator or protective clothing may not be available for the different types of chemicals, and when it is, workers often refuse to wear the awkward gear, or they may not be adequately trained in respirator use or maintenance.

The pesticide categories most often associated with acute pesticide poisonings are organophosphates and carbamates. Both inhibit the activities of the enzyme cholinesterase, which is necessary for the transmission of nerve impulses. Organophosphates bind irreversibly to acetylcholinesterase, blocking the breakdown of acetylcholine. Carbamates bind to acetylcholinesterase in a reversible fashion. Blocking acetylcholinesterase results in unopposed acetylcholine at high concentrations in the synaptic region, leaving the cholinergic system "turned on." See Table 5 for signs and symptoms. For accurate diagnosis, a serum cholinesterase determination is helpful, but treatment of a clinical syndrome should not be delayed while awaiting laboratory results.

For most pesticides, medical monitoring is available only through history-taking, physical examination, and laboratory testing, as indicated in Table 5. However, for cholinesterase-inhibiting pesticides, biologic monitoring is available. In biologic monitoring, preexposure cholinesterase levels must be determined as a baseline. Periodic determinations should then be performed to watch for lowered levels. Declining levels of cholinesterase can be an early indication of chronic

TABLE 4. Reported Associations Between Pesticides and Health Risks to Farmers*

Health Risk	Type of Pesticide	Study Group and/or Location
Systemic poisoning[a,b]	Parathion residues	Orchard workers and crop workers
Dermatitis[c]	Organophosphates, carbamates	13 states
Skin cancer[c]	Organophosphates, carbamates	13 states
Neurologic and behavioral abnormalities, persistent eye problems[d]	Mevinphos, phosphamidon	Farm workers (California)
Inhibition of cholinesterase (plasma and red blood cell)[e,f]	Organophosphates	Corn and peach pickers, cotton field workers (North Carolina)
CNS symptoms[g,h]	Organophosphates	Farm workers (New Jersey) and farmers (Nebraska)
Behavioral effects[i]	Organophosphates	Farm workers
Infertility, sterility[j]	Halogenated hydrocarbon: dibromochloropropane (DBCP)	Male field workers
Chromosome aberrations[k]	Variety of pesticides	Agricultural workers
Dysmenorrhea[l]	Organochlorines	Migrant workers (Colorado)
Pulmonary fibrosis (fatal)[m]	Dipyridyl: paraquat	Agricultural workers
Lymphoma[n]	Chlorophenoxy compound: 2,4-D	Wheat farmers (Kansas)
Dermatitis[o]	Organosulphite: Omite: CR	Orange pickers (California)
Liver damage[p]	Organochlorines	Agricultural workers
Eye injuries[q]	Variety of pesticides	Rural communities
Distal symmetric sensori-motor neuropathy[r]	Organophosphates	Agricultural workers

* Adapted from Cordes DH, Rea DF: Health hazards of farming. American Family Physician 38:233–243, 1988, with permission.
a. Milby TH, Ottoboni F, Mitchell HW: Parathion residue poisoning among orchard workers. JAMA 189:351, 1964.
b. Quinby GE, Lemmon AB: Parathion residues as a cause of poisoning in cropworkers. JAMA 166:740, 1958.
c. Morgan DP, Lin LI, Saikaly HH: Morbidity and mortality in workers occupationally exposed to pesticides. Arch Environ Contam Toxicol 9:349–382, 1980.
d. Whorton MD, Obrinsky DL: Persistence of symptoms after mild to moderate acute organophosphate poisoning among 19 farm field workers. J Toxicol Environ Health 11:347–354, 1983.
e. Wicker GW, Williams WA, Guthrie FE: Exposure of field workers to organophosphorus insecticides: Sweet corn and peaches. Arch Environ Contam Toxical 8:175–18222, 1979.
f. Wicker GW, Williams WA, Bradley JR, Jr, Guthrie FE: Exposure of field workers to organophosphorus insecticides: Cotton. Arch Environ Contam Toxicol 8:433–40, 1979.
g. Quinones MA, Bogden JD, Louria DB, Nakah AE, Hansen C: Depressed cholinesterase activities among farm workers in New Jersey. Sci Total Environ 6:155–159, 1976.
h. Spigiel RW, Gourley DR, Holcslaw TL: Organophosphate pesticide exposure in farmers and commercial applicators. Clin Toxicol Cons 3:45–50, 1981.
i. Levin HS, Rodnitzky RL: Behavioral effects of organophosphate in man. Clin Toxicol 9:391–403, 1976.
j. Whorton MD, Meyer CR: Sperm count results from 861 American chemical/agricultural workers from 14 separate studies. Fertil Steril 42:82–86, 1984.
k. Yoder J, Watson M, Benson WW: Lymphocyte chromosome analysis of agricultural workers during extensive occupational exposure to pesticides. Mutat Res 21:335–340, 1973.
l. Chase HP, Barnett SE, Welch NN, Briese FW, Krassner ML: Pesticides and U.S. farm labor families. Rocky Mt Med J 70:2731, 1973.
m. Fitzgerald GR, Barniville G, Black J, Silke B, Carmody M, O'Dwyer WF: Paraquat poisoning in agricultural workers. Ir Med J 71:336–342, 1978.
n. Hoar SK, Blair A, Holmes FF, et al: Agricultural herbicide use and risk of lymphoma and soft-tissue sarcoma. JAMA 256:1141147, 1986.
o. Saunders LD, Ames RG, Knaak JB, Jackson RJ: Outbreak of Omite-CR-induced dermatitis among orange pickers in Tulare County, California. J Occup Med 29:409–413, 1987.
p. Hunter J, Maxwell JD, Stewart DA, Williams R, Robinson J, Richardson A: Increased hepatic microsomal enzyme activity from occupational exposure to certain organochlorine pesticides. Nature 237(355):399–401, 1972.
q. Blake J: Eye hazards in rural communities. Practitioner 214(1283):641–645, 1975.
r. Johnson MK: The delayed neurotoxicity caused by some organophosphorus esters: Mechanisms and challenge. Crit Rev Toxicol 3:289, 1975.

TABLE 5. Pesticides: Categories, Acute Effects, and Symptoms

Category	Compounds	Effects	Signs and Symptoms	Tests to Order
Organophosphates	Parathion, malathion, diazinon, methyl parathion, mevinphos, carbophenothion, EPN, methamidophos, azinphos-methyl, methiadathion, dichlorvos, chlorpyrifos, phosmet, fenthion	Irreversible inhibitors of cholinesterase activity; impair CNS function	Parasympathetic hyperactivity: headache, dizziness, weakness, blurred vision, sweating, nausea and vomiting, ataxia, stomach cramps, diarrhea, salivation, chest tightness, pinpoint sized pupils, muscle twitching, neuromuscular paralysis, pulmonary edema	Plasma and RBC cholinesterase level; urinary metabolites
Carbamates	Aldicarb, carbaryl propoxur, carbofuran, methomyl, bendiocarb	Reversible inhibitors of cholinesterase activity; impair CNS function	Same as for organophosphates	Plasma and RBC cholinesterase levels; urinary metabolites (for some)
Organochlorines	Aldrin, endrin, heptachlor, lindane, endosulfan, BHC, gamma BHC, methoxychlor. Restricted use: dieldrin, chlordane, DDT	Nervous system stimulators	Nervous system excitability and dysfunction; nausea and vomiting after ingestion	Urinary levels or metabolites
Nitrophenols (herbicides)	Dinitrophenol, dinitro-o-cresol, dinosam, dinoprop, dinoterbon, dinosulfon, binapacryl, dinobuton, dinopenton, dinocap, dinoseb	Toxic to the liver, kidney, and nervous system	Yellow staining of skin and hair; general hypermetabolic state: profuse sweating, headache, thirst, malaise, lassitude, warm flushed skin, tachycardia, fever, apprehension, convulsions	Blood and urine levels
Pentachloro-phenols	PCP, Dowicide EC-7, penchlorol, Pentacon, penwar, Veg-I-Kill, and as an ingredient in many other weed killers, defoliants, wood preservatives, germicides, fungicides, and molluscicides	Toxic to the liver, kidney, and CNS; irritating to skin, eyes, and upper respiratory mucous membranes	Irritation of nose, throat, eyes, and skin; contact dermatitis; chloracne; profuse sweating; headache; weakness; nausea; fever; tachycardia; tachypnea; chest pain; abdominal pain; thirst; declining mental alertness; weight loss	Blood, urine, adipose tissue levels by gas-liquid chromatography
Dipyridyls (herbicides, defoliants, desiccants)	Paraquat, diquat	Liver, lung, and kidney damage (paraquat affects the lungs, skin, and eyes; diquat affects the gastrointestinal tract, kidney, and liver)	When ingested: lung fibrosis; 1 ounce of paraquat is fatal; when inhaled: eye irritation, nose bleeds, discolored and irregular nails, gastrointestinal irritation, vomiting, skin irritation; cough; dyspnea; tachypnea; pulmonary edema	Blood and urine levels; later phase: bilirubin and hepatocellular enzymes

Continued on next page.

TABLE 5. Pesticides: Categories, Acute Effects, and Symptoms *(Cont.)*

Category	Compounds	Effects	Signs and Symptoms	Tests to Order
Anticoagulants (rodenticides)	Warfarin, coumafuryl, zoocoumarin (RAX) dicumarol	Slows down body's clotting mechanism	Large doses: hematuria, nosebleed, hematomata, melena, anemia, abdominal pain, back pain	Prothrombin time
Pyrethrum		Allergic contact dermatitis; allergic rhinitis; asthma	Dermatitis: itching, papules, vesicles, erythema. Rhinitis: nasal congestion, sore throat. Asthma: wheezing, cough, chest tightness, dyspnea	Skin test
Chlorophenoxy compounds (herbicides; several hundred commercial products include one or more chlorophenoxy compounds)	2,4-D; 2,4,5-TP; 2,4-DEP; MCPA; MCPB; MCPP	Mildly to severely irritating to skin, eyes, and respiratory and gastrointestinal linings	Irritation of skin, nose, eyes, throat and bronchi; cough; dizziness; ataxia; when ingested: irritation of mouth and throat; chest pain; fibrillary muscle twitching; skeletal muscle tenderness; myotonia; peripheral neuropathy. 2,4-D: nausea, vomiting, abdominal pain, diarrhea, paresthesias, weakness	Blood and urine levels

Source of information for table: Recognition and Management of Pesticide Poisonings, 3rd ed. Washington, D.C., U.S. Environmental Protection Agency, 1982.

TABLE 6. Pesticides with Potential for Reproductive Toxicity Based on Animal Studies

Male	Female	
Ethylene dibromide	Benomyl	Endrin
Dibromochloropropane	Bromoxynil	Ethylene bis dithiocarbamates EBDCs:
Chlordecone	Captafol	Maneb, Nabam, Zineb, Metiram
Carbaryl	Captan	Folpet
Triphenyltin	Carbaryl	Lindane
Ordram	Cyanazine	Naled
Chlorbenzilate	Dimethoate	Oxydemetonmethyl
Fenchlorophos	Dinocap	Pentachlorophenol
	Dinoseb	Thiram
	Diuron	Triadimefon
	Endothall	Warfarin

Adapted from Rosenberg J: Pesticides. In LaDou J (ed): Occupational Medicine. Norwalk, CT, Appleton & Lange, 1990.

overexposure and depletion of cholinesterase. A worker with depletion of cholinesterase $< 70\%$ of baseline should be removed from the worksite temporarily, and should have his work practices evaluated for safety and to minimize further exposures. Declining levels indicate an increased health risk in the event of further exposure. It is also important to have baseline comparisons, because there are individual variations in "normal" levels of circulating cholinesterase.[74] Routine biologic monitoring is important for workers who handle organophosphates or carbamates regularly. This would include those who work as applicators, mixers, loaders, flaggers, and those who maintain equipment.

The general treatment for pesticide poisoning can follow the guidelines suggested by the EPA, which are included in Appendix III.

PREVENTION, PERSONAL PROTECTION, AND DECONTAMINATION

The first priority in prevention of occupational diseases in farming is clearly education. Farm workers and rural physicians need to recognize potential hazards in order to avoid them. Once these hazards have been recognized, avoidance of unsafe procedures may be the primary preventive measure. In addition to avoidance, the addition of control measures such as adequate ventilation can go a long way towards preventing serious injury and death. Silos and animal waste storage areas should not be entered by a lone farmer, but the buddy system should be used. Ideally, an oxygen supply system should be available for rescues, should they be necessary. A worker should never enter an enclosed space such as a silo or animal waste confinement area to rescue a fallen co-worker without supplied air and other experienced rescue workers outside. It should be stressed that common cartridge respirators do not protect the worker in a low oxygen environment and are therefore unsuitable for entry into a confined space, where the oxygen levels may be lower than required to sustain life.

It is wise to follow routine and practical decontamination procedures after the use of any agricultural chemical. The McKennan Poison Control Center in Sioux Falls, SD, has organized practical tips for the decontamination of clothing, and they are included in Appendix II.

Even simple personal protective equipment can prevent many injuries. Respirators are recommended for use with many agricultural chemicals. Education with regard to the proper fit, selection, and maintenance is imperative. Elbow-length rubber gloves should be used for most chemical applications. Because cloth and leather gloves retain chemicals, they should not be worn while using agricultural chemicals. Rubber boots with high tops are recommended when handling chemicals. The pants should be worn over the boot, rather than tucked inside. This will prevent spills into the boot. Goggles and/or face shields are imperative. Eye injuries are an extremely common, preventable injury resulting from chemical use. Eye protection should be worn by agricultural workers, because many work practices put the worker at risk for eye injury. Certainly, eye protection should be worn when using any chemical. Local county extension offices can be helpful in supplying farm safety information and education.[35]

APPENDIX I

Recommendations for Those Working In or Near Conventional Silos*

1. Avoid entry for 2 weeks after filling the silo. (The risk is greatest 1 to 2 days after filling.) Consider alternative sources of feed such as a second silo, a silage pile, or standing forage.
2. If the silo must be entered within 1 to 4 days after filling, first ventilate it thoroughly.
   a. Leave the doors open down to the level of the silage after filling has been completed.
   b. Run the blower 1 hour before entry and during the entire time anyone is inside the silo.
3. Avoid descending into low places in the silo; gas may settle there in toxic concentrations and may not be removed by ventilation.
4. Never jump down from the top or a chute door considerably higher than the level of the silage. Concentrated gas may be present just above the silage and may cause sudden collapse before escape is possible. If entry is necessary, consider using a self-contained breathing apparatus, wearing a lifeline, and having one or two rescuers available nearby.

5. Avoid ascending the silo chute if 1- or 2-day-old silage is present at any level in the silo. Consider using the exposed external ladder and looking down from above.
   a. If ascent must be done through the chute, first check carefully for gas at the base of the chute or the floor of the silo room.
   b. Use a good light to examine the chute carefully for gas leaking out around the doors.
6. When a silo is only partially filled and the doors have been left closed, never open the door just above the silage without first checking for silo gas by using a good light and looking down from above.
7. When the silo is entered immediately after filling has been completed, exposure may still occur in the silo or silo chute from gas originating in 1- to 2-day-old-silage.
   a. Check the direction of airflow in the chute.
   b. Check for silo gas in the chute.
   c. Leave the blower running at all times.
   d. Avoid using silage cut 1 to 2 days previously during "topping off."
8. Workers should learn to recongize silo gas by sight and smell.
9. Family members unfamiliar with silo gas should not work near a silo or in attached building within two weeks after filling of the silo.
10. Children should never be allowed to play near a silo.
11. If coughing, choking, wheezing, shortness of breath, or light-headedness develops while workers are in the chute or in the silo, these symptoms are probably due to exposure to silo gas. Workers should immediately leave the area and consult a physician. Strenuous exercise should be avoided for at least 24 hours. Preventive therapy may decrease the risk or severity of subsequent lung injury.
12. If shortness of breath, rapid breathing, coughing, or chest pain develops within a few hours or days after exposure to silo gas, lung injury may have occurred. This disorder may progress rapidly and can be fatal. Exposed workers should immediately report to the nearest hospital emergency room.
13. If coughing, wheezing, shortness of breath, or fever develops between 1½ and 6 weeks after exposure to silo gas, this illness may reflect a delayed lung injury due to nitrogen dioxide. Although the symptoms may suggest bronchitis or pneumonia, antibiotics do not cure the disease. Be certain that the physician is informed of the previous exposure to silo gas.

---

* From Douglas WW, Hepper NGH, Colby TV: Silo-fillers' disease. Mayo Clin Proc 64:291–304, 1989, with permission.

APPENDIX II

Laundering Contaminated Clothing*

What water temperature should be used? Can you wash contaminated clothing with other clothing? Is there a difference between soaps? Must I always use bleach? What is the best method for handling and washing chemical-contaminated clothing?

These are questions that are heard more and more often by county extension offices and poison centers as chemical use becomes widespread. Chemicals are classified on the labels as to their inherent toxicity (i.e., danger, poison, warning, caution.) Use these key words in determining how aggressive you need to be when laundering contaminated clothing.

Clothing that has been contaminated by highly concentrated chemicals (i.e., saturation) needs to be discarded. However, ease of chemical removal through laundering is more often related to the formulation of the chemical and not the concentration. Chemicals soluble in water are much more easily removed than nonwater-soluble chemicals.

Recommendations for Laundering
1. Wash contaminated clothing separately from the family wash.
2. Pre-soak all clothing in a suitable container prior to washing.
3. Pre-rinse clothing when transferred to automatic washer.
4. Use multiple washings to wash contaminated clothing (two or three times.)
5. Use hot water (140° F) and a full water level.
6. Wash a few garments at a time; do not overload washer.
7. Wash garments daily; do not leave them lying around to contaminate other articles and humans!
8. Rinse machine after using by running it through the whole wash cycle and adding soap and/or bleach as before.
9. If possible dry clothes on the line to prevent contaminating the dryer.
10. Protect yourself! Wear rubber gloves when handling contaminated clothing.

It is important to use a lot of soap and hot (very hot) water. Research has proven that heavy duty detergents are most effective in removing chemicals, especially the nonwater-soluble variety. Bleach and ammonia can be used in addition to soap though they don't contribute to the removal of chemical. **Never** use both at the same time. Ammonia and bleach, when mixed together, give off a toxic gas that can be fatal.

Wearing disposable outer garments is recommended because they add an extra layer of protection and help prevent underlying clothes from becoming contaminated. Laundering, therefore, is much simplified and safer for all concerned!

---

* From McKennan Poison Control Center, Sioux Falls, South Dakota, with permission.

APPENDIX III

Emergency Medical Treatment for Acute Pesticide Poisoning

ORGANOPHOSPHATES	CARBAMATES	CHLORINATED HYDROCARBONS
Irreversible Cholinesterase Inhibitors	Reversible Cholinesterase Inhibitors	BHC
azinphos – Guthion ®		Chlordane
chlorpyrifos – Duraban ®	aldicarb – Temik ®	chlorphenzilate – Acaraben ®
DDVP – Vapona®	carbaryl – Sevin ®	dicofol – Kelthane ®
demeton – Systox ®	carbofuran – Furadan ®	endosulfan – Thiodan ®
diazinon – Spectracide ®	bendiocarb – Ficam-W ®	endrin – Hexadrin ®
dicrotophos – Bidrin ®	metalkamate – Bux ®	Heptachlor
dimethoate – Cygon ®	methiocarb – Mesurol ®	Kepone
disulfoton – Di-Syston ®	methomyl – Lannate ®	Lindane
malathion – Cythion ®	oxamyl – Vydate ®	methoxychlor – Mariate ®
mevinophos – Phoadrin ®	propoxur – Baygon ®	Mirex
monocrotophos – Azodrin ®	Zectran ®	toxaphene – Torakil ®
parathion – methyl parthion		
phorate – Thimet ®		

Symptoms of Poisoning

1. MILD – headache, dizziness, weakness, anxiety, miosis, impairment of visual acuity.

2. MODERATE – nausea, salivation, lacrimation, abdominal cramps, vomiting, sweating, slow pulse, muscular tremors.

3. SEVERE – diarrhea, pinpoint and non-reactive pupils, respiratory difficulty, pulmonary edema, cyanosis, loss of sphincter control, convulsions, coma, and death.

Constriction of pupils.
Salivation.
Profuse sweating.
Lassitude.
Muscle incoordination.
Nausea.
Vomiting.
Diarrhea.
Epigastric pain.
Tightness in chest.

(Twenty minutes to four hours)
Nausea.
Vomiting.
Restlessness.
Tremor.
Apprehension.
Convulsions.
Coma.
Respiratory failure.
Death.
DO NOT INDUCE EMESIS IF THE INGESTED POISON IS PRINCIPALLY A HYDROCARBON SOLVENT (e.g. kerosene).

Therapy

1. Support respiration. Keep airways clear. Use artificial respiration with oxygen if indicated for cyanosis. Death from pesticide poisoning is usually due to respiratory failure.

2. Decontamination as indicated. Remove contaminated clothing. Wash skin, hair and fingernails with soap and water. Sponge with alcohol. Cleanse eyes. If ingested lavage stomach with 5% sodium bicarbonate if not vomiting.

3. Draw 5 ML heparinized blood for cholinesterase determination. Save samples of first urine and first/early vomitus for possible laboratory analysis.

4. Consult insecticide label under "ACTIVE INGREDIENTS" for specific chemicals involved.

5. When mixtures of organophosphates and chlorinated hydrocarbons are involved (e.g. endrin-methyl parathion), give specific treatment for organophosphates first and indicated support therapy and decontamination.

ANTIDOTES	ANTIDOTE	TREATMENT
1. Adults: After cyanosis is overcome, use Atropine sulfate, 2–4 mg. intravenously. Repeat dose at 5 to 10 minute intervals until signs of atropinization appear. Maintain for 24 hours or longer if necessary.	1. Adults: After cyanosis is overcome, use Atropine sulfate, 2–4 mg intravenously. Repeat dose at 5 to 10 minute intervals until signs of atropinization appear. Maintain for 24 hours or longer if necessary.	1. Gastric lavage with 2–4 L tap water. Catharsis with 30 gm (1.0 oz) sodium sulphate in one cup of water.
2. Children: Atropine sulfate in proportion to body weight: app. 0.05 mg/kg.		2. Barbituates in appropriate dosages repeated as necessary for restlessness or convulsions.
3. Support atropine treatment with 2-PAM (Pralidoxime chloride) (Protopam Chloride Ayerst).	2. Children: Atropine sulfate in proportion to body weight – approximately 0.05 mg/kg.	3. Avoid oils, oil laxatives and epinephrine (adrenalin). Do not give stimulants.
a. Adult Dose: 1 gm, slowly, intravenously. b. Infants: 0.25 gm, slowly, intravenously.	Note: 2-PAM is contraindicated in carbamate insecticide poisoning. Also avoid morphine, aminophylline, theophylline, phenothiazine tranquilizers and barbituates.	4. Give calcium gluconate (10% in 10 ml ampules) intravenously every four hours.
Note: Contraindicated are morphine, aminophylline, theophylline, penothiazine, tranquilizers and barbituates.		

Nearest Poison Control Center Telephone No. _____

Note: A complete wall chart, bearing these steps along with other guidelines, is available for $3 from the Superintendent of Documents, U.S. Government Printing Office, Washington, D.C. 20402. The order number is S/N 008-045-00023-2.

REFERENCES

1. Aherin RA: Enclosed environments of silos and grain storage structures. Ann Am Conf Gov Ind Hyg 2:129–135, 1982.
2. Alexandersson R, Kolmondon-Hedman B, Hendenstierna G: Exposure to formaldehyde: Effects on pulmonary functions. Arch Environ Health 37:279–824, 1982.
3. American Conference of Governmental and Industrial Hygienists: Chloropicrin in Documentation of Threshold Limit Values and Biological Exposure Indices. Cinncinati, OH, ACGIH, 1990.
4. American Conference of Governmental Industrial Hygienists: 1990 Recommended Threshold Limit Values. Cinncinati, OH, ACGIH, 1990.
5. Bergner H, Constantinidis P, Martin JH: Industrial pentachlorophenol poisoning in Winnipeg. Can Med Assoc J 92:448–451, 1965.
6. Berlin M: Mercury. In Friberg L, et al (eds): Handbook on the Toxicology of Metals, 2nd ed. Vol II, Specific Metals. Amsterdam, Elsevier, 1986, pp 418–445.
7. Cockcroft DW, Dosman JA: Respiratory health risks in farmers. Ann Intern Med 95:380–382, 1981.
8. Close LG, Catlin FI, Cohn AW: Acute and chronic effects of ammonia burns of the respiratory tract. Arch Otolaryngol 106:151, 1980.
9. Comley HH: Cyanosis in infants caused by nitrates in well water. JAMA 129:112, 1945.
10. Commins BT, Raveney FJ, Jesson MW: Toxic gases in silos. Ann Occup Hyg 14:275–283, 1971.
11. Cordes DH, Foster Rea D: Health hazards of farming. AFP 38:233–243, 1988.
12. Correa P, Haenzel W, Cuello C, et al: A model for gastric cancer epidemiology. Lancet ii:58–60, 1975.
13. Craft BF: Solvents and related compounds. In Rom WN (ed): Environmental and Occupational Medicine. Boston, Little, Brown, 1983.
14. Cuello C, Correa P, Haenszel W, et al: Gastric cancer in Columbia. 1. Cancer risk and suspected environmental agents. J Natl Can Inst 57:1015–1020, 1976.
15. Davis A, Schafer LJ, Bell ZG: The effects on human volunteers of exposure to air containing gasoline vapor. Arch Environ Health 1:548–554, 1960.
16. Donahoe WE: Cyanosis in infants with nitrates and drinking water as cause. Pediatrics 3:308–311, 1949.
17. Donham KJ, Horvath EP: Agricultural occupational medicine. In Zenz C (ed): Occupational Medicine, 2nd ed. Chicago, Year Book Medical Publishers, 1988.
18. Donham KJ, Gustafson KE: Human occupational hazards from swine confinement. Ann Am Conf Ind Hyg 2:137–144, 1982.
19. Donham KJ, Knapp LW, Monson R, Gustafson K: Acute toxic exposure to gases from liquid manure. J Occup Med 24:142–145, 1984.
20. Donham KJ, Rubino M, Thedell TD, Kammermeyer J: Potential health hazards to agricultural workers in swine confinement buildings. J Occup Med 19:383–387, 1977.
21. Donham KJ, Zavala DC, Merchant JA: Acute effects of the work environment on pulmonary functions of swine confinement workers. Am J Ind Med 5:367–375, 1984.
22. Donham KJ, Zavala DC, Merchant JA: Respiratory symptoms and lung function among workers in swine confinement buildings: A cross-sectional epidemiologic study. Arch Environ Health 39:96–101, 1984.
23. Ferrant M: Methemoglobinemia: Two cases in newborn infants caused by nitrates in well water. J Pediatr 29:585–592, 1946.
24. Fortenberry JD: Gasoline sniffing (review). Am J Med 79:740–744, 1985.
25. Douglas WW, Hepper NG, Colby TV: Silo-fillers' disease. Mayo Clin Proc 64:291–304, 1989.
26. Frasier P, Chilvers C, Beral V, et al: Nitrate and human cancer: A review. Int J Epidemiol 9:3–11, 1980.
26a. Goldsmith M: As farm workers help keep America healthy, illness may be their harvest. JAMA 262:3207–3213, 1989.
27. Gosslin RE, et al: Clinical Toxicology of Commercial Products, Section III, 5th ed. Baltimore, Williams & Wilkins, 1984, pp 193–195.
28. Gosslin RE, et al: Clinical Toxicology of Commercial Products, Section III, 5th ed. Baltimore, Williams & Wilkins, 1985(a), pp 202–203.
29. Gosslin RE, et al: Clinical Toxicology of Commercial Products, Section III, 5th ed. Baltimore, Williams & Wilkins, 1984(b), pp 375–379.
30. Gosslin RE, et al: Clinical Toxicology of Commercial Products, Section III, 5th ed. Baltimore, Williams & Wilkins, 1984(c), pp 379–383.
31. Gray RE, et al: Pentachlor phenol intoxication: Report of a fatal case, with comments on the clinical course and pathologic anatomy. Arch Environ Health 40:161–164, 1985.
32. Hagley SR, South DL: Fatal inhalation of liquid manure gas. Med J Aust 2:459–460, 1983.

33. Hamilton A, Hardy HL: Fungicides in Industrial Toxicology, 3rd ed. Acton, MA, Publishing Sciences Group, 1974, p 365.
34. Hansbrough JF, Zapata-Sirvent R, Dominic W, et al: Hydrocarbon contact injuries. J Trauma 25:250–252, 1985.
35. Harris-Oines P: Farm Chemicals. Sioux Falls, SD, The McKennan Poison Center, 1985.
36. Harrisson JWE, et al: Acute poisoning with sodium flouroacetate (compound 1080). JAMA 149:1522, 1952.
37. Heydon JL, Kagan AN: Metal fume fever. NZ Med J 103:52, 1990.
38. Hendrick DJ, Lane DJ: Occupational formalin asthma. Br J Ind Med 34:11–18, 1977.
39. Herzstein J, Cullen MR: Methyl bromide intoxication in four field workers during removal of soil fumigation sheets. Am J Ind Med 17:321–326, 1990.
40. Hoeffler HB, Schweppe HI, Greenberg SD: Bronchiectasis following pulmonary ammonia burn. Arch Pathol Lab Med 106:151, 1980.
41. Horvath EP, Guillermo AD, Barbee RA, Dickie HA: Nitrogen dioxide induced pulmonary disease. J Occup Med 20:103–110, 1978.
42. Inship MJ, Piotrowski JK: Review of the health effects of methylmercury. J Appl Toxocol 5:113–133, 1985.
43. Johnson CJ, Bonrud PA, Dosch TL, et al: Fatal outcome of methemoglobinemia in an infant. JAMA 257:2796–2797, 1987.
44. Johnson CJ, Kross BC: Continuing importance of nitrate contamination of ground water and wells in rural areas. Am J Ind Med 18:449–456, 1990.
45. Jones AT, Jone RC, Longley: Environmental and clinical aspects of bulk wheat fumigation with aluminum phosphide. Am Ind Hyg Assoc J 25:376, 1964.
46. Juhasaz L, Hill MJ, Nagy G: Possible relationship between nitrates in drinking water and incidence of stomach cancer. IARC Sci Pub 31:619–623, 1980.
47. Keskinen H, Kalliomaki PL, Alanko K: Occupational asthma due to stainless steel welding fumes. Clin Allergy 10:151, 1980.
48. Kross BC: Technical workshop report: Working group III: Environmental health strategies for agriculture. Am J Ind Med 18:517–522, 1990.
49. Laconture P, McGuigan M, Lovejoy FH: Gasoline ingestion after the great blizzard (letter). N Engl J Med 298:1037, 1978.
50. Lewis R: Metals. In LaDou J (ed): Occupational Medicine. Norwalk, CT, Appleton & Lange Publishers, 1990.
51. Lintovitz TL: Myocardial sensitization following inhalation abuse of hydrocarbons. In Weaver NK (ed): The Petroleum Industry. Occup Med State Art Rev 3:567–568, 1988.
52. Lunau FW: Ozone in arc welding. Ann Occup Hyg 10:175, 1967.
53. Machado B, Cross K, Snodgrass WR: Accidental hydrocarbon ingestion cases telephoned to a regional poison center. Ann Emerg Med 17:804, 1988.
54. Marraccini JV, Thomas GE, Ohgley JP, et al: Death and injury caused by methyl bromide, an insecticide fumigant. J Forensic Sci 28:601–607, 1983.
55. May JJ, Pratt DS, Tallones L, et al: A study of dust generated during silo opening and its physiologic effects on workers. In Dosman JA, Cockcroft DW (eds): Principles of Health and Safety in Agriculture. Boca Raton, FL, CRC Press, 1989, pp 76–79.
56. Meister RT: Farm Chemicals Handbook, 75th ed. Willoughby, OH, Meister Publishing Company, 1989.
57. Merchant JA, Donham KJ: Health risks from animal confinement units. In Dosman JA, Cockcroft DW (eds): Principles of Health and Safety in Agriculture. Boca Raton, FL, CRC Press, 1989, pp 58–60.
58. Morse DL, Woodbury MA, Rentmeester K, Farmer D: Death caused by fermenting manure. JAMA 245:63–64, 1981.
59. Miller EC, Miller JA: Carcinogen and mutagens that may occur in foods. Cancer 58:1975–1802, 1986.
60. Mirvish SS: Effects of vitamins C and E on N-nitroso compound formation, carcinogenesis and cancer. Cancer 58:1842–1850, 1986.
61. Morrissey WL, Gould IA, Carrington CB, Gaensler EA: Silo filler's disease. Respiration 32:81–92, 1975.
62. Murphy SD: Toxic effects of pesticides. In Klassen CD, Amdur MO, Doull JD (eds): Cassarett and Doull's Toxicology: The Basic Science of Poisons, 3rd ed. New York, Macmillan, 1986, p 565.
63. Murphy SD: Toxic effects of pesticides. In Klassen CD, Amdur MO, Doull JD (eds): Cassarette and Doull's Toxicology: The Basic Science of Poisons, 3rd ed. New York, Macmillan, 1986, pp 568–569.

64. National Institute of Occupational Safety and Health: Occupational Diseases, A Guide to Their Recognition. DHHS (NIOSH) Publication No. 77-181:412–414, 1977.
65. Norwood WD, Wisehart DE, Earl CA, et al: Nitrogen dioxide poisoning due to metal cutting with oxyacetylene torch. J Occup Med 8:301–306, 1966.
66. Osbern LN, Crapo RO: Dung lung: A report of toxic exposure to liquid manure. Ann Intern Med 95:312–314, 1981.
67. Parreggiani L: Encyclopedia of Occupational Health and Safety, 3rd ed. Geneva, International Labour Office, 1983.
68. Peters HA, Levine RL, Matthews CD, et al: Carbon disulfide-induced neuropsychiatric changes in grain storage workers. Am J Ind Med 3:373–391, 1982.
69. Pratt DS, May JJ: Feed-associated respiratory illness in famers. Arch Environ Health 39:43–48, 1984.
70. Procter NH, Hughes JP, Fishman ML: Chemical Hazards of the Workplace, 2nd ed. Philadelphia, J.B. Lippincott, 1988.
71. Reczek EB: Agricultural chemical hazards in commercial mushroom growing operations. In Principles of Health and Safety in Agriculture. Boca Raton, FL, CRC Press, 1989.
72. Rettig BA, Klein DK, Sniezek JE: The incidence of hospitalizations and emergency room visits resulting from exposure to chemicals used in agriculture. The Nebraska Medical Journal July:215–219, 1987.
73. Rosenberg J: Solvents. In LaDou J (ed): Occupational Medicine. Norwalk, CT, Appleton & Lange Publishers, 1990.
74. Rosenberg J: Pesticides. In LaDou J (ed): Occupational Medicine. Norwalk, CT, Appleton & Lange, 1990, pp 401–431.
75. Ross DS: Welder's metal fume fever. J Soc Occup Med 24:125–129, 1974.
76. Sjogren B: Effects of gases and particles in welding and soldering. In Zenz C (ed): Occupational Medicine: Principles and Practical Applications, 2nd ed. Chicago, Year Book Medical Publishers, 1988, pp 1053–1060.
77. Sobonya R: Fatal anhydrous ammonia inhalation. Hum Pathol 8:293, 1977.
78. Ulfvarson U: Survey of air contaminants from welding. Scand J Work Environ Health (7 Suppl 2):7, 1981.
79. United States Environmental Protection Agency: Recognition and Management of Pesticide Poisonings, 4th ed. EPA Publication No. 540/a-88-001, 1989.
80. Weaver NK: Gasoline toxicology: Implications for human health. In Malconi C, Selikoff IJ (eds): Living in a Chemical World: Occupational and Environmental Significance of Industrial Carcinogens. New York, The New York Academy of Sciences (Vol 534), 1988.
81. Weisenburger DD: Environmental epidemiology of non-Hodgkin's lymphoma in eastern Nebraska. Am J Ind Med 18:303–305, 1990.
82. Wharton DM, Channing RM: Sperm counts from 861 American chemical/agricultural workers from 14 separate studies. Fert Ster 42:82–86, 1984.
83. Whorton DRM, et al: Infertility in male pesticide workers. Lancet ii:1259–1261, 1977.
84. Wilson R, et al: Acute phosphine poisoning aboard a grain freighter. JAMA 244:148, 1980.
85. Wood S, et al: Pentachlorophenol poisoning. J Occup Med 25:527–530, 1983.
86. Wright JL: Lung disease in farm workers: Pathologic reactions. In Dosman JA, Cockcroft DW (eds): Principles of Health and Safety in Agriculture. Boca Raton, FL, CRC Press, 1989, pp 26–29.
87. Zaebst D, Morelli-Schroth P, Bade L: Summary of recent environmental assessments of exposure to grain fumigants at export, inland and country elevators. In Dosman JA, Cockcroft DW (eds): Principles of Health and Safety in Agriculture. Boca Raton, FL, CRC Press, 1989.

MARC SCHENKER, MD, MPH
THOMAS FERGUSON, MD, PhD
THOMAS GAMSKY, MD, MPH

RESPIRATORY RISKS ASSOCIATED WITH AGRICULTURE

Marc Schenker, MD, MPH
Associate Professor and Division
Chief
Occupational and Environmental
Medicine, and
Director, U.C. Agricultural Health
and Safety Center at Davis
University of California, Davis
Davis, California

Thomas Ferguson, MD, PhD
Occupational and Environmental
Medicine Fellow
Division of Occupational and
Environmental Medicine
Davis, California

Thomas Gamsky, MD, MPH
Divison of Pulmonary Medicine
Veteran's Administration Hospital
Martinez, California

Reprint requests to:
Marc Schenker, MD, MPH
Division of Occupational and
Environmental Medicine
University of California, Davis
Davis, CA 95616-8648

Although respiratory disease associated with agricultural endeavors was reported by Ramazzini in 1713,[77] it has been only within the 20th century that careful clinical evaluation of respiratory disease among this working population was attempted. Large gaps still exist in our knowledge of the epidemiology of respiratory hazards in agriculture, particularly among populations such as migrant or seasonal workers. Farmers and other agricultural workers are exposed to a variety of natural and man-made toxic materials including dusts, noxious gases, microbial products and toxins (endotoxins, fungal proteins), and a variety of chemicals such as pesticides and fertilizers. In addition, farmers may be involved in processes during agricultural operations that generate potential respiratory toxins such as diesel exhaust, welding gases, hydrogen sulfide, and ammonia. Thus, exposures to potential respiratory toxins in a farm environment can be diverse and are not limited to sources associated with primary processes of cultivation or livestock confinement.

The focus of this chapter is to review the respiratory health effects associated with agricultural work. In particular, we will focus on epidemiologic evidence of respiratory disease among agriculture workers and suggestions for further studies.

OBSTRUCTIVE AIRWAYS DISEASE

Because agricultural workers are exposed to many dust-generating processes, it is not

TABLE 1.   Respiratory Diseases Associated with Agricultural Work

Syndrome	Work Processes/Locations	Suspect Agent
Obstructive Lung Disease		
Asthma and bronchitis	Grain storage	Storage mites (Europe), (?) endotoxins, unknown
	Swine, cattle, and poultry confinement	Animal danders, bacterial and fungal antigens, unknown
	Fertilizer application	Ammonia
	Pesticide application	Inhibition of acetylcholine esterase
	Animal waste storage	Hydrogen sulfide, ammonia, bacterial or fungal antigens
Restrictive Lung Disease		
Interstitial lung disease	Grain storage	Crystalline silica contamination
	Vineyard	Copper sulfate, (?) silicates
Hypersensitivity pneumonitis	Silage storing	Variety of fungal agents including *Micro-*
	Bird breeding	*polyspora* sp, *Thermoactinomyces*
	Mushroom cultivation	sp, *Penicillium* sp, *Graphium* sp, and *Aurobasidium* sp
Organic Dust Toxic Syndrome	Silo uncapping	Unknown, (?) endotoxin
	Handling wood chips	

surprising that acute obstructive airway dysfunction has been documented in this industry (Table 1). Examples of dusts that may be respiratory irritants in the agricultural environment include pollens, grain particles, animal danders, and bacterial and fungal cell-wall components.[14,25,38,53]

Documented decreases in peak expiratory flow rates (PEFR) have been demonstrated for grain elevator workers in the United States and Canada.[63] Similarly, grain industry workers in Australia had decreases in forced vital capacity (FVC) and forced expiratory volume in one second (FEV_1) within 1 week of starting work.[35] Grainhandlers with higher dust exposure or a previous history of bronchial responsiveness were more likely to exhibit respiratory symptoms.[35] In a study of American grainworkers, do Pico and coworkers[18] found an adverse dose-related acute respiratory effect from grain dust exposure across the work shift that was not related to smoking habit, atopic status, or age. In a "nested" case-control study of grainworkers, exposure to grain dust at concentrations greater than 5 mg/M^3 was associated with a more rapidly declining pulmonary function.[24] Broder and collaborators[7] observed that when grain workers in Canada experienced temporary layoffs, there was a corresponding decrease in respiratory symptoms.

While the precise etiology for the acute respiratory symptoms related to work in the grain handling industry has not been elucidated, there is evidence from studies of European grain-storing farmers to suggest that allergic reactions to insects may be one cause of acute symptomatology. Allergy to storage mites is a documented cause of allergic rhinitis and occupational asthma among certain European farmers.[72,73] The predominant symptom among farmers was rhinoconjunctivitis, but a significant proportion also reported allergic symptoms.[73] There was nearly a 60% prevalence of storage mite-specific IgE demonstrated in grain-storage workers who complained of work-related cough, wheezing, or breathlessness versus 9% in symptomless farm workers.[2] However, a study of Canadian grainworkers showed no increased reactivity to allergy testing with grain dust mite or grain dust extract, and it is unlikely that the reduction in FEV_1 observed in these Canadian workers is related to storage mite allergy.[45] It is possible that differences in storage conditions, especially moisture content, may lead to conditions that favor growth of these mites, and this in turn may produce a greater antigenic exposure for European workers than for workers who handle grain stored under drier conditions.[2] Thus, the etiology of grain dust-related respiratory symptoms and airflow obstruction is due to more than a single agent, and the condition may indeed be related to the many constituents found in this complex mixture.[6]

While most studies of acute respiratory disease in agriculture are commodity-specific, limited data from large population based studies suggest that chronic respiratory disease morbidity and mortality may be increased in this industry. Analysis of Social Security records suggests that agricultural workers have increased rates of respiratory disease disability, and mortality studies have shown an increase in chronic obstructive disease mortality in agriculture.[48,71] These observations are particularly notable in view of the lower prevalence of cigarette smoking among farmers and farm workers than in the general population.

Bronchitis and Other Chronic Airway Obstruction

Several studies have reported an increased prevalence of chronic respiratory symptoms among farmers exposed to biologic and physical agents. Studies of chronic respiratory symptoms in agricultural workers have been limited by the lack of a uniform definition of chronic respiratory disease and the lack of a universal reporting system.[68] Despite these limitations, several studies have documented chronic airway obstruction in agricultural populations.

Hog confinement workers are exposed to dusts with especially high concentrations of animal dander, bacterial and fungal proteins, and endotoxins.[16] In a study of hog farmers versus other farmers, there was increased frequency of respiratory symptoms, including cough, sputum production, and chronic bronchitis, but no significant corresponding differences in lung function.[33] Others have reported a slight decrease in FVC for swine-producing farmers versus nonfarming controls.[19] Dosman and coworkers[20] evaluated over 1800 Canadian farmers and found an increased prevalence of chronic bronchitis as well as slight reductions in both FVC and FEV_1 relative to a nonfarming control group.

Other studies have not confirmed these results. A study of male farmers and farm workers in England and Wales, for example, found no difference in the prevalence of chronic bronchitis symptoms compared with controls from industry.[32] This group of farmers was less likely to smoke but showed a slight reduction in FEV_1 and forced expiratory flow from 25 to 75% (FEF_{25-75}), which was more common among silage and dairy workers.

Chronic respiratory symptoms were not more prevalent in Canadian farmers exposed to grain dust compared with community controls.[45] While slight reductions in FVC and FEV_1 were recorded for former farmers relative to nonfarmers in this study group, this was felt to be secondary to grater involvement with livestock confinement. There was a strong relationship between respiratory symptoms and smoking.

In a survey of Yugoslavian farmers, Milosevic[49] observed increased prevalence of bronchitis among nonsmoking workers who reported their occupation as farmer or cattle breeder compared to those workers who reported their occupation as craftsmen. The prevalence of chronic bronchitis was also increased for smokers employed in cattle breeding or farming but not for tractor drivers. The results of this study were somewhat compromised by the high prevalence of smoking in the study group.

Occupational Asthma

Occupational asthma may result from many exposures occurring in the agricultural workplace. In general, causal agents consist of organic antigens contained in dusts from plant or animal sources, although chemical irritants may cause or exacerbate asthma. The prevalence of asthma among farmers and farm workers is unknown, and most reports have focused on single commodities or exposures, such as coffee bean, mushroom, and wood dusts. Many of the reported etiologies occur in the production of agricultural products, such as among production workers for vegetable gums, teas, and spices. For some agents, such as grain dusts, it may be difficult to separate chronic bronchitis with reduced FEV_1 from occupational asthma. For other agents, such as cotton dust, bronchoconstriction may occur via nonimmunologic mechanisms. The decrease in FEV_1 following cotton dust exposure has been shown to be dose-related to endotoxin concentration.[53]

In summary, while most studies of farmers have not demonstrated consistent objective evidence of chronic lung injury, there is ample evidence that the prevalence of respiratory symptoms is increased for several groups of agriculture workers. This is apparent for both grain handling/storage workers as well as for livestock confinement workers. While agriculture workers generally have a lower prevalence of smoking than the general public, this observation appears to be independent of smoking status. However, the interaction between smoking and agriculture exposure may vary, with some agricultural dust exposures having an additive effect with smoking on pulmonary function but a greater than additive effect (synergism) on respiratory symptoms.[12,31] It is hoped that future studies will elucidate more precisely the respiratory risks associated with these endeavors and their interaction with cigarette smoking, thus providing a sound basis for strategies to prevent acute and chronic respiratory symptoms among agricultural workers.

RESTRICTIVE PULMONARY DISEASE

Aside from the chronic effects of hypersensitivity pneumonitides, such as farmer's lung, restrictive lung disease has not been an outcome generally associated with agricultural work. The paucity of data concerning this subject is partially a result of the low incidence of reported disease, the difficulty of diagnosis, the difficulties in recognizing a link between exposures and disease, and the lack of long-term epidemiologic studies.

Restrictive lung disease in agricultural workers has been observed among workers chronically exposed to organic dusts.[66] These hypersensitivity pneumonitides were originally classified according to the source of dust exposure (farmer's lung, maple bark disease, bagassosis, suberosis, "vegetable dust" pneumoconiosis, etc.). The offending substances were found to be complex mixtures of inhaled endotoxins, single-cell organisms, chemicals, inorganic particles, and insects. The discovery of common cellular pathophysiologic mechanisms for multiple disease states (including activation of pulmonary alveolar macrophages and T lymphocytes) has led recent investigators to rename these disorders as "organic dust diseases."[66] The acute clinical course is often fulminant in nature and the patient seeks medical care, thus enabling detection of disease by surveillance mechanisms. The diagnosis can be verified by the exposure history, clinical course, and the demonstration of serum precipitins to offending substances such as actinomycetes.

While chronic inhalation of organic dust represents a known risk for restrictive lung disease, recent studies indicate that inorganic dust may be hazardous as well. Data from industrial hygiene measurements of fibrogenic dust in the breathing zones of agricultural employees have found levels that consistently exceed standards set for nonagricultural industries. Recent studies include California agricultural operations,[44,60] European and Russian agricultural operations,[21,42] sugar cane harvesting,[4] bean processing in the U.S.,[52] and grain elevator operations.[25,52]

Crystalline silica (including quartz) is virtually ubiquitous in the earth, constituting over 12% of the earth's land mass, and it may represent up to 20% of soil dust in California agricultural operations.[60] Quartz dust inhalation is a significant risk for restrictive lung disease, both acute and chronic, as demonstrated in cohort studies of exposed workers in nonagricultural settings.[58] High ambient levels of respirable quartz (< 5 μm diameter particles) have been detected for agricultural settings as varied as tillage in Europe[42] and California grape workers.[60] Inorganic agents including silica also may be used as diluents or carriers for pesticides, but the extent of exposure and hazard from this source is unknown.

Screening for restrictive lung disease usually relies on clinical history, results of radiologic studies, and the demonstration of a "restrictive defect" on pulmonary function testing. The clinician's history and physical examination provide only modest insight into early restrictive lung disease, because symptoms and examination findings are often nonspecific or absent. Thus, for screening purposes, the diagnosis of restrictive lung disease is heavily dependent on radiographic studies and pulmonary function determinations. Since radiographic studies are rarely employed in asymptomatic individuals, spirometry may be the best objective screening tool for detection of restrictive lung disease in an exposed population. While the term "restrictive defect" most accurately refers to a reduced total lung capacity, with the widespread use of spirometry the term has been operationally defined as a reduced FVC with relatively preserved FEV/FVC (FEV%), compared to expected values.[30] As such, the use of this term is nonstandardized and has less than optimal specificity. A "restrictive defect" has been measured in up to 10% of individuals with reversible obstructive disease and documented in an agricultural setting for a farmer with the "reactive airways syndrome" after massive exposure to silage byproducts.[28]

The diagnosis of "agricultural pneumoconiosis" and its differential diagnosis from idiopathic pulmonary fibrosis therefore requires at least a demonstration of restrictive lung function and a positive work exposure history. Confirmation of cases can be accomplished by the biopsy of lung tissue, followed by x-ray dispersion techniques or scanning electron microscopy to demonstrate mineral content. Given the labor-intensive and costly nature of this diagnostic regimen, the lack of specific clinical findings in diseased individuals, the lack of access to medical care, and the migrant nature of many individuals with high exposures to inorganic agricultural dusts, it is not surprising that agricultural pneumoconioses are infrequently diagnosed.

Recent studies of agricultural workers suggest that restrictive lung disease may be more common than previously suspected. Large cross-sectional spirometric studies of pulmonary function in Canadian farmers,[20] Canadian swine producers,[19] Canadian grain handlers,[34] and California grape workers[27] have found restrictive or mixed restrictive/obstructive pulmonary function compared to controls. Cross-shift or short-term longitudinal studies have found reduced FVC and/or restrictive lung disease in grain workers in Canada[8,34] and in Wisconsin and Minnesota.[18]

In addition to pulmonary function studies, some radiologic studies have found evidence of restrictive lung disease in agricultural populations. These include a Bulgarian farming community,[78] tractor drivers in the Russian forestry service,[21] and Danish fruit growers.[41] Other reports, such as a cross-sectional study of Canadian grain handlers,[8] have found no increase in radiologic evidence of restrictive lung disease.

Relatively few case-reports of agricultural pneumoconiosis exist. Pulmonary fibrosis and heavy deposits of silicates as determined by x-ray dispersion radiography have been found in several career farmers,[26,29] and silicosis has been diagnosed in a railroad worker with a heavy 11-year exposure to silica-laden wheat dust.[52] In northern California, an autopsy series of seven individuals, including six agricultural workers, demonstrated heavy pulmonary deposition of silicates and interstitial fibrosis.[70] In addition, the pulmonary silicate type matched regional soil type, suggesting that environmental silica dust was responsible for interstitial lung disease in these agricultural workers.

Interstitial lung disease due to pesticide inhalation has been reported. Paraquat has been the best studied ("pesticide lung").[41] An animal model has been devised documenting pesticide binding in the lung, followed sequentially by characteristic fibrotic pathologic changes.[41] Pulmonary fibrosis following accidental ingestion of paraquat is well-described.[9] Epidemiologic studies have not consistently shown pulmonary effects from nonparenteral exposures, but there have been case reports of restrictive lung function following percutaneous exposure to paraquat.[40] Pathologic lesions in affected workers, and in a rat model following prolonged low-dose skin application, included medial hypertrophy of the pulmonary arteries. One exposed worker also had interstitial fibrosis on lung biopsy.

Two case reports of a silicosis-like disease were reported in vineyard workers in Portugal ("vineyard sprayer's lung") who were working with copper sulfate. Similar histologic lesions were produced experimentally in animals inhaling copper sulfate.[59] Animal models have also aided in defining the pathophysiology of silicosis. An altered regulation of collagen accumulation has been implicated causally in fibrotic lung disease from chronic inhalation.[74]

In summary, restrictive lung disease is a recognized hazard in agriculture. While diseases due to organic agents have been well described, the extent of restrictive lung disease due to inorganic agents and some chemicals in agriculture is at present unknown. The dearth of reported cases of "agricultural pneumoconiosis" suggests that this hazard may be slight, but diagnostic biases and the migrant nature of the exposed population may make the rarity of case reports misleading. Data from recent studies indicate that agricultural workers may be at greater risk from inorganic agents than previously thought. Clinicians should become more aware of possible toxic respiratory exposures in agricultural work and of the possible link between these exposures and resultant restrictive lung disease, which is often indistinguishable from idiopathic or infectious disease without a careful occupational history and/or mineralogic analysis. Employers should be advised to reduce employee exposure wherever practical. More research is needed to quantitatively and qualitatively analyze agricultural exposures and the relationship between exposures and subsequent development of respiratory symptoms and pulmonary function abnormalities.

HYPERSENSITIVITY PNEUMONITIS

"Farmer's lung" is probably the most well known respiratory disease of farmers. A variety of airborne organic dusts have been associated with development of this form of hypersensitivity pneumonitis, or allergic alveolitis, in agricultural workers. Farmer's lung is most commonly associated with exposure to moldy hay. This dust contains a variety of antigenic substances, including spores and cell wall components from thermophilic actinomycetes.[37] During enclosed feeding of livestock there may be high exposures to dusts from decomposing feedstuffs. Other agricultural workers with documented risk for hypersensitivity pneumonitis (and the associated exposures) include malt workers (sprouting barley), sugar cane workers (moldy cane fibers), mushroom workers (compost), and bird breeders (bird feces and dander).[37]

The acute symptoms of hypersensitivity pneumonitis typically occur within 4 to 8 hours of heavy exposure. Symptoms may include fever, chills, cough, myalgias, and arthralgias. These manifestations may entirely resolve if there are no further exposures. Commonly, the symptoms become progressively worse with increasing exposure, and the affected worker becomes increasingly symptomatic. Continued exposure may lead to a progressive syndrome characterized by cough, dyspnea, weakness, anorexia, and severe restricted lung function. Similar acute symptoms may also be found in organic dust toxic syndrome (Table 2).

Minimal objective findings may be present in acute hypersensitivity pneumonitis. The chest x-ray is commonly normal in an initial episode, but a more severe case or progressive exposure may lead to alveolar filling and eventually a reticular nodular infiltrate. Repeated exposure may result in interstitial fibrosis, which can be severe with persistent exposure. Pulmonary function testing in chronic disease reveals a restrictive pattern with reductions in lung volume and diffusing capacity. The demonstration of IgG antibodies to one of the farmer's lung antigens (*Micropolyspora faeni* or *Thermoactinomyces*) is more a measure of exposure than an index of disease,[46] and the test has very low specificity for the diagnosis of hypersensitivity pneumonitis.

Once diagnosed, the worker should be removed from exposure and measures taken to prevent further injury. Treatment is largely supportive, because most workers have spontaneous regression of symptoms with removal from the offending exposure. Corticosteroids have been advocated, but efficacy has not been demonstrated. A randomized controlled study of Finnish farmers with the diagnosis of hypersensitivity pneumonitis found that while the steroid-treated

TABLE 2. Hypersensitivity Pneumonitis (HP) Versus Organic Dust Toxic Syndrome (ODTS)

Characteristics	Hypersensitivity Pneumonitis	Organic Dust Toxic Syndrome
Symptoms	Chills, dyspnea, myalgias, arthralgias, cough	Chills, headache, myalgias, cough
Time course	4–6 hours postexposure	4–6 hours post *high*-level exposure
Clinical findings	Fever, rales, abnormal CXR, ↓ DLCO, + serum precipitins	Fever
Alveolitis	Lymphocytic	Neutrophilic
Course	Acute syndrome has variable course depending on severity. Chronic syndrome may be progressive, leading to restrictive interstitial lung disease	Resolves spontaneously without long-term sequelae
Prevalence estimates	5–8% of exposed	30–40% of exposed

CXR = chest x-ray; DLCO = single breath diffusing capacity.

group reported some subjective benefit initially, there was no significant change in lung function compared to control patients.[50]

Unfortunately, exposure often continues after the diagnosis of hypersensitivity pneumonitis in the agricultural setting, because there is financial incentive or necessity for these individuals to continue working. In one study fully two-thirds of patients returned to farming and cattle feeding after the diagnosis of farmer's lung disease.[50] One long-term evaluation of patients with the diagnosis of farmer's lung disease found that patients who continued to work in farm environments and had recurrences of symptoms were most likely to have abnormal pulmonary function and chest x-ray abnormalities.[5]

Although hypersensitivity pneumonitis has been studied for over 25 years,[57] the precise pathologic mechanism of the illness is not known. Because over 85% of patients with acute farmer's lung disease have precipitating antibodies to the fungi found in moldy hay, it was felt that the acute process was secondary to an allergic alveolitis induced by such an exposure.[22,57] This is supported by the finding of an intense lymphocytic alveolitis in patients with acute farmer's lung disease who undergo bronchoalveolar lavage (BAL).[64] However, the precise role of the lymphocytosis in the development of disease is not known, because many patients will have persistence of BAL lymphocytosis without evidence of clinical disease,[10] and asymptomatic dairy farmers may have BAL lymphocytosis.[11]

In summary, hypersensitivity pneumonitis can be induced by a variety of organic dust exposures in the agricultural environment. The precise mechanism of disease is not known but appears to involve an immune-mediated response to respirable fungal or other antigens. Treatment is largely supportive, and there is no evidence to support steroid use. Since this syndrome can be progressive and lead to a severe restrictive pulmonary disease, farmers at risk should be encouraged to avoid exposure to contaminated materials.

ORGANIC DUST TOXIC SYNDROME

The term "pulmonary mycotoxicosis" was used to describe a syndrome that resembled farmer's lung disease in symptoms but lacked positive antibody status.[23] This syndrome has been described in relation to handling of moldy hay, grain handling, or cleaning up moldy wood chips, and has recently been renamed "organic dust toxic syndrome."[17] It is distinct from farmer's lung disease primarily by virtue of the lack of reactivity to farmer's lung antigen and BAL findings. The results of biopsy and bronchoalveolar lavage suggest that this disease entity is secondary to an acute inflammatory response triggered by inhaled dusts.[46] Often the only significant objective findings are fever and an elevated white blood cell count.[62]

A recent cross-sectional study of Swedish farmers found that 44% of farmers interviewed had experienced at least one attack of this disorder and that it was most commonly associated with grain handling.[62] The mechanism of injury is not known but appears to be in some way related to direct injury secondary to toxin inhalation. Since recent studies of silo unloading have demonstrated very high levels of organic dusts containing fungal and bacterial components, these components may play a role in the development of the acute syndrome.[51,53] The syndrome is usually short-lived and resolves spontaneously within a few days with only supportive measures.[62,67]

INFECTIOUS AGENTS

A variety of bacterial diseases including anthrax, brucellosis, mycobacterial infections, psittacosis, Q-fever, and tularemia have been spread by respiratory

TABLE 3. Respiratory Infectious Diseases Associated with Agricultural Work

Bacterial Disease	Source	Agent
Q fever	Livestock—sheep, cattle	*Coxiella burnetii*
Anthrax	Livestock	*Bacillus anthracis*
Brucellosis	Cattle, pigs	*Brucella* sp.
Psittacosis	Turkeys	*Chlamydia psittaci*
Tularemia	Sheep	*Francisella tularensis*
Mycobacterial disease	Poultry, cattle	*Mycobacterium avium-intracellulare* complex
Leptospirosis	Cattle, sheep	*Leptospira interrogans*
Fungal Disease		
Coccidiomycosis	Farming contaminated soil, Southwest U.S., Mexico	*Coccidioides immitis*
Histoplasmosis	Ranching, poultry waste	*Histoplasma capsulatum*

means among agricultural workers (Table 3).[69] Human psittacosis is probably the most common of these diseases but is typically associated with workers eviscerating poultry for market rather than farmers involved only in cultivation.[61] Psittacosis typically occurs following direct inhalation of the bacteria from fecal material of infected birds, leading to an acute illness characterized by fever, headache, and a hacking nonproductive cough.[69] Chest x-ray may reveal an interstitial pneumonitis, but this is nonspecific and the disease can only be confirmed by serologic testing.

Fungal agents may also cause respiratory disease in agricultural workers, and coccidiomycosis is probably the most well-documented fungal cause of disease in this population.[55,56] *Coccidioides immitis* is a dimorphic fungus that is endemic to the semi-arid regions of the southwestern U.S. and may be transmitted by inhalation of fungal spores from infected soils. In a survey of 100 patients who developed coccidiomycosis in Fresno, California, it was found that 50% had been employed in farm labor just prior to the onset of illness.[36] Since farmers are often involved in activities that disrupt the integrity of the topsoil and thus disperse the fungal spores, one might expect that this occupational group should be at risk for acquiring pulmonary coccidiomycosis. Histoplasmosis has not been as carefully studied with regard to occupation, but there appears to be an increased risk for agricultural workers.[39] Those farmers and others who are exposed to poultry waste also may be at an elevated risk for pulmonary histoplasmosis. Fortunately, fungal respiratory infections in immunocompetent hosts are often self-limited and resolve spontaneously without long-term sequelae. In rare cases dissemination may occur, leading to fungemia, meningitis, and occasionally death.

Although a variety of infectious biologic agents have been associated with pulmonary infection among agricultural workers, serious infections are apparently relatively rare. Nevertheless, physicians caring for agricultural workers should be alert for possible associations between respiratory infection and employment in agricultural endeavors.

OTHER SPECIFIC PULMONARY TOXINS

Agricultural workers may be exposed to a multitude of potential acute respiratory toxins and to a variety of hazardous conditions. Some potential toxins to the respiratory system include hydrogen sulfide, fumigants such as phosphide and phosgene, ammonia, oxides of nitrogen from decomposing silage, herbicides, and pesticides. The toxicity of these compounds is discussed in greater detail elsewhere in this issue and thus will be only briefly discussed here.

The confined spaces used for storage of animal excrement provide an anaerobic environment that favors the production of hydrogen sulfide. Agricultural workers who have inadvertently entered these environments have developed acute toxicity, including respiratory failure and death.[15,54] These environments may also contain toxic levels of ammonia, which can act as an acute respiratory irritant at low concentrations and cause pulmonary edema with very high exposures.[15]

Another common exposure to ammonia occurs when agricultural workers are inadvertently exposed to anhydrous ammonia concentrates used for fertilizer. Anhydrous ammonia inhaled under these conditions can expose the upper airway to concentrations that overwhelm the normal host defense mechanisms and lead to severe scarring and occasionally bronchiectasis.

Oxides of nitrogen are formed during natural fermentation of silage in an enclosed space, and a syndrome of pulmonary edema with progressive bronchiolitis obliterans has been described among silo unloaders.[43] The low solubility of nitrogen dioxide facilitates the entry of this gas deep into the lung, thus resulting in alveolar injury. Prevention of disease depends upon recognition of the hazard and avoidance of entry into confined spaces containing silage until adequate ventilation has been achieved.

Agricultural workers may also be at increased risk for cancer, including lung cancer, from exposure to pesticides and herbicides or to other agents in the agricultural environment. While most studies of cancer in farmers have observed lower lung cancer rates and increases in several nonrespiratory malignancies,[3] there is some concern that specific exposures could predispose this group to respiratory cancer. Etiologic studies of this population are difficult, because the lower smoking prevalence is associated with a lower rate of lung cancer than for the general population. One retrospective cohort study found a two-fold increased risk for lung cancer among pesticide workers that could not be attributed to differences in smoking habits,[1] but a study of pesticide applicators in Sweden was unable to demonstrate increased lung cancer risk.[76] A case-control study of orchardists exposed to arsenic-containing pesticides in Washington state found no excess mortality from lung cancer.[75] Finally, a case-control study of lung cancer patients in Canada found that farmers who developed lung cancer reported a more extensive exposure to herbicides, grains, and diesel exhaust than siblings who did not develop lung cancer.[47]

One rather unique occupational exposure is exposure of agricultural workers to biogenic silica during harvesting and field preparation. Biogenic silica is generated when sugar cane and rice fields are burned, and industrial hygiene surveys confirm that amorphous silica particulate is present during harvesting.[4] These fibers are of respirable size and air concentrations may exceed 300,000 fibers/cubic meter. It remains to be seen whether these fibers are potentially toxic, but there are two reports of mesothelioma among sugar cane workers,[13,65] and one study showed an increased relative risk for the development of lung cancer among sugar cane workers.[65]

CHILDREN AND RESPIRATORY RISKS

Historically, farming has been a family endeavor with all members participating in agricultural activities, from field preparation to harvest or livestock feeding. Thus, members of farm families may assist in a wide range of agricultural activities from a very young age. Very young children may also be exposed to respiratory hazards from living and playing in the farm environment. In addition, many farm workers such as migrant and seasonal workers may not have access to day care facilities and may need to have all members of their family participate in work activities.

It is of particular concern that young children and adolescents may be exposed to these work environments, because occupational standards for exposures are based upon adult exposures. Children also may be at increased risk for injury because they are less likely to heed written advisories or react appropriately to noxious warning properties of certain toxins, and adult supervision may not be readily available. Finally, there are physiologic differences between the respiratory system of children relative to adults (e.g., increased lung surface area to volume, increased minute ventilation) that may place these young workers at increased risk for injury from respiratory toxins. Few clinical or epidemiologic data exist on respiratory illnesses among children due to agricultural exposures.

SUMMARY AND RECOMMENDATIONS

Respiratory risks associated with agriculture reflect the diversity of exposures for this population, ranging from organic and inorganic dusts to numerous chemicals and biologic agents. Although clinical studies have documented the existence of many respiratory symptoms and diseases from agricultural exposures, there are limited epidemiologic studies on the incidence of these outcomes. In addition, the wide variety of agricultural practices and associated factors such as climate suggests that disease risk factors and occurrence may vary widely in different locations. A priority for research in agricultural-related respiratory disease should be epidemiologic studies of agricultural populations, with specific attention to identifying activities or processes associated with increased respiratory symptoms.

Physicians caring for agricultural workers should be alert for respiratory symptoms and attempt to familiarize themselves with the processes in which their patients are involved. Worksite evaluations, although time-consuming, may help the clinician better assess exposures and provide insight for rational recommendations regarding treatment or preventive interventions. In many instances, simple recommendations such as wearing dust masks or minor engineering controls may alleviate symptoms and thus decrease the potential for development of impairment. Likewise, identification of high-risk processes may aid the worker in developing preventive strategies that will minimize exposure to respiratory toxins. These workers also should be queried regarding other family members involved in agriculture activities and advisories should be made regarding the possible increased susceptibility of younger workers. Children must be adequately supervised, and this group should not be placed in situations where there is increased risk for exposure to respiratory toxins.

Physicians providing care for agricultural workers should also keep in close contact with agencies and organizations providing education services for this group, such as county agricultural commissioners and university agricultural extension services. The recent establishment of two regional Agricultural Health and Safety Centers in the United States sponsored by the National Institute for Occupational Safety and Health will help facilitate health education services for these workers.

REFERENCES

1. Barthel E: Increased risk of lung cancer in pesticide-exposed male agricultural workers. J Toxicol Environ Health 8:1027–1040, 1981.
2. Blainey AD, Topping MD, Ollier S, Davies RJ: Respiratory symptoms in arable farmworkers: Role of storage mites. Thorax 43:697–702, 1988.
3. Blair A, Axelson O, Franklin C, et al: Carcinogenic effects of pesticides. In Baker SR, Wilkinson CF (eds): The Effect of Pesticides on Human Health. Princeton, Princeton Scientific Publishing Company, 1990, pp 201–260.
4. Boeniger M, Hawkins M, Marsin P, Newman R: Occupational exposure to silicate fibres and PAHs during sugar-cane harvesting. Ann Occup Hyg 32:153–169, 1988.
5. Braun SR, do Pico GA, Tsiatis A, et al: Farmer's lung disease: Long-term clinical and physiologic outcome. Am Rev Respir Dis 119:185–191, 1979.
6. Broder I: Overview of adverse pulmonary effects of grain dust. In Dosman JA, Cockcroft DW (eds): Principles of Health and Safety in Agriculture. Boca Raton, FL, CRC Press, 1989, pp 97–103.
7. Broder I, Mintz S, Hutcheon MA, et al: Effect of layoff and rehire on respiratory variables of grain elevator workers. Am Rev Respir Dis 122:601–608, 1980.
8. Chan-Yeung M, Schulzer M, MacLean L, et al: Epidemiologic health survey of grain elevator workers in British Columbia. Am Rev Respir Dis 121:329–338, 1980.
9. Copland GM, Kolin A, Schulman HS: Fatal pulmonary intra-alveolar fibrosis after paraquat ingestion. N Engl J Med 291:290–292, 1974.
10. Cormier Y, Belanger J, Laviolette M: Prognostic significance of bronchoalveolar lymphocytosis in farmer's lung. Am Rev Respir Dis 135:692–695, 1987.
11. Cormier Y, Belanger J, Beaudoin J, et al: Abnormal bronchoalveolar lavage in asymptomatic dairy farmers: Study of lymphocytes. Am Rev Respir Dis 130:1046–1049, 1984.
12. Cotton DJ, Graham BL, Li KLR, et al: Effects of grain dust exposure and smoking on respiratory symptoms and lung function. In Dosman JA, Cockcroft DW (eds): Principles of Health and Safety in Agriculture. Boca Raton, FL, CRC Press, 1989, pp 138–143.
13. Das PB, Fletcher AG, Deodhare SG: Mesothelioma in an agricultural community of India: A clinicopathological study. Aust NZ J Surg 46:218–226, 1976.
14. Donham KJ: Hazardous agents in agricultural dusts and methods of evaluation. Am J Ind Med 10:205–220, 1986.
15. Donham KJ, Knapp LW, Monson R, Gustafson K: Acute toxic exposure to gases from liquid manure. J Occup Med 24:142–145, 1982.
16. Donham KJ, Popendorf W, Palmgren U, Larsson L: Characterization of dusts collected from swine confinement buildings. Am J Ind Med 10:294–297, 1986.
17. do Pico GA: Report on diseases. Am J Ind Med 10:261–265, 1986.
18. do Pico GA, Reddan W, Anderson S, et al: Acute effects of grain dust exposure during a work shift. Am Rev Respir Dis 128:399–404, 1983.
19. Dosman JA, Graham BL, Hall D, et al: Respiratory symptoms and alterations in pulmonary function tests in swine producers in Saskatchewan: Results of a survey of farmers. J Occup Med 30:715–720, 1988.
20. Dosman JA, Graham BL, Hall D, et al: Respiratory symptoms and pulmonary function in farmers. J Occup Med 29:38–43, 1987.
21. Dynnik VI, Khizhniakova LN, Baranenko AA, et al: Silicosis in tractor drivers working on sandy soils at forestries. (Russian: English abstract) Gig Tir Prof Zabol 12:26–28, 1981.
22. Emanuel DA, Wenzel FJ, Bowerman CI, Lawton BR: Farmer's lung: Clinical, pathologic and immunologic study of twenty-four patients. Am J Med 37:392–401, 1964.
23. Emanuel DA, Wenzel FJ, Lawton BR: Pulmonary mycotoxicosis. Chest 67:293–297, 1975.
24. Enarson DA, Vedal S, Chan-Yeung M: Rapid decline in FEV-1 in grain handlers. Am Rev Respir Dis 132:814–817, 1985.
25. Farant JP, Moore CF: Dust exposures in the Canadian grain industry. Am Ind Hyg Assoc J 39:177–194, 1978.
26. Fennerty A, Hunter AM, Smith AP: Silicosis in a Pakistani farmer. Br Med J 287:648–649, 1983.
27. Gamsky TE, McCurdy SA, Samuels SJ, Schenker MB: Pulmonary function among California Hispanic farmworkers (abstract). Am Rev Respir Dis 141:A590, 1990.
28. Gilbert R, Auchincloss JH: Reactive airways dysfunction syndrome presenting as a reversible restrictive defect. Lung 167:55–61, 1989.
29. Glyseth B, Stettler L, Mowe G, et al: A striking deposition of mineral particles in the lungs of a farmer: A case report. Am J Ind Med 16:231–240, 1984.

30. Gold WM, Boushey HA: Pulmonary function testing. In Murray JF, Nadel JA (eds): Textbook of Respiratory Medicine. Philadelphia, W.B. Saunders, 1988, pp 667–668.
31. Greaves IA Schenker M: Tobacco smoking. In Brain JD, Beck BD, Warren J, Shaikh R (eds): Variations in Susceptibility to Toxic Agents in the Air: Identification, Mechanisms and Policy Implications. Baltimore, MD, Johns Hopkins University Press, 1987, pp 182–203.
32. Heller RF, Hayward DM, Farebrother MTB: Lung function of farmers in England and Wales. Thorax 41:117–121, 1986.
33. Holness DL, O'Blenis EL, Sass-Kortsak A, et al: Respiratory effects and dust exposures in hog confinement farming. Am J Ind Med 11:571–580, 1987.
34. Hutcheon M, Broder I, Corey P, et al: Restrictive ventilatory defect in grain elevator workers. In Gee JBL, Morgan WKC, Brooks SM (eds): Occupational Lung Disease. New York, Raven Press, 1984, pp 192–193.
35. James AL, Zimmerman MJ, Ee H, et al: Exposure to grain dust and changes in lung function. Br J Ind Med 47:466–472, 1990.
36. Johnson WM: Occupational factors in coccidiomycosis. J Occup Med 23:367–374, 1981.
37. Jones A: Farmer's lung: An overview and prospectus. Ann Am Gov Ind Hyg 2:171–182, 1982.
38. Lacey J: Collection, detection, and identification of agents in farm dust implicated in respiratory disease. Am J Ind Med 10:311–313, 1986.
39. Larsh HW: Histoplasmosis. In DiSalvo A (ed): Occupational Mycoses. Philadelphia, Lea & Febiger, 1983, pp 29–43.
40. Levin PJ, Klaff LJ, Rose AG, Ferguson AD: Pulmonary effects of contact exposure to paraquat: A clinical and experimental study. Thorax 34:150–160, 1979.
41. Lings S: Pesticide lung: A pilot investigation of fruit growers and farmers during the spraying season. Br J Ind Med 39:370–376, 1982.
42. Louhelainen K, Kangas J, Husman K, Terho EO: Total concentrations of dust in the air during farm work. Eur J Respir Dis 152:73–79, 1987.
43. Lowry T, Schuman LM: 'Silo-filler's disease'—A syndrome caused by nitrogen dioxide. JAMA 162:153–160, 1956.
44. Maddy K, Shimer D, Smith C, et al: Employee exposure to pesticide residue and nuisance dust during the mechanical shaking and sweeping of almond harvest during August and September 1984. California Dept Food Ag, Div Pest Manage, Environ Prot Worker Safety. Pub #HS-1283. Jan 11, 1985.
45. Manfreda J, Cheang M, Warren CPW: Chronic respiratory disorders related to farming and exposure to grain dust in a rural adult community. Am J Ind Med 15:7–19, 1989.
46. Marx JJ, Guernsey J, Emanuel DA, et al: Cohort studies of immunologic lung disease among Wisconsin dairy farmers. Am J Ind Med 18:263–268, 1990.
47. McDuffie HH, Klaasen DJ, Cockcroft DW, Dosman JA: Farming and exposure to chemicals in male lung cancer patients and their siblings. J Occup Med 30:55–59, 1988.
48. Milham S: Occupational mortality in Washington state, 1950–1971, Vol. 1, NIOSH Res Rept. HEW Publ No. (NIOSH) 76-175-A, Cincinnati, OH, 1976.
49. Milosevic M: The prevalence of chronic bronchitis in agricultural workers of Slavonia. Am J Ind Med 10:319–322, 1986.
50. Monkare S, Haahtela T: Farmer's lung—a 5-year follow-up of 86 patients. Clin Allergy 17:143–151, 1987.
51. Morey PR: Practical aspects of sampling for organic dusts and microorganisms. Am J Ind Med 18:273–278, 1990.
52. Nicas M: Silica exposure in agricultural operations. In The State of the Workplace. California Dept Health Serv (HESIS) 3(2):8–11, 1989.
53. Olenchock SA, May JJ, Pratt DS, et al: Presence of endotoxins in different agricultural environments. Am J Ind Med 18:279–284, 1990.
54. Osbern LN, Crapo RO: Dung lung: A report of toxic exposure to liquid manure. Ann Intern Med 95:314–315, 1981.
55. Pappagianis D: Coccidiomycosis (San Joaquin or Valley fever). In DiSalvo A (ed): Occupational Mycoses. Philadelphia, Lea & Febiger, 1983, pp 13–28.
56. Pappagianis D: Epidemiology of coccidiomycosis. In Current Topics in Medical Mycology, Vol. 2. New York, Springer-Verlag, 1988, pp 199–238.
57. Pepys J, Jenkins PA, Festenstein GN, et al: Farmer's lung. Thermophilic actinomycetes as a source of "farmer's lung hay" antigen. Lancet ii:607–611, 1963.
58. Peters JM: Silicosis. In Merchant JA (ed): Occupational Respiratory Diseases. USDHHS, Publ Health Serv, CDC, NIOSH, Sept 1986, Pub No 86-102, pp 219–237.

59. Pimentel JC, Marques F: 'Vineyard sprayer's lung': A new occupational disease. Thorax 24:678–688, 1969.

60. Popendorf WJ, Pryor A, Wenk HR: Mineral dust in manual harvest operations. Ann Am Conf Gov Ind Hyg 2:101–115, 1982.

61. Pullen MM: Human chlamydial infections (ornithosis) in an agricultural environment: Case studies. Ann Am Conf Gov Ind Hyg 2:155–159, 1982.

62. Rask-Andersen A: Organic dust toxic syndrome among farmers. Br J Ind Med 46:233–238, 1989.

63. Revsbech P, Andersen G: Diurnal variation in peak expiratory flow rate among grain elevator workers. Br J Ind Med 46:566–569, 1989.

64. Reynolds HY, Fulmer JD, Kazimieroweski JA, et al: Analysis of cellular and protein content of bronchoalveolar lavage fluid from patients with idiopathic pulmonary fibrosis and chronic hypersensitivity pneumonitis. J Clin Invest 59:165–175, 1977.

65. Rothschild H, Mulvey JJ: An increased risk for lung cancer mortality associated with sugar cane farming. J Nat Cancer Inst 68:755–760, 1982.

66. Rylander R: Introduction: Organic dusts and disease. Am J Ind Med 17:1–2, 1990.

67. Rylander R: Lung diseases caused by organic dusts in the farm environment. Am J Ind Med 10:221–227, 1986.

68. Samet JM: Definitions and methodology in COPD research. In Hensley MJ, Saunders NA (eds): Clinical Epidemiology of Chronic Obstructive Pulmonary Disease. New York, Marcel Dekker, 1989, pp 1–22.

69. Schnurrenberger PR: Agricultural respiratory hazards—Occupational zoonoses. Ann Am Conf Gov Ind Hyg 2:145–154, 1982.

70. Sherwin RP, Barman ML, Abraham JL: Silicate pneumoconioses of farm workers. Lab Invest 40:576–582, 1979.

71. Singleton JA, Beaumont JJ: COMS II. California Occupational Mortality, 1979–1981. Adjusted for Smoking, Alcohol, and Socioeconomic Status. Sacramento, CA, CA Dept Health Serv, Health Data and Statistics Branch, Health Demographics Section, 1989.

72. Terho EO, Husman K, Vohlonen I, et al: Allergy to storage mites or cow dander as a cause of rhinitis among Finnish diary farmers. Allergy 40:23–26, 1985.

73. Van Hage-Hamsten M, Johansson SGO, Hoglund S, et al: Storage mite allergy is common in a farming population. Clin Allergy 15:555–564, 1985.

74. Vuorio EI, Makela JK, Vuorio TK, et al: Characterisation of excessive collagen production during development of pulmonary fibrosis induced by chronic silica inhalation in rats. Br J Exp Path 70:305–315, 1989.

75. Wicklund KG, Daling JR Allard J, Weiss NS: Respiratory cancer among orchardists in Washington State, 1968 to 1980. J Occup Med 30:561–564, 1988.

76. Wiklund K, Dich J, Holm L-E, Eklund G: Risk of cancer in pesticide applicators in Swedish agriculture. Br J Ind Med 46:809–814, 1989.

77. Wright WC (transl): Diseases of farmers. In Ramazzini B: De Morbis Artificum (1713). New York, Hafner Publishing Company, 1964, pp 338–351.

78. Zolov C, Bourilkov T, Babadjov L: Pleural asbestosis in agricultural workers. Environ Res 1:287–292, 1967.

EVAN W. KLIGMAN, MD
WAYNE F. PEATE, MD, MPH
D. H. CORDES, MD, MPH

OCCUPATIONAL INFECTIONS IN FARM WORKERS

From the Department of Family
and Community Medicine
University of Arizona College
of Medicine
Tucson, Arizona

Reprint requests to:
Evan W. Kligman, MD
Section of Family Medicine
Department of Family and
Community Medicine
University of Arizona College
of Medicine
Tucson, AZ 85724

For 6.5 million farm workers in the United States, occupational infections may cause acute illnesses, prolonged disease and, infrequently, disability.[6] Farming activities that place workers at greatest risk for infection include plowing, planting, and working with soil and plant products. Exposure to pathogens during earth moving is another source of possible infection. Husbandry activities with associated risk include exposure to potentially infected animals, their byproducts, or excreta, and caring for animals in confinement.

Of 150 zoonoses and helminthic infections occurring throughout the world, about 40 have importance as etiologic agents of agricultural and farming occupational infections. Of these 40, about half are definite risks to U.S. farmers and therefore discussed in this chapter.

Factors increasing the susceptibility of farm workers to infection include temperature extremes, stress, fatigue, poor general health, dust exposure, and contaminated water supply.

Occupational infections affect thousands of farm workers each year, despite the fact that hazardous exposures to zoonoses and other biological agents can be well controlled in the workplace and nearly all occupation-related infections are preventable. Even after exposure, susceptible workers can often still receive prophylaxis to prevent the onset of clinical disease. Most clinical infections can also be treated effectively to prevent serious complications, if diagnosed and properly managed early in their course.

Awareness of common sources of infections and the specific type of farm work settings that put the worker at risk for particular infections can help physicians make an earlier diagnosis in the infected worker; minimize individual disability; prevent the transmission of infection to co-workers, the worker's family, and the public; and help set in motion the steps necessary to improve safeguards against further infection on the farm or other relevant workplace environment. The preventive approach emphasized in this chapter is equally important for family physicians, other physicians, and other members of the health care team who work in settings caring for farm workers and their families.

In this report, we will review occupational infections resulting from contact with or exposure to animals (and their byproducts or excreta), including breeding of animals, and exposure related to groundbreaking, earth moving, and gardening (e.g., cultivation of plants, gardens and crops). Special emphasis will be given to incorporation of risk assessment into the routine history and physical, and implementation of a general prevention and control program for occupational infections.

The incidence of the 11 most common infections that can be acquired during farm work is shown in Table 1.[3]

PREVENTION AND CONTROL

Prevention and control of occupational infections in agricultural workers are challenging tasks for the physician and health care team. Unlike other high risk occupations such as manufacturing and mining, most farm operations lack adequate supervision, suffer from poor sanitation, including inadequate toilet and hand-washing facilities, and are distant from medical care. Collective response to hazards is unlikely. However, occupational infections are largely preventable by using simple measures and current technology. These measures can be grouped into five categories: (1) personal protection; (2) preventive services such as immunization, chemoprophylaxis, and screening; (3) education; (4) revisions in the workplace; and (5) animal control measures.

Personal protective gear should be worn to prevent contact with contaminated secretions and excretions and physical trauma such as lacerations, abrasions, bites and scratches. The farm worker should be advised to treat aborted fetal products with as much caution as health care workers approach blood products because of the risk of brucellosis and Q fever. Unfortunately, personal protection is often

TABLE 1.   Incidence of Eleven Most Common Agricultural Acquired Infections*

Infectious Disease	1989	1980–1989
Anthrax	0	5
Ascariasis	NA[†]	NA
Brucellosis	95	1479
Encephalitis	981	8589
Leptospirosis	93	637
Tetanus	63	721
Tularemia	152	2305
Rabies	1	10
Rocky Mountain spotted fever	NA	NA
Q fever	NA	NA
Staph infections	NA	NA

* Adapted from CDC Summary of Notifiable Diseases in the U.S., MMWR 39:3, 1989.
† NA = not available as a reportable infection.

neglected for reasons of inconvenience, expense, and poor fit. Physicians should always ask if the worker has protection, if it is worn, and if not—why?

The following are specific examples of infectious agents and protective measures:

1. Goggles and glasses prevent inoculation of conjunctivae (brucellosis, leptospirosis).

2. Gloves made of heavy mesh (such as Kevlar) will protect fish and meat processors (erysipeloid); gloves, aprons, and boots deter entry of infective material through open wounds when handling infected animals and their byproducts (anthrax, brucellosis, leptospirosis, tetanus, tularemia while dressing rabbits, and vesicular stomatitis).

3. Respirators prevent infection with anthrax spores, Q fever in dusty environments, and aerosolized Brucella in pens.

4. Insect repellents on exposed skin (the most effective is diethyltoluamide) and repellents on clothing prevent exposure to ticks (Rocky Mountain spotted fever [RMSF] and Lyme disease) and mosquitoes (viral encephalitis).

Examples of **preventive services** effective in the prevention and control of certain occupational infections of farm workers include:

1. Immunization of high risk workers for anthrax, rabies, tularemia (systemic not ulceroglandular), and Q fever; and immunization of all workers against tetanus.

2. Skin testing as an indicator of prior infection (brucellosis).

Education is the cornerstone of prevention. Examples include:

1. Instruction in proper and timely wound care is one of the most effective measures to decrease zoonotic infections such as rabies, tetanus, and pasteurellosis. Vigorous wound cleansing has been shown to decrease rabies transmission by 50%.[10] Broken skin *must also* be protected from later inoculation. The usual dressings rarely tolerate the heavy physical abuse encountered on the farm or in an abattoir. An effective, inexpensive, and durable method that prevents dressing failure is to use a conforming, semi-adhesive bandage. Patients should be instructed to air dry wounds while on work breaks and at home. Sufficient dressing changes and tape should *always* be offered.

2. Food storage and ingestion: Remind the worker to always keep hot foods hot and cold foods cold due to *E. coli* gastroenteritis and to wash hands well before eating and after defecating to avoid oral transfer of contaminants, such as brucellosis. Offer caution about the ingestion of raw milk (brucellosis, Q fever, *Staphylococcus aureus*), undercooked meats (anthrax, echinococcosis, tularemia) and contaminated water (*E. coli* gastroenteritis, leptospirosis).

3. Recommend the proper disposal of infected carcasses and offal, i.e., deep burial for tularemia and anthrax (add lime), and *Echinococcus*; and isolation of infected animals to avoid spread of brucellosis, cowpox, sheep pox, and vesicular stomatitis.

4. Install precautionary placards regarding the appearance of anthrax pustules and about avoidance of meat processing if skin lesions on hands—to prevent *Staphylococcus aureus* infection and erysipeloid.

5. To prevent infection of family members, advise when appropriate the daily laundry of infected clothes at work to stop spread of anthrax.

Revisions in the workplace can be effective. Woolsorters' disease, or inhalation anthrax, was eliminated in Great Britain in the 1930s by the introduction of government mandated wool disinfection.[12] Some other examples include:

1. Installation of proper ventilation (dusty goat wool—anthrax) and wet operations to decrease dust (Q fever).

2. Pen and paddock sanitation: working barn cleaners and other measures (brucellosis, pasteurellosis). Drainage of stagnant ponds (anthrax, leptospirosis).

3. Disinfection of hair, hides, hoofs, and bone meal (anthrax).

4. Installation and periodic restocking of convenient *first aid kits* with sufficient antiseptic in vehicles and outbuildings.

5. Introduction of privies (ascariasis) and potable water (ceramic filters for springs and streams or portable container).

6. Work site rodent control (leptospirosis). On many farms felines (toxoplasmosis) are important in rodent control; prohibiting hunting is impractical. Pregnant workers with unknown *Toxoplasma gondii* titers should avoid cuts, practice adequate hand-washing, and wear gloves during contact with soil.

7. Tick control (Q fever, Rocky Mountain spotted fever, and Lyme disease).

Animal control measures are the neglected stepsisters in the prevention of zoonoses that affect humans. Consult a veterinarian for advice regarding the following:

1. Animal vaccines (anthrax, leptospirosis, rabies for cats and dogs; not economically feasible for livestock).

2. Infected animal and carcass isolation and burying.

3. Sanitation and prevention of infected animals urinating in water supply (leptospirosis).

4. Serologies and ring test milk (brucellosis).

5. Deworming of dogs (echinococcosis).

6. Antibiotics to eliminate carrier state (psittacosis).

INCORPORATING RISK ASSESSMENT INTO A ROUTINE HISTORY AND PHYSICAL

Social/Occupational History.   The physician seeing a farmer for a persistent cough (Q fever, etc.) should inquire routinely about work activities. Careful inquiry about farm work and animal processing and transport may be the key that unlocks the diagnosis in the patient with fever and vague constitutional complaints (brucellosis) and may be life-saving in inhalation anthrax. In addition to asking "What's new?," physicians should inquire about work with sick animals, work with animals behaving unusually, delivery of aborted fetuses, introduction of new animals, and paddocks (brucellosis) or processes (anthrax).[13] The health of other workers and family members who may have been ill should be determined. Finally it is important to ask the worker, *"What do you think is the cause?"*

Nutritional History.[9]   Investigate unexplained nutritional deficits, consumption of raw milk and undercooked meats (echinococcosis, etc.), and contaminated wells (leptospirosis).

Home and Worksite.   Consider the location: Mexican border (rabies from unimmunized canines); Northern New Mexico and Arizona, Southern Utah (plague); Alaska, Central United States (echinococcosis).

Facilities: toilets, privies, and handwashing.

Hobbies.   Hunting (Lyme disease, plague) and skinning rabbits (tularemia) are possible risks. Also imported yarn (anthrax).

Animal exposures.   Direct bites: ticks—RMSF, Lyme disease; dog and cat bites—pasteurellosis and rabies; mosquito—viral encephalitis; scratches—brucellosis, etc.

Indirect: semen, artificial inseminators (brucellosis), urine (leptospirosis), parturition products, etc.

Pets: birds—psittacosis; dogs—echinococcosis; cats—toxoplasmosis.

Seasonal onset of symptoms is relevant to Lyme disease and mosquito-borne infections (viral encephalitides), which are prevalent in summer and early fall.

Past History. Prior infection with brucellosis confers active and cross-immunity to other brucella species. In tetanus, second infections are possible.

Prior Studies. Previous serologies (several abattoirs mandate preplacement testing for brucellosis), skin testing (brucellosis) and chest films (echinococcosis—hydatid cysts) can be revealing and establish a base line.

Immunization Status. Check for tetanus, rabies, tularemia, and anthrax immunization history.

History of Unusual or Painful Skin Lesions. Causes of characteristic lesions are:

Petechiae	Rocky Mountain spotted fever (RMSF)
Red ulcerated papule	Tularemia
Erythema (chronicum migrans)	Lyme disease
Painless black eschar	Anthrax
Painful black eschar	Consider *Staphylococcus aureus*
Extremely painful given size	not anthrax
of lesion	Erysipeloid

ELEVEN MOST COMMON INFECTIONS

Anthrax

Anthrax remains the classic occupational disease of agriculture. It was the first identified occupational infection caused by a bacteria. Its discovery led to the founding of a new field—occupational hygiene, and work history remains the cornerstone to early diagnosis, which is essential in the rapidly progressing and fatal (if misdiagnosed) pulmonary infection.[14] The causative agent is *Bacillus anthracis,* a gram positive rod. Common names are "malignant pustule," "wool-sorters' disease," and "ragpickers disease." Anthrax has an infrequent and sporadic incidence in the U.S.

Bacillus anthracis forms durable spores that persist at risk settings such as soil, hair, hides, bone, and fertilizer for years. Direct skin contact, particularly in abattoir, meat and hide processors, and gardeners, and inhalation, especially dusty goat wool, are two common modes of exposure. Other exposures include contact with tissues of dying animals, biting flies, and contaminated animal products such as hoofs. Ingestion of the bacteria causes intestinal and oropharyngeal disease.

Signs and Symptoms. Depending on site of contact, there are four categories of clinical signs and symptoms:

1. **Cutaneous anthrax** or **malignant pustule,** which in spite of the name is rarely fatal if treated adequately, is transmitted through broken skin. Itching develops, followed by a small brownish red papule that crowns into a vesicle with surrounding erythema and induration. This lesion ulcerates and forms a 2–5 cm painless black eschar ("anthrax" meaning coal or charcoal in Greek). After 3–4 days and if pain is present, consider staphylococcus in the differential or a secondary infection by *Staphylococcus aureus.* Other zoonoses should also be considered. If the disease disseminates, regional lymphadenopathy may present, leading to the rare septicemia with associated fever, myalgias, nausea, vomiting,

malaise, and lowered blood pressure, with potential spread to meninges. A history of occupational exposure is critical. The eschar's location is characteristically on exposed areas of the face and arms. Multiple papules occur in 4–10% of cases.[12]

2. **Inhalation anthrax (woolsorters' disease)** is unusual but has a higher case fatality rate than cutaneous anthrax. It begins with a prodrome similar to a viral upper respiratory infection, resulting from the inhalation of spores and leading to nonspecific symptoms, including an initial dry cough. Later, bloody sputum, fever, and malaise develop, followed by multiplication in the mediastinal lymph nodes. Radiography may reveal a hemorrhagic necrotizing lymphadenitis with spread to the surrounding mediastinum. Pulmonary edema, dyspnea, hypoxia, chest pain, bacteremia, high fever, and death can occur in 2–3 days. It must be differentiated from pneumonic plague. Hemorrhagic meningoencephalitis can also develop.

3. **Gastrointestinal** or **ingestion anthrax** is an animal disease unusual in man, especially in the temperate latitudes. It results from ingestion of inadequately cooked meat contaminated with *B. anthracis* and is characterized by gastroenteritis, abdominal pain, vomiting, fever with prostration, and bloody diarrhea. Occasionally, septicemia, mesoadenitis, peritonitis, and intestinal perforation develop. Close observation for 14 days is advised.[12]

4. **Anthrax meningitis** usually begins with a primary oropharyngeal mucosal lesion followed by fever, chills, lymphadenopathy and edema.

Diagnostic Tests. Diagnostic tests include a white blood cell count, which will be normal in cutaneous anthrax but often elevated in more severe varieties, and a Gram stain of a vesicle smear, unfixed with methylene blue, identifying bacilli with red capsules. In pulmonary anthrax, a hemorrhagic mediastinal widening on chest x-ray with possible pulmonary infiltrate and the presence of *B. anthracis* on sputum are seen. In anthrax meningitis, *B. anthracis* can be isolated in cerebrospinal fluid (CSF), which is often hemorrhagic. *B. anthracis* may also be cultured from other specimens or identified by immunofluorescence. A four-fold increase in enzyme-linked immunosorbent assay (ELISA) or electrophoretic immunotransblot (ETIB) titer between acute and convalescent phase serum specimens should be obtained more than 2 weeks apart. Anthrax ELISA titer greater than 64 or an ETIB reaction to the protective antigen and/or lethal factor bands in one or more serum samples may be obtained after onset of symptoms.

Treatment. Treatment of cutaneous anthrax should be initiated with parenteral penicillin G, 2–6 million units daily in divided doses for 1 weeks, oral tetracycline, 250–500 g every 6 hrs, or erythromycin. Skin defects often require plastic surgery. Incision and drainage are contraindicated because dissemination can result. Purulence is unusual unless secondary infection develops. For pulmonary anthrax, parenteral penicillin G, 12–24 million units daily, should be administered. The roles of steroids and anthrax serum are controversial. The patient should be isolated if in a hospital.

Prevention and Control. Prevention and control measures should take into consideration that risk is greatest when untreated hair, hides, bone meal, and hoofs are handled. Spores can be killed by processing, dyeing, or disinfection of wool with gamma radiation. Workplace hygiene should include drainage of stagnant ponds, dust control, and the wearing of gloves and respirators. A chart should be placed on workplace walls with precautions and pictures of typical cutaneous lesions. When opening bales of hides, ventilation should blow down and out, away from workers. Prophylactic antibiotics should be considered for high-risk workers exposed to animals that died of *B. anthracis*. Proper cooking, workplace personal protection, and proper disposal of infected carcasses with deep burial and lime are other useful measures. A human anthrax vaccine is recommended for high-risk workers and is available from the Michigan Department of Public Health, Division of Bio Products, Lansing, MI. It is effective in preventing cutaneous and inhalation anthrax. Annual vaccination of animals and area disinfection with 5–10% activated hypochloride solution should also be considered.

Ascariasis

Ascariasis or roundworm is most often caused in humans by *Ascaris lumbricoides,* and rarely *Ascaris suum.* It occurs in rural areas of the southeastern U.S., especially in areas of poor public and private hygiene. Ascariasis should be considered if an eosinophilic pulmonary infiltration presents in a farmer or in children, who are often part of the work force on a seasonal or part-time basis and who may contaminate a farm household through poor hygienic practices. Not a notifiable disease in the U.S., ascariasis has a 50% prevalence in many developing countries.

Infection is usually by the fecal-oral route, ingestion of soil contaminated by human feces or inadequately cooked food. Eggs deposited in feces are ingested by humans and hatched in the intestine. The larvae then enter the lymphatic and vascular systems.

Signs and Symptoms. Clinical signs and symptoms can be **nutritional** (malnutrition with large worm burden), **pulmonary** (Löffler's syndrome with eosinophilic leukocytosis secondary to cellular immune response causing wheeze, cough, fever, and shifting pulmonary infiltrates during larval migrations; commoner in reinfections), **gastrointestinal** (abdominal discomfort; obstruction with heavy infestation; appendix, bile, and pancreatic duct blockage possible with only one adult worm, leading to liver abscesses, cholangitis, pancreatitits, and cholecystitis), **larva migrans** (symptoms secondary to larval migration through viscera, with eye, brain, and heart damage with *Ascaris suum*—a rare zoonosis in humans).

Diagnostic tests. Diagnostic tests may identify: eosinophilic leukocytosis; eggs in stool; larvae in sputum and gastric washings; and worms in stool, nose, mouth, and vomitus. Gastrointestinal obstruction may be seen on radiologic flat plates, indicating an abdominal emergency. Chest x-rays may reveal migrating pulmonary infiltrates in Löffler's syndrome.

Treatment. Fatalities are unusual except in inadequately treated ascaric bowel obstruction. Treatment options include pyrantel pamoate 11 mg/kg for a maximum of 1 g (1 dose) or mebendazole 100 mg twice a day for 3 days (contraindicated in pregnancy).

Prevention and Control. Prevention and control measures include avoiding contact with human waste, proper disposal of human feces, installation of privies in the field, encouraging hand washing after defecation and before eating and keeping finger nails short and clean. For personal protection, gloves should be worn by persons working with feces. In all cases, others who need treatment (family and co-workers) should be identified and instructed in proper hygiene.

Brucellosis

Common names for brucellosis include: Neopolitan fever, Gibralter fever, Malta fever, Mediterranean fever, undulant fever, and Bang's disease.

An occupational history is the key to timely diagnosis. Livestock producers and meatpackers comprise most of the 100–200 cases reported annually in the

U.S. (thousands worldwide). Of these cases, only 10% are attributed to ingestion of contaminated dairy products, such as unpasteurized milk and Mexican and Italian cheeses.[4,11] A third to a half of those in the high-exposure occupations acquire an asymptomatic infection.[2]

Human brucellosis is contracted from **exposure to the secretions and excretions of animals,** through direct contact in 70% of cases, such as milking and handling aborted fetal tissue and placentas. Bull semen has infected artificial inseminators.[11] Other modes of exposure include contaminated food and water ingestion, and incubation of aerosolized contaminants. The gram negative bacilli *Brucella abortus* (cattle, seldom hogs), *B. melitensis* (goats and sheep; the most severe cause of brucellosis in man), *B. suis* (hogs, seldom cattle, caribou, reindeer, and hares), or *B. canis* (dogs, foxes) enter the lymphatics through broken skin or the oropharynx and spread to the bloodstream. Infection by one species of *Brucella* gives the host immunity to other members of the genus.

Signs and Symptoms. Clinical signs and symptoms begin with an acute stage that often mimics influenza, i.e., spiking fevers, chills, myalgias, arthralgias, weakness, fatigue, night sweats, headache, and occasional diarrhea; later constipation, abdominal pain, anorexia, weight loss, and irritability. Chronic complications may mimic subacute bacterial endocarditis, neuritis, orchitis, osteomyelitis, particularly suppurative spondylitis, cholecystitis, and meningoencephalitis. Even the febrile phase is frustratingly unpredictable, with intermittent fevers occurring for up to a month followed by remission for 2 days to 2 weeks, with recurrences or "undulations" for months to years. It is not surprising that neurosis is sometimes diagnosed.

Diagnostic Tests. Diagnostic tests should include a leukocyte count with characteristic mild lymphocytosis and elevation in sedimentation rate. Case classification depends on isolation of *Brucella* species by culture or a four-fold or greater increase in *Brucella* agglutination titer between acute and convalescent phase serum taken more than 2 weeks apart. False positives can occur after skin testing with *Brucella* antigen, yersinia or salmonella infection, tularemia, and cholera immunization. Skin testing for *Brucella,* like tuberculosis, indicates prior infection.

Treatment. Treatment is recommended with oral tetracycline 500 mg a day for 3 weeks, and repeated for relapses. Cardiac, meningeal, and bone involvement require additional measures, including streptomycin or rifampin combined with trimethoprim-sulfamethoxazole, or one of the tetracyclines and chloramphenicol, with or without streptomycin.[8] A suggested regimen is oral rifampin 600–900 mg and doxycycline 200 mg daily for 6 weeks. Oral prednisone 20 mg three times a day for 5–7 days is of value for toxemia. Fatalities are unusual.

Prevention and Control. Prevention and control measures include: wearing gloves and goggles or glasses when working with animal products, especially placentas during animal abortions. High-top boots and aprons should be considered. Adequate hand washing is essential. Avoidance of eating, drinking, and smoking in the work area is encouraged, although sometimes impractical in an agricultural environment. Unpasteurized milk should be avoided. Aged cheeses are usually free of *Brucella.* With early disease identification (animal serologies and a ring test of cow's milk), diseased stock can be segregated and eradicated. Adequate sanitation in animal areas, particularly pens (maintain working barn cleaners) and slaughterhouses where airborne transmission is possible, should be attempted. Farmers and abattoir workers need to be educated about transmission of *Brucella* and the hazards of working with unprotected broken skin. An information placard can be placed in high-risk work areas to provide instruction in proper wound cleaning. First aid kits should be installed in barns, abattoirs, and farm vehicles.

Encephalitis, Viral

Sixteen different virus groups found in the U.S. are causative agents for viral encephalitis. The arbovirus group, most likely to cause infection in farm workers, consists of over 450 arthropod-borne viruses. St. Louis encephalitis is the most common cause of epidemic encephalitis in the U.S., followed by Eastern (EEE) and Western equine encephalitis (WEE). Though 2000 cases of viral encephalitis are reported in the U.S. annually, 40 to 60% of cases go unreported. Two-thirds of persons infected with the Western equine virus are males infected by mosquitoes in rural agricultural areas.

At risk occupations include agricultural and forestry workers and farmers in small valleys with deciduous hardwood trees. Significant outbreaks occur in summers.

Common modes of exposure are arthropod-borne mosquito or tick bites from birds to horses to humans, woodland mosquitoes bred in discarded tires, and woodland animals, squirrels for example, which are reservoirs for California encephalitis. Other animal sources include horses, rats, dogs, and birds.

Signs and Symptoms. Clinical signs and symptoms include lethargy, fever, headache, and disorientation. Presentations vary from mild febrile illness to full blown encephalitis with coma and meningeal signs.

Diagnostic Tests. Diagnostic tests include a lumbar puncture where a cloudy CSF is present, and elevated protein and white cell count. Rarely are CSF viral cultures positive. Mortality can exceed 30% for some virus groups, and many survivors have some form of neurologic sequelae. No specific treatment is available. Supportive measures are indicated.

Prevention and Control. Prevention and control measures include protective clothing, insect repellents, surveillance of human case findings, mosquito trapping, and insecticide spraying in high incidence areas. Inactivated WEE and EEE vaccines are currently available from the U.S. Army Medical Research Institute for Infectious Disease, Fort Detrick, MD and are indicated for farm workers under continued and extensive exposure.[1]

Leptospirosis

The causative agent, *Leptospira interrogans,* has over 170 serotypes. Common names include Weil's disease, aseptic meningitis, pretibial fever, swineherd's disease, swamp fever, and mud fever. **High-risk occupations** include veterinarians, trappers, farmers working in rice fields or sugar cane fields, milkers, and meat inspectors. Persons working with cattle or swine, abattoir workers, hunters, and persons swimming in contaminated water are also at risk. Infections in the U.S. are more commonly found in southern and western states during the summer and winter months. One hundred cases are reported annually in the U.S. Many cases probably go unreported because of variability in signs and symptoms and subclinical infections among farm workers commonly exposed to usual sources.

Common modes of exposure include contaminated urine from infected domestic farm animals, such as cats, dogs, cattle, swine, and sheep, and wild animals, such as rodents and raccoons. Contact with infected excreta and soil, water, or mud contaminated with urine, as well as rodent or dog bites are other sources of infection. Leptospires from these sources enter the human host through abrasions in the skin, conjunctiva, or oral mucosal membranes. After entry, they disseminate via blood to multiple organs, including the liver, kidneys, meninges, myocardium, and muscle.

Signs and Symptoms. Clinical signs and symptoms include chills, fevers, myalgias, headache, nausea, vomiting, jaundice, skin rash, conjunctival suffusion, bradycardia, stiff neck, and muscle tenderness, commonly in the calves, thighs, and lumbar areas. More severe infections can cause hemoglobinuria, nephritis, meningitis, and rarely central and/or peripheral neurologic manifestations.[9,13,16] There is a 3–6% case-fatality rate, with the highest mortality rate in patients who develop jaundice and in the elderly (15 to 40%). Recovery is usually complete. Complications include psychiatric disturbances, chronic lethargy, and intrauterine fetal infection and death in pregnancy.

Diagnostic Tests. Diagnostic tests include a wound culture, microscopic agglutination or indirect hemagglutination tests, immunoglobulin M ELISA (positive in recent infection), multiple blood and urine cultures, abnormal renal and liver tests, and thrombocytopenia.

Treatment. Treatment includes oral doxycycline 100 mg twice a day for 7 days, tetracycline 500 mg every 6 hours for 7 days, or penicillin G 1.2 g IV four times a day. Antibiotics must begin within the first 2–4 days.

Prevention and Control. Prevention and control measures include animal vaccines for cattle and pigs (2 doses required), rodent control, avoidance of contact with contaminated water, wearing of protective gloves and boots, and early identification and treatment of infected animals. Infection control in livestock requires good environmental sanitation and immunization. Infected animals should be prevented from reaching water and urinating in water used by humans. To prevent infection acquired from sporadic exposure to rodent or wildlife carriers, chemoprophylaxis with doxycycline should be considered.[17]

Q Fever

The causative agent of "Q" or "Query" fever is *Coxiella burnetii* (the disease was designated "Q fever" in the original 1937 report pending further knowledge to substantiate a better name). Other names include Australian Q fever, Brisbane fever, and nine-mile fever. Occupations at risk include abattoir and livestock workers, dairy workers, veterinarians, farmers, ranchers, and hide and wool handlers. **At-risk settings** include farms with pregnant cattle, sheep, and goats, and areas where farmers are in contact with these animals or their byproducts, or assist in the birthing of lambs. The prevalence of Q fever is uncertain since all states are not required to report cases. The incidence of disease is probably greater than that reported because of mild symptoms in most cases.

Exposure occurs through airborne or direct contact with animals (or byproducts), or ingestion of unpasteurized dairy products. Common animal vectors include ticks and fomites from small mammals, birds, ruminants, goats, and sheep. Inhalation of aerosolized particles from contaminated material such as infected placentas, post partum discharge, and feces can cause a primary atypical pneumonitis. Organisms can live in water and milk for long periods of time.

Signs and Symptoms. Clinical signs and symptoms include acute fever, malaise, headache, and weakness following an incubation period of 2–4 weeks. A transient pneumonitis with cough, chest pain, and inspiratory rales is common.

With a prolonged course greater than 3 weeks, granulomatous hepatitis with jaundice can occur. A chronic form can develop as late as 20 years after an acute illness and is often associated with infective endocarditis.

Diagnostic Tests. Diagnostic tests include Q-fever-specific complement-fixing immunoglobulin G antibody (greater than 1:200) and/or an indirect fluorescent antibody of specific immunoglobulin M antibody.

Treatment. Treatment includes tetracycline 500 mg every 6 hours or chloramphenicol 500 to 750 mg every 6 hours. Rapid recovery is usual with early treatment. Individuals affected with complications such as endocarditis require prolonged antibiotic treatment. Overall, the case-fatality rate is under 10%.

Prevention and Control. Prevention and control measures include aerosol reduction of ticks and spraying of cattle. Killed vaccines are available for high-risk workers, e.g., dairy workers, woolsorters, and tanners. Other preventive measures are pasteurization of milk by the flash method (71°C for 15 sec), wearing personal protective gear when handling infected animals, and respiratory protection when working in dusty environments contaminated with organisms.

Rabies

The causative agent is a rhabdovirus, of the genus *Lyssavirus* and is classified as a neurotropic virus. Monoclonal antibodies have demonstrated several serotypes in recent years. Common names include hydrophobia and lyssa. Over 30,000 doses of post-exposure prophylaxis are administered in the U.S. each year. Two human cases have been reported in the U.S. in the past decade. However, tens of thousands of deaths occur worldwide. There are 4,500–7,000 animal cases reported in the U.S. every year. Human rabies is no longer always fatal, but recovery requires intensive management and is most successful in the previously immunized.

At-risk settings for rabies include livestock producing areas, especially equine and bovine, rural environments with exposure to wild animals, and border areas with Mexico. Rabies is not present in Hawaii or U.S. Pacific territories. Agricultural workers with a history of a bite, hydrophobia/aerophobia, and a variable prodrome should alert a clinician. Rabies is exclusively a mammalian disease found especially among carnivores, such as skunks, raccoons, foxes, bats, cats, and dogs, and not among rodents or lagomorphs.

The virus enters through a bite, pre-existing wound, mucous membrane, or, rarely, corneal implants. Virus inhalation has occurred among spelunkers exploring bat-colonized caves. The rhabdovirus multiplies in the muscle or other tissue (cornea), travels along peripheral nerves, ascends the spinal cord to the brain, replicates further, and then passes through the efferent nerves of the salivary glands and into the saliva. The incubation period varies from 10 days to less than 1 year, usually 1–2 months, depending on proximity of the inoculation site to the head.

Signs and Symptoms. Early prodromal clinical symptoms are variable and may include discomfort and paresthesias at the virus-inoculation site, apprehension, headache, irritability, malaise, hydrophobia, aerophobia, and fever. Excess salivation, severe progressive encephalitis, and ascending paralysis with hyperreactivity to external stimuli, with spastic skeletal muscle contraction, follow; then dysphagia, delirium, convulsions, respiratory failure, and death occur—except in a few intensively supported cases. Diagnostic testing involves identification of a rabies-neutralizing antibody titer more than or equal to 5 (complete neutralization) in the serum or CSF of an unvaccinated individual.[1]

Treatment. Treatment begins with immediate, thorough, and vigorous wound cleansing, which has been shown to decrease virus transmission by 50%.[10] Copious irrigation of the wound is recommended using a large heavy duty syringe, Waterpik TM device, or IV bag with a blood pressure cuff wrapped around. The post-exposure immunization protocol is indicated if the individual is bitten by a domestic animal that is rabid or that becomes so in the 10-day isolation period. The protocol is also necessary when the animal is not captured or a captured animal behaves unusually. Individuals bitten by any wild animal, except rodents and lagomorphs, require the protocol.

A contaminated wound should not be sutured. If suturing is unavoidable for cosmetic or functional reasons, the wound should be infiltrated with rabies immune globulin (RIG) first. Isolation precautions should be followed. It is important to also provide tetanus immunization and treatment for other infectious agents common to animal bites (such as *Pasteurella*). Providers can consult with the Centers for Disease Control **Rabies Hotline** 1-404-332-4555 and their local health department for further information.

Prevention and Control. Prevention and control measures include immunization of dogs and cats, especially along the border of Mexico where unimmunized strays and feral animals are found, and among those exposed to wild animals, particularly in border ranches. Immunization of livestock is not economically feasible. However, wild animal reservoirs should be removed where there is frequent human exposure. New employees in high-risk settings should be required to prove their immune status with adequate titers. See Table 2 for post-exposure immunization recommendations with human cell diploid vaccine (HCDV) and RIG for bites.

Rocky Mountain Spotted Fever

The causative agent is *Rickettsia rickettsii*. **High-risk occupations** include farmers, trappers, and foresters. About half of all U.S. cases occur in the southeastern U.S., with the remaining 50% throughout the country. Only 3% of cases are now reported from the Rocky Mountain area. Ninety-five percent of cases occur between April 1 and September 30. The incidence has been declining in recent years. About 592 cases were reported in 1987, making RMSF one of the most common zoonoses in the U.S. Though there is a 4% overall mortality, the vast majority of cases are cured if treatment is begun before the sixth day. Risk

TABLE 2. Treatment of Bites

Animal	Condition	Human Treatment
Wild	Rabid, unless fluorescent antibody neg.	HDCV* (or RVA*) and RIG*
Domestic canine, feline, or livestock	Healthy and under observation	None
Domestic canine, feline, or livestock	If rabies develops	HDCV (or RVA) and RIG
Domestic canine, feline, or livestock	Rabid or suspect	HCDV (for RVA) and RIG
Lagomorphs (hares, rabbits), rodents		Rarely need prophylaxis

* HCDV: Human diploid cell virus. RIG: rabies immune globulin. RVA: rabies vaccine absorbed, available from the Michigan Department of Public Health for those unable to tolerate the human serum albumin in HCDV.

factors for an increased mortality rate include age over 20 years, jaundice, and neurologic, cardiac, or renal complications. **Exposure** commonly occurs as a bite from an infected tick or contamination of skin with tick tissue, juices, or feces. Animal sources include rabbits, field mice, and dogs.

Endothelial cell damage is caused by the invading intracellular pathogen, resulting in platelet aggregation, coagulation defects, and problems with fibrinolytic pathways. The incubation period is usually between 2 and 7 days.

Signs and Symptoms. Clinical signs and symptoms include abrupt headache, nausea, conjunctival injection, rigors, high fever, myalgias, marked weakness, abdominal pain, a nonproductive cough, a maculopapular or petechial rash beginning on the extremities and spreading to trunk, myocardial vasculitis, and pulmonary edema. Thrombocytopenia, anemia, hyponatremia, and elevated liver enzyme tests are also commonly found.

Diagnostic Tests. Diagnostic tests include complement-fixation, indirect hemagglutination, or indirect fluorescent antibody tests. A positive Weil-Felix reaction (Proteus OX-19, OX-2) is confirmatory.

Treatment. Treatment includes oral tetracycline 25–50 mg/kg/day in divided doses every 6 hours or chloramphenicol in a loading dose of 50 mg/kg followed by 50 mg/kg/day in divided doses every 6 hours.

Prevention and Control. Prevention and control measures include avoidance of contact with ticks, wearing protective clothing, using insect repellents, and removal of ticks daily with tweezers. No vaccine is currently available.

Staphylococcal Infections

Staphylococcus aureus, a gram positive coccus, is the most common causative agent of staphylococcus infection among farm workers. Common manifestations are food poisoning or skin lesions. Livestock workers, especially on dairy farms, are particularly at risk. The bacteria is widespread, causing frequent infections that are not reportable. Humans are the most common reservoir of infection. The mode of exposure is often direct contact with an infected human, usually by hand contamination of nasal or rectal carriers. Dairy animals are the more likely animals to be infected, with *Staphylococcus aureus* transmitted in milk or the normal flora of the respiratory tract and skin.

Signs and Symptoms. Clinical signs and symptoms include gastroenteritis, which can be sudden in onset and often occurs with severe nausea, cramping, vomiting, diarrhea, and hypotension. Hypothermia can occur, with symptoms usually persisting less than 2 days. Skin infection can present as impetigo, folliculitis, furuncles, carbuncles, abscesses, or infected lacerations. Complications (when the bacteria become blood-borne) include pneumonia, lung abscess, septicemia, osteomyelitis, endocarditis, meningitis, and brain abscess.

Diagnostic Tests. Diagnostic tests include wound culture or culture of vomitus or feces.

Treatment. Treatment with penicillin G is ineffective in most skin infections caused by coagulase-positive strains. These strains require nafcillin IV or oral dicloxacillin 250–500 mg every 6 hrs for 10–14 days in minor infections. Often gastroenteritis is treated only with supportive measures. **Prognosis** is excellent with early treatment. Fatalities are rare.

Prevention and Control. Prevention and control measures include sound animal hygiene methods, early detection and treatment of mastitis in dairy herds, early detection and treatment of skin lesions in animal handlers and food handlers, milk pasteurization, sanitary preparation and storage of animal food products, and selected use of antibiotics to prevent development of resistant strains.

Tetanus

The causative agent of tetanus, or "lockjaw," is the bacillus *Clostridium tetani.* **High-risk occupations** include livestock and cattle producers and farmers susceptible to open wounds. Person-to-person transmission does not occur. In 1990, there were 95 cases reported in the U.S. Over a million cases occur worldwide every year, mostly in neonates.

Contamination of an open, even trivial, wound with infected soil or feces can cause disease. Clostridium spores can remain in soil for years. Also reservoirs of the bacteria can exist in the intestine of animals and humans as normal flora. Spores introduced into the body grow anaerobically. *C. tetani* produces an exotoxin that either enters peripheral motor neurons or becomes blood-borne.

The incubation period ranges from 3 to 21 days (average is 10 days), shorter with increased severity of contamination. Dead tissue or foreign bodies in wounds will increase the growth of *C. tetani,* with a resultant increase in toxin production.

Signs and Symptoms. Clinical signs and symptoms can include muscle spasms, abdominal rigidity induced by sensory stimulation, trismus, risus sardonicus, opisthotonos, spastic/contracted skeletal muscle, tonicoclonic convulsions, respiratory failure, and death.

Diagnosis. Diagnosis is usually made by clinical findings and history of lack of immunization, because *C. tetani* is very difficult to isolate from wounds, and antibody responses are often undetectable.

Treatment. Treatment should include penicillin G IV 12–24 million units daily in divided doses and immunization. Tetracycline is an alternative antibiotic. Surgical debridement may also be helpful. Intensive supportive measures are essential, because there is a 50–90% case-fatality rate. Infection does not confer long-term immunity and second infections are possible.

Prevention and Control. Prevention and control measures include adherence to the recommended tetanus immunization protocol for all workers (primary series with boosters every 10 years), tetanus immune globulin (TIG) for all major and contaminated wounds, and the thorough cleansing of all wounds.

Tularemia

The causative agent is *Francisella tularensis.* **High-risk occupations** include trappers, hunters, farmers, sheep shearers, and other employees who handle wild rabbits, squirrels, foxes, muskrats, or deer meat and/or the pelts of these animals. Outbreaks have been reported following the processing of certain agricultural products. Animal sources include sheep, hares, and rabbits. Less than 200 cases are reported each year in the U.S. Winter and summer are peak seasons for onset of infection, representing animal tissue contact or insect-vector–borne disease, respectively. One of the most common zoonoses in the U.S., most cases are reported in west north-central and west south-central states.

Tularemia is highly infectious, with **four major modes of exposure:** (1) arthropod vectors (hard-bodied ticks and deerflies); (2) contact exposure to infectious animal tissue, mud, crushed ticks, or contaminated water (the organism can invade through unbroken or broken skin or an oculoglandular syndrome can develop if material is rubbed or sprayed into eyes); (3) airborne transmission; and (4) ingestion of infectious agents. In general, transcutaneous infections cause ulceroglandular syndromes, inhalation or bacterial spread cause pulmonary syndromes, and bacilli ingestion cause enteric syndromes.

Signs and Symptoms. Clinical signs and symptoms can be clustered among four major syndromes: (1) the **ulceroglandular syndrome** (70 to 80% of cases) involves erythematous macules on the skin or mucous membrane within 2 days after inoculation that evolve into pruritic papules, which then ulcerate on the fourth day. High fevers up to 41°C and local lymphadenopathy, chills, sweats, myalgia, headache, and hepatosplenomegaly may develop. Lymph nodes may suppurate; (2) the **oculoglandular syndrome** includes intense conjunctival inflammation, enlarged preauricular, submandibular, and anterior cervical nodes; (3) the **pulmonary syndrome** is associated with tracheitis, bronchitis, pneumonia, pleural effusions, pleuritic chest pain, cough, dyspnea, hemoptysis, and patchy infiltrates with hilar adenopathy on chest x-rays, but rarely lung abscesses; and (4) the **enteric syndrome** causes exudative pharyngitis with gray membrane. Rarely, primary GI tract lesions develop, causing abdominal pain, nausea, vomiting, and diarrhea.

Diagnostic Tests. Diagnostic tests involve isolation by culture and animal inoculation. In the agglutination test, antibodies appear by the 10th to 14th day and rapidly rise (a 1:160 titer is possible). The Foshay skin test gives a positive specific delayed hypersensitivity response during the first week of illness.

Treatment. Treatment is with intramuscular streptomycin 500 mg twice a day for one week, or gentamicin. Oral tetracycline or chloramphenicol can also be administered in less severe infections. Infection is rarely fatal.

Prevention and Control. Prevention and control measures include minimizing exposure to infected animals and vectors, avoiding contact with sick or dead wild animals, wearing rubber gloves when dressing wild rabbits, and cooking meat from game animals thoroughly. A live vaccine is available providing protection to systemic infection but not ulceroglandular manifestations.

Other Occupational Infections

See Table 3 for other occupational infections of farm workers.

CONCLUSION

Farm workers in the U.S. are exposed to a number of high-risk occupational settings where infections from zoonotic and helminthic agents can cause illnesses or disability. Effective prevention and control measures are available for 21 infections that pose definite health risks to these workers. In addition, health care providers should maintain a reasonable index of suspicion that an occupational source or setting may be responsible for clinical signs and symptoms. Incorporating appropriate risk-assessment questions and diagnostic tests into the routine history and physical examination will assist in the early diagnosis of occupational infections.

TABLE 3. Other Common Occupational Infections in Farm Workers

Disease Name	At-Risk Settings/Occupations	Exposure Mode	Signs and Symptoms	Diagnosis	Treatment	Prevention and Control
Echinococcosis (parasite)	Livestock and sheep herding; Southwest and Central U.S., Alaska	Ingesting eggs from dog feces	Cysts in liver, lungs, kidneys, bone, spleen, CNS; hemoptysis, cough	CXR = coin lesion, cyst; ultrasound; serology	Surgical removal of cysts; mebendazole, abendazole	Routinely deworm dogs; deep bury or burn dead sheep; avoid feeding uncooked mutton to dogs
Erysipeloid (bacteria)	Fish or meat processing; sheep, swine, poultry workers; rabbit skinners; butchers	Contamination of hand/finger lesions with organism	Raised red-purple macule/papule; itching; swelling; rarely septic arthritis, endocarditis, splenomegaly	Culture needle aspirate; blood cultures; skin biopsy	Self-limiting; resolves in 3 weeks; penicillin VK or erythromycin 500 mg QID X 7 days	Wear gloves, long sleeves; install protective handles and shields
Escherichia coli gastroenteritis (bacteria)	Livestock, poultry workers; rural and poor areas, e.g., migrant farm workers	Ingesting contaminated water, food, waste	Severe cramps, diarrhea, nausea, vomiting, dehydration, possible hemolytic–uremic syndrome	Stool gram stain and culture	Rehydrate orally or by IV; cephalosporin, trimethoprim/sulfamethoxazole, ciprofloxacin, norflaxacin, bismuth-subsalicylate, or loperamide	Hand washing; proper food preparation and cleaning; potable water in rural areas
Lyme disease (bacteria)	Livestock producers in deciduous areas; tick habitats; deer farmers; contact with tick vectors (horses, dogs, cattle)	Tickbite	Erythema migrans rash, arthralgias, stiff neck, fatigue, meningitis, myocarditis, neuropathy	IgM, IgG antibodies in serum or CSF	Penicillin G or ceftriaxone IV	Vector control; wear light clothes; careful removal of ticks; diethyltoluamide spray/permethrin
Orf virus disease (sheep pox)	Sheep and goat herding; animal sheds; feed bunks	Contact with animal reservoirs, carcasses (e.g., lips, mouth, eyes, skin)	Pustular dermatitis on fingers; fever; ulcerated vesicles	Clinical findings	Self-limited; resolves usually in 1 month	Isolate infected animals; wear protective gloves; environmental sanitation

Disease	Occupational exposure	Mode of transmission	Clinical findings	Diagnosis	Treatment	Prevention
Pasteurellosis (bacteria)	Cat and dog breeders; livestock and poultry producers	Bites and scratches; occasionally respiratory	Cellulitis; swelling and pain; sepsis; respiratory infection	Culture wound site; blood culture	Penicillin G, or tetracycline, or amoxclavil, or cephalosporin	Wear gloves, long pants, and sleeves; clean all wounds thoroughly; keep animal pens and kennels clean
Plague (bacteria)	Contact with wild rodents, coyotes, rabbits; veterinarians; western U.S.	Flea bite or direct hand contact with diseased animal	Regional lymphadenitis, bubo; fever, chills, septic shock, pneumonia	Fluorescent antibody staining, lymph node aspirate	Streptomycin 1 g IM BID X 10 days; tetracycline or chloramphenicol	Killed vaccine for high-risk workers; isolate infected workers
Pseudocowpox (virus)	Dairy cow milkers and handlers	Teats and udders of infected milking cows	Hard wart-like nodules on hands and forearms	Clinical findings	Self-limited; resolves usually in 1 month	Isolate infected animals; wear protective gloves; environmental sanitation
Toxoplasmosis (parasite)	Abattoir workers; cat veterinarians; cat breeders	Ingesting oocysts passed in feline feces, or cysts in infected uncooked meat, or contaminated water	Often asymptomatic; fever, chills, lymphadenitis, myalgias, pharyngitis, hepatosplenomegaly, maculopapular rash	Sabin-Feldman dye tests; IgG antibody titers over 1:1000; lymph node biopsy	Pyrimethamine 100 mg orally, then 20 mg/day for 4–5 weeks, plus a sulfonamide	Eliminate feral cats; feed cats only processed food; prevent cats from hunting
Vesicular stomatitis (virus)	Cattle ranchers; swine and wild animal workers; pastures, milking shed with mechanical apparatus[18]	Oral ulcers of infected animals; spread possible by sandflies, mosquitos	Fever; vesicular enathemas in hand, mouth, lips; headache; myalgias; flu-like symptoms	Elevated antibody titers during second week of symptoms	Self-limited; supportive measures	Isolate infected animals; wear protective gloves; mosquito control

REFERENCES

1. Benenson AS: Control of Community Diseases in Man, 15th ed. Washington, DC, American Public Health Association, 1990.
2. Buchanan TM, et al: Brucellosis in the United States 1960–1972; An abattoir-associated disease. Medicine 53:427–439, 1974.
3. Centers for Disease Control: Summary of notifiable diseases in the U.S. MMWR 38:3, 1989.
4. Centers for Disease Control: Case definitions for public health surveillance. MMWR 39:7–8 (No. RR-13), 1990.
5. Centers for Disease Control: Rabies in case definitions for public health surveillance. MMWR 39:29, 1990.
6. Cordes DH, Rea DF: Health hazards of farming. AFP 38:233–244, 1988.
7. Donham KJ: Zoonotic disease of occupational significance in agriculture: A review. Int J Zoonoses 12:163–191, 1985.
8. Drugs of choice for bacterial infections. Medical Letter 817:44–46, 1990.
9. Faine S: Leptospirosis—still here. Med J Aust 144–145, 1986.
10. Fekety R: Rabies prevention: The latest guidelines. PA Drug Update, October 1982.
11. Fox MD, Kaufman AF: Brucellosis in the United States, 1965–1975. J Infect Dis 136:312, 1977.
12. Kebedjeiv GN: Anthrax. In Encyclopedia of Occupational Health and Safety. Geneva, International Labour Office, 1983, pp 163–165.
13. Mumford C, Dudley N, Terry H: Leptospirosis presenting as a flaccid paralysis. Postgrad Med J 66:218–220, 1990.
14. Raffle PAB: Anthrax. In Raffle PAB, Lee WR, McCallum RI, Murray R (eds): Hunter's Diseases of Occupations. London, MacMillan, 1987, pp 718–724.
15. Rubenstein E, Federman DD (eds): Scientific American Medicine. Section 7—Infectious Disease, 1990.
16. Smart KS, Wilks CR, Jackson KB, et al: Human leptosporisis in Victoria. Med J Aust 1:460–463, 1983.
17. Takafuji ET, Kirkpatrick JW, Miller RN, et al: An efficacy trial of doxycycline chemoprophylaxis against leptospirosis. N Engl J Med 310:497–500, 1984.
18. Webb PA, Monath TP, Reif JS, et al: Epizootic vesicular stomatitis in Colorado, 1982: Epidemiologic studies along the Northern Colorado front range. Am J Trop Med Hyg 36:183–189, 1987.

LESLIE BOYER HASSEN, MD

REPTILE AND ARTHROPOD ENVENOMATIONS

From the Section of Emergency
  Medicine
University of Arizona Health
  Sciences Center
Tucson, Arizona

Reprint requests to:
Leslie Boyer Hassen, MD
Clinical Toxicology Office
Section of Emergency Medicine
University of Arizona Health
  Sciences Center
1501 N. Campbell Ave.
Tucson, AZ 85724

Venomous arthropods are found in the fossil record dating back to the Silurian Period, over 400 million years ago[39]; so it seems safe to assume that envenomation has been an occupational hazard since the days when farmers first tilled the earth. Over the centuries of recorded history, venomous creatures have been credited with tremendous medicinal powers and blamed for evil of biblical proportions. Bites and stings have been the inspiration of popular myth and the cause of widespread fear. Envenomations have been treated with analgesics, sedatives, narcotics, antihistamines, steroids, epinephrine, antivenin, surgery, cryotherapy, electric shock, and prayer.

Broadly, venom may be seen as having three essential purposes for the survival of the animal involved. The first of these, **defense,** is readily apparent in any bite or sting that causes immediate local pain; examples would include scorpion sting and snake bite, both of which usually cause enough pain to discourage the advances of even the largest human or animal attacker. The second purpose, **prey immobilization,** is vital to the survival of small predators whose prospective meal might otherwise be prone to successful flight; examples of this include black widow spider bite and bark scorpion sting, both of which provide neurotoxins. Third, many venoms contain enzymes analogous to mammalian pancreatic secretions, which may **begin the digestive process** before the meal is consumed. A digestive function is most frequently cited in the case of snakes, whose low surface-area-to-volume-ratio meals are swallowed whole; but this may also explain the function of enzymes found in the venom of many arthropods.

Care of the envenomated patient varies with the geographic origin of the accident, because tremendous differences exist among the toxins produced by creatures of different regions. Fortunately, although accidental and deliberate importation of exotic species do occasionally result in domestic bites and stings, the vast majority of patients presenting for medical care have been bitten or stung by indigenous fauna. Both the differential diagnosis and the approach to treatment of envenomation may thus usually be targeted specifically toward a defined subset of creatures. This chapter will focus on reptiles and arthropods native to the United States.

DIFFERENTIAL DIAGNOSIS OF ENVENOMATION

Not every bite and sting injury results in envenomation. In some cases other complications may predominate. Anaphylaxis or another hypersensitivity response may occur alone or in combination with more specific envenomation reactions. Local infection, most often by skin contaminants but occasionally with less well-known animal flora, may be introduced via a bite and may be difficult to distinguish from the underlying inflammatory response. Also, although the effects may not be evident acutely, certain arthropods serve as vectors for spirochetes, rickettsia, and protozoa that may later cause chronic, systemic disease. Reptile bites may cause significant local trauma from laceration or deposition of broken-off teeth. Finally, the consequences of misguided "first aid" activities may cause more injury than the bite itself, with complications of incision, burn, frostbite, or ischemia.

In most cases, arthropod bites and stings are readily distinguished from those of larger creatures; and, among the arthropods, different patterns of systemic as well as local presentation will help to define the specific cause (Table 1). The

TABLE 1. Summary of Physical Findings by Type of Envenomation

Type of Animal	Local findings	Systemic findings
Pit vipers	Fang marks, erythema, edema, ecchymosis, bullae, tenderness, lymphangitis; long-term atrophy, and contracture	Shock, acidosis, coagulopathy, nausea, vomiting, central nervous system depression, rhabdomyolysis, renal impairment
Coral snakes	Mild edema, paresthesias, tenderness	Lethary, muscle weakness, fasciculations, salivation, cranial nerve palsies, convulsions, respiratory failure, shock
Gila monster	Bite mark, embedded teeth, erythema, edema, ecchymosis, tenderness, lymphangitis	Hypotension, weakness, diaphoresis, shock
Widow spiders	Minimal erythema, edema, tenderness	Muscle fasciculation and spasm; severe abdominal, back, and leg tenderness
Brown (violin) spiders	Tenderness, erythema, lymphangitis, induration with central blister or necrotic ulcer; long-term scarring	Malaise, rash, hemolysis
Bark scorpion	Minimal erythema, edema, may have positive "tap test"	Neuromotor hyperactivity, respiratory impairment, hypertension, pulmonary edema, salivation
Other U.S. scorpions	Edema, erythema, tenderness	Usually none
Centipedes	Edema, erythema, tenderness	Usually none

differential diagnosis must often be carefully considered, however, as small, unpaired marks and clustered shallow lacerations from a glancing snakebite are easily confused with arthropod bites and excoriations.

Trauma, infection, and certain dermatologic conditions may mimic envenomation. All suspected envenomation sites should be inspected for evidence of teeth, cactus spines, splinters, or other foreign bodies. Cellulitis, abscess, and the vesiculobullous diseases should be considered in the differential diagnosis whenever the cause of injury is in doubt.

Physical examination of the patient with systemic presenting signs should include a full survey of the skin, with special attention to hands, feet, and— particularly among users of outhouses—the buttocks and genital region. The absence of cutaneous findings does not rule out bite or sting, but diagnosis may be aided by the discovery of tiny marks, erythema, edema, or local tenderness. Limbs should be examined for evidence of lymphangitis proximal to the site of injury. Vital signs and pulmonary and neurologic status should be considered fully. Repeated evaluation over several hours' time is often necessary to differentiate envenomation from other causes of wound or illness.

Consider consulting your regional Poison Control Center or clinical toxicology service when the diagnosis is in doubt, when conservative measures fail to control the patient's symptoms, when intensive care is necessary, or when considering the use of specific antivenin.

REPTILES

Pit Vipers

Crotalids, or pit vipers, are snakes of the family Crotalidae. American members of the pit viper family include rattlesnakes, pigmy rattlesnakes, massasaugas, copperheads, and cottonmouth moccasins (Table 2). Generally, a crotalid may be recognized by its facial pits (infrared sensory organs located between eye and nostril), elliptical pupils, paired fangs, and broad, somewhat triangular head.[40]

Crotalus and *Sistrurus* species (rattlesnakes) are distinguished by rattles on the end of the tail. Copperheads and cottonmouths are pit vipers without rattles. The *Agkistrodon* venoms are similar to those of rattlesnakes but less potent, and venom yields are typically smaller.[32] The clinical effects are, therefore, usually of a lesser order than seen in bites by rattlesnakes.

TABLE 2. Partial List of Venomous Creatures Native to the United States

Pit vipers	Rattlesnakes	*Crotalus* species
(*Crotalidae*)	Pygmy rattlesnakes and massasaugas	*Sisturus* species
	Copperheads and cottonmouth moccasins	*Agkistrodon* species
Coral snakes	Eastern coral snakes	*Micrurus fulvius* ssp.
(*Elapidae*)	Arizona coral snake	*Micruroides euryxanthus*
Lizards	Gila Monster	*Heloderma suspectum*
Spiders	Widow spiders	*Latrodectus* sp.
	Brown spiders (violin spiders)	*Loxosceles* sp.
Scorpions	Bark scorpions	*Centruroides exilicauda*
	Other scorpions	*Centruroides, Vejovis, Hadrurus, Androctonus* sp.
Centipedes	Giant Desert Centipede	*Scolopendra heros*

Pit vipers are found wild in all of the lower 48 states, although their number and variety is greater in southern than in northern latitudes of the U.S. They are most active during warm months, with roughly 90% of bites occurring between April and October.

All pit vipers are venomous, although venom quantity, composition, and potency vary greatly among species and among individual snakes. The venom is a complex poison. It is 90% water, with a variety of enzymes, nonenzymatic proteins and peptides, and other, still-unidentified, substances.[46] Physiologic effects include increased capillary permeability, procoagulant and anticoagulant activities, and a broad variety of tissue-degradative enzymatic changes.[32]

Presentation. Puncture marks from the upper, venom-injecting fangs of pit vipers classically are paired, but single-fang injuries and multiple bites are commonly observed. A group of small scratches left by the snake's tiny lower teeth may sometimes also be identified on close inspection. Over minutes to hours following the bite, local signs may progress to include tenderness, edema, erythema, bleeding, ecchymoses, hemorrhagic bullae, and lymphangitis.[32] Rarely, a true compartment syndrome may threaten nerve and muscle.

Dramatic local symptoms are typical in, for instance, bites by Western and Eastern diamondback rattlesnakes (*C. atrox* and *C. adamanteus*). Patients may develop severe swelling and purpura of the entire extremity, accompanied by shock from volume loss.[16,32]

Systemic reactions to pit viper bite vary from none at all (in up to a quarter of crotalid bites there is no significant envenomation) to life-threatening. There may be hypotension, weakness, sweating or chills, perioral or peripheral paresthesias, nausea and vomiting, and fasciculations. Central nervous system depression may be significant even in the absence of shock. Coagulopathy is common and may involve thrombocytopenia, hypofibrinogenemia, and greatly increased prothrombin and partial thromboplastin times. Severe envenomation may lead to hemoconcentration, lactic acidosis, hypovolemic shock, pulmonary edema and hemorrhage.[32,34]

Management. If poisonous snakebite is suspected, the principle behind early management is rapid, safe transport to the nearest medical facility while minimizing absorption of venom. Transport should not be delayed to perform first aid measures, and potentially injurious maneuvers such as electric shock and tourniquet placement should be avoided.

Insofar as possible, the victim should be kept calm. If equipment is available to apply direct suction over the fang marks, this should be done without incising the skin. The bitten area should be immobilized with a sling or splint. A constriction band may be applied immediately proximal to the bite site; this should be loose enough to allow a finger between band and skin. The band may require frequent adjustment to maintain proper tension; it must not be allowed to tighten and become a tourniquet.

Initial medical assessment should include inquiry into the timing and circumstances of the bite, nature of first aid used, and any identifying characteristics of the snake involved. After cardiovascular stability is assured, a careful physical exam should be done, and the extent of local edema and lymphangitis should be recorded with a skin-marking pen.

Initial laboratory evaluation should include complete blood count, platelet count, prothrombin and partial thromboplastin times, fibrinogen, creatine phosphokinase (CPK), and urinalysis. In moderate and severe cases, blood should

TABLE 3.   Grade of Envenomation by Pit Viper

Grade of Envenomation	Local Findings	Systemic Findings	Laboratory Findings
None	Fang marks only	None	Unaffected
Minimal	Confined to or around the bite area	None	Unaffected
Moderate	May extend beyond the bite area, but are generally less than an entire extremity	May be significant	Slightly changed (low fibrinogen and platelets, hemoconcentration, mild coagulopathy)
Severe: any one or a combination of local and systemic findings	Involving the entire extremity or part	Serious (e.g., shock, CNS depression)	May be dramatic

be sent for type and hold at the time of admission. Tests should be repeated daily or as indicated for patient management. For moderate and severe envenomations, they may need to be done every 3 to 4 hours for the first 12 or more hours.

After examination and laboratory assessment, the presenting grade of envenomation may be determined (Table 3). Repeated assessment of patient status and grade of envenomation is essential, because signs, symptoms, and laboratory abnormalities may progress over many hours' time.[3]

Early management includes the placement of an intravenous line and infusion of isotonic crystalloid solution. The wound should be cleansed and the limb loosely immobilized and slightly elevated. Tetanus prophylaxis and analgesic should be given if indicated.

Before mixing antivenin or placing a skin test, determine whether its use is indicated in the particular patient. Bear in mind that 25% of all crotalid bites are "dry," with no or trivial envenomation and no need for antivenin. Patients who do not need antivenin should be exposed neither to the skin test antigen nor to antivenin, as immediate hypersensitivity reaction and delayed serum sickness are potential sequelae.

The exact indications for antivenin remain controversial, because controlled studies demonstrating long-term outcome of comparable injuries with and without its use have never been done. It is clear from both clinical and laboratory experience, however, that early treatment with antivenin reduces ongoing venom injury significantly. The decision to use antivenin is influenced by grade of envenomation, rapidity of change in symptoms, time since the bite, and body part involved.

In the U.S., Wyeth Crotalid Polyvalent is the only available antivenin active against pit viper venom. In general, moderate and severe envenomations should be treated with antivenin in increments of 5–10 vials at a time. Minimal envenomation frequently can be managed without antivenin; however, rapid progress of injury or high-risk bite site may indicate its use nevertheless.

Before administering antivenin, check allergy history, particularly to horse serum products. With epinephrine and antihistamines available at the bedside, administer the manufacturer's skin test solution as directed in the package insert. If history or skin test suggests allergy, prophylaxis with H1 and H2 receptor blockers, such as dephenhydramine and cimetidine, may be used prior to antivenin administration; check with your regional poison control center or clinical toxicologist for assistance.

Antivenin should be administered slowly at first, then faster (up to about 10 vials per hour) if no reaction occurs. It is generally given in increments of 5–10 vials until local injury is static and coagulopathy has been reversed; the entire dose should ideally be given during the first few hours. The use of antivenin more than 24 hours following envenomation is currently limited to reversal of coagulopathy.

In general, pit viper bite victims should be observed for a minimum of 6 hours; envenomated patients should be admitted to the hospital. Cryotherapy, tourniquet application, and wound excision should be avoided, because these tend to contribute to morbidity. Fasciotomy, except in cases of frank tissue necrosis or true compartment syndrome, is almost never indicated.[42]

A regional Poison Control Center should be notified of all bites, for informational purposes. For moderate-to-severe bites, or those with complicating factors, ask for the "Toxicologist On Call."

Coral Snakes

United States coral snakes are brightly colored reptiles with broad circumferential rings of red and black separated by bands of yellow. The head is solid black from the eyes to the snout. Several similarly colored nonvenomous species mimic the coral snake's stripes, but in most of these harmless snakes the yellow bands are separated on each side by a black ring.[32,40] Thus the mnemonic rhyme: "Red on yellow kill a fellow; red on black venom lack."

Coral snakes are unlikely to bite unless they are roughly handled. Arizona coral snakes have small mouths with short fangs that do not readily accommodate a human finger, and the webbing between fingers is reported to be the most vulnerable. Eastern coral snakes, somewhat larger, may bite a hand or foot. When they do strike, coral snakes may hang on firmly until they are forcibly removed.[14,40]

Micrurus fulvius ssp.   The Eastern coral snake ranges across the American South from central Texas to Florida and as far north as North Carolina. Eastern coral snake venom is a very potent neurotoxin, and untreated bites carry a significant risk of mortality.

Micruroides euryxanthus.   This small cylindrical snake is found across southern Arizona and in the southwest corner of New Mexico. Subterranean, small, and inoffensive, it is rarely implicated in significant envenomations. No deaths have ever been reported following its bite.

Presentation.   In contrast with the pit vipers', coral snake envenomations commonly result in very little local injury. The bite itself is usually associated with pain, although this may be slight; and there may be mild edema locally. Paresthesias may be noted around the bite area, and weakness of the extremity may follow over several hours. Often, local symptoms are absent.

Systemic symptoms of Eastern coral snake bite, which may be delayed for many hours, include lethargy, nausea, vomiting, muscle weakness, and fasciculations. Tongue fasciculations may occur, with dysphagia and sialorrhea. Over the course of hours, there may be extraocular nerve palsies, convulsions, descending bulbar paralysis, respiratory failure, shock, and sometimes death.[3,14,32,34]

Reports of envenomation by the Arizona coral snake are rare. Three cases described by Shaw and Campbell[37] showed a pattern of local pain over 15–120 minutes, with drowsiness, nausea, and weakness hours later. Neurologic symptoms included lacrimation, difficulty focusing the eyes, and incoordination.

Management.   As with pit vipers, early management of coral snake bite is geared toward rapid transport to the nearest medical facility while minimizing absorption of venom. The victim should be kept calm, and the bitten area should be immobilized. A constriction band may be applied immediately proximal to the bite site; as before, it must not be allowed to become a tourniquet.

Neurologic effects of Eastern coral snake envenomation may be severe, and they may develop many hours after the initial bite. Observation for at least 12 hours is important, and preparations should be made to administer antivenin promptly in the event of local or systemic neurologic changes. Although it is unlikely that the bite of the Arizona coral snake will result in significant envenomation, observation for approximately 12 hours is recommended because of the potential for similar neurologic effects. If skin penetration has occurred, local wound care and tetanus prophylaxis are indicated.

Unlike pit viper envenomations, coral snake bites are not associated with a characteristic laboratory profile. Routine blood chemistries and gases should be followed as necessary for supportive care.

Antivenin against Eastern coral snake venom is the mainstay of treatment for bites by *Micrurus* species. The usual starting dose is three to five vials, intravenous; up to 20 may be needed.[14,24,34] Precautions should be taken to recognize and treat hypersensitivity reactions, as with the administration of crotalid antivenin (see preceding section). All envenomated patients should be monitored in an intensive care setting, with intravenous hydration and, if necessary, ventilatory support.

No antivenin exists against the venom of the Arizona coral snake. Antivenin against *Micrurus* venom fails to neutralize *Micruroides* venom. Monitoring and supportive care should be provided for the first 12 hours for all patients, longer for those who are symptomatic.[34]

Gila Monsters

The Gila monster *(Heloderma suspectum)* is one of only two known venomous lizard species. (The other is the closely-related Mexican beaded lizard [*H. horridum*], whose range does not include the United States.) It has a stout body, usually under 20 inches long, covered with beads of black and pink, orange, or yellow.[40]

Gila monsters are most active in March, April, and May; but they may surface from their burrows on occasions year-round. Overall, they are active outside their burrows only about 190 hours out of the entire year![19] Their range reaches across the state of Arizona, from southwestern New Mexico to southern Nevada.

The venom-introduction apparatus of the Gila monster is different from that of pit vipers in that the teeth are grooved rather than hollow. In addition, the venom glands are paired on either side of the lower, rather than the upper, jaw. Delivery of venom into a wound is time-related, with more venom injected during prolonged pumping of the jaw. It is **not** true that the lizard must flip upside-down to inject venom!

Venom from the Gila monster has been demonstrated to contain serotonin, amine oxidase, phospholipase A, kallikrein, protease, and hyaluronidase activity. High hyaluronidase activity may explain the tissue edema commonly seen; relatively low proteolytic activity is consistent with the small amount of tissue breakdown usually noted.[32]

Presentation. Clinical signs of Gila monster bite depend in part upon the nature of the bite. Brief, slashing bites are common; in these cases the animal either withdraws or is flung off by the victim before an appreciable amount of venom has been injected.

In many cases, however, the creature is able to hold fast after a bite. There ensues a period of firm jaw contraction and sometimes grinding that is notoriously difficult to escape. During this time (which may last a few seconds, or over 10 minutes) envenomation may be ongoing and more severe.

Local manifestations of Gila monster bite include tooth marks or embedded teeth, pain, edema, erythema, lymphangitis, and lymphadenitis. Systemic signs may include weakness, dizziness, diaphoresis, hypotension, and shock. A few fatalities have been reported; most of these were complicated by alcohol, drugs, or preexisting illness.[19]

Management. Other than removal of the animal from the victim, there are no proven first aid measures for treatment of Gila monster bite. The part should be loosely immobilized and the patient transported to an emergency room as quickly as possible.

In the emergency room, the bite site should be examined carefully for puncture marks, erythema, edema, and lymphangitic streaking. When foreign body is suspected, x-rays may demonstrate the presence of shed teeth. Local infiltration with lidocaine may help to define the location of indistinct puncture sites. The wound should be cleaned thoroughly, and tetanus prophylaxis should be given if indicated.

Initial laboratory evaluation should include complete blood count, urinalysis, blood coagulation profile, and electrolytes; these should be repeated periodically over several days as clinically indicated.

No antivenin against Gila monster venom is commercially available at this time. Supportive care for envenomation includes loose immobilization of the part at or just above heart level, volume and pressor support for hypotension, and pain management with acetaminophen or narcotics. Systemic signs usually resolve by 24 hours; discharge is possible when pain and local signs are stable.

ARTHROPODS

The phylum *Arthropoda* includes insects, crustaceans, horseshoe crabs, and millipedes, in addition to the venomous species described here. This discussion will focus on spiders, scorpions, and centipedes, which are responsible for most clinically significant envenomations within the U.S.

Mortality from arthropod envenomation is fortunately very low in the U.S. today. Many mild cases can be cared for at home, and moderate reactions in otherwise healthy adults can often be managed without hospital admission. Severe local and systemic consequences are possible, however. Details will be presented by genus.

Widow Spiders *(Latrodectus species)*

Widow spiders are cosmopolitan in distribution. *Latrodectus mactans,* the black widow, is found in every state of the U.S. except Alaska. The female, responsible for all envenomations, is shiny black with a characteristic red "hour glass" marking on the ventral abdomen. She spins an irregular web in sheltered corners of fields, gardens, barns, garages, and outbuildings, where she is most likely to bite when the web is disturbed. In regions where outdoor privies are in common use, human envenomations are likely to involve the buttocks or genital area.[5,20]

Unlike many other arthropod venoms, that of the widow spiders appears to lack locally active toxins capable of provoking inflammation. It does contain several toxic components, including a potent neurotoxin, alpha-latrotoxin, which induces neurotransmitter release from nerve terminals by acting as a calcium ionophore.[21]

Presentation.   The initial bite may be sharply painful or may be unrecognized. Local reaction is commonly trivial, with only a tiny papule or punctum visible on exam. The surrounding skin may be slightly erythematous and slightly indurated.

Within 30 to 60 minutes of the bite, however, neuromuscular symptoms can become dramatic, as involuntary spasm and rigidity affect the large muscle groups of the abdomen and limbs; abdominal pain and rigidity may closely mimic an acute abdomen. Associated signs include fasciculations, weakness, ptosis, priapism, vomiting, fever, salivation, perspiration, and bronchorrhea. Respiratory muscle weakness, combined with pain, may lead to respiratory arrest; hypertension with or without seizures may complicate management in elderly or previously hypertensive individuals. Pregnancy may be complicated by uterine contractions and, potentially, premature delivery.[3,11,22,31,33]

Management.   Local care should include routine cleansing, intermittent application of ice, and tetanus prophylaxis. Pain and muscle spasm may be managed initially with slow intravenous infusion of calcium gluconate 10% solution at 10 cc/dose. The effects of calcium infusion, while occasionally dramatic, are often fleeting. An alternative muscle relaxant is methocarbamol, 15 mg/kg IV over 5 minutes followed by a similar dose in drip form over 4 hours' time. Spasms and pain not relieved by these measures may respond to diazepam or to meperidine hydrochloride. Careful observation of respiratory status is vital when using benzodiazepines or narcotics.[13]

Laboratory evaluation should include complete blood count, urinalysis, electrolytes, and blood glucose. In the presence of severe muscle spasm, CPK may be elevated. Abdominal films and stool hemoccult exam, both of which should be normal following widow spider envenomation, may help with differential diagnosis of abdominal pain. A pregnancy test should be done where clinically indicated.

Antivenin active against *Latrodectus* venom is available in the United States from Merck, Sharp & Dohme. It should be used in cases involving respiratory arrest, seizures, uncontrolled hypertension, or pregnancy; it should not be used routinely in less severe settings because of the risks of allergic reaction or delayed serum sickness following use of the equine product. When antivenin is used, preliminary skin testing is advised to minimize the chance of unanticipated severe allergic reaction; even after a negative skin test, the patient should remain under direct observation during treatment. The usual therapeutic antivenin dose is one to two vials, via intravenous infusion.

Although the worst pain usually occurs during the first 8 to 12 hours following a bite, symptoms may remain severe for several days. All symptomatic children, pregnant women, and patients with a history of hypertension should be admitted to the hospital. Discharge is usually possible within 1 to 3 days, when hypertension and muscle spasm have subsided.

Brown or Violin Spiders *(Loxosceles* species)

At least five species in the genus *Loxosceles* have been associated with necrotic arachnidism in the U.S., including *L. reclusa* (the true brown recluse spider). The brown spiders are about 1 centimeter in body length, 2 to 3 centimeters in leg length, and brown in color. Characteristically, they are marked with a dark, violin-shaped spot centered anteriorly, such that the neck of the violin extends backward across the cephalothorax.[7,11]

Loxosceles spiders are native to all of the southernmost states of the U.S.; in the center their territory extends as far north as southern Wisconsin. They are most active at night from April to October, emerging from woodpiles and closets to hunt insects and other spiders. Naturally unaggressive, they are not prone to bite humans unless threatened or trapped among bedsheets or clothing.

The venom is a hemolysin and cytotoxin, with a variety of enzymatic activities whose combined effect may bring about dermonecrosis and hemolysis. The pathogenesis is not well understood but is known to be dependent upon the function of both complement and polymorphonuclear leukocytes.[2,36]

Presentation.   The clinical spectrum of loxoscelism runs from mild and transient skin irritation to severe local necrosis accompanied by dramatic hematologic and renal injury. Isolated cutaneous lesions are the most common presentation; many bites resolve spontaneously without medical intervention.

Local symptoms usually begin at the moment of the bite itself, with a sharp stinging sensation; although it is not uncommon for patients to report no awareness of having been bitten at all. The stinging usually subsides over 6 to 8 hours, being replaced by aching and pruritus as the lesion becomes ischemic from local vaso-spasm. The site then becomes edematous, with an erythematous halo surrounding an irregular violaceous center. In more severe cases, serous or hemorrhagic bullae may arise at the center, and a black eschar forms over several days. After 2 to 5 weeks, this eschar sloughs, leaving an ulcer, through skin and adipose tissue, of variable size and depth. The ulcer may persist for many months, leaving a deep scar.[1,30,45]

Systemic involvement is less common but may occur with all *Loxosceles* species. Fever, chills, scarlatiniform rash, weakness, leukocytosis, arthralgias, nausea, and vomiting may all occur. There may be hemolytic anemia with hemoglobinuria, usually beginning within 24 hours of envenomation and resolving within a week. The anemia is usually Coombs' negative and may be severe. Thrombocytopenia and disseminated intravascular coagulation have been reported. In severe cases, hemoglobinuria and proteinuria have led to renal failure and even to death.[9,10,27]

Management.   Treatment of loxoscelism depends upon the severity of the lesion. Most mild envenomations will respond to application of local ice compresses, elevation of the affected extremity, and loose immobilization of the part. Necrotic lesions may need debridement after erythema has subsided around the central eschar; this can be followed with skin grafting when the wound is stable.

In the past, efforts have been made to treat brown spider bites with corticosteroids, antihistamines, immediate surgical incision, and prophylactic antibiotics, none of which has shown particular clinical effectiveness. Recently, dapsone (a leukocyte inhibitor) has gained popularity for the prevention of lesion progression; clinical efficacy has been reported, although animal studies generally have not demonstrated efficacy. Dapsone may be administered orally as 25 to 100 mg twice daily. It should not be used in patients with glucose-6-phosphate dehydrogenase deficiency; potential side-effects include methemoglobinemia, hemolysis, and idiosyncratic bone marrow suppression.[12,15]

A basic laboratory evaluation should be performed for patients with moderate-to-severe local signs or any systemic signs of envenomation. This should include peripheral blood count, basic coagulation screening, and urinalysis in all cases; liver and renal function tests are indicated in severe poisonings. Frequency of follow-up testing depends upon the course and severity of envenomation.

Cutaneous loxoscelism can usually be managed on an outpatient basis; severe necrotic or infected lesions may require hospitalization. Patients with systemic symptoms should be considered for admission when there is evidence of coagulo-pathy, hemolysis, and hemoglobinuria, or rapid progression of other systemic signs. Discharge is appropriate when renal and hematologic status is stable. Follow-up visits should be scheduled for examination and debridement of the ulcer; skin grafting is sometimes necessary.

Bark Scorpion *(Centruroides exilicauda)*

The only scorpion native to the U.S. whose venom is potentially life-threatening is the bark scorpion, *Centruroides exilicauda* (also called *C. sculpturatus*). It may be straw-colored, yellow or light brown in color; and it reaches up to 7.5 cm in length. Called the "bark" scorpion because of its predilection for hiding in the bark of trees, it may also be found in cracks and crevices under rocks or in woodpiles. The bark scorpion is found only in the southwestern U.S. and northwestern Mexico. It is a nocturnal predator, feeding mostly upon other small arthropods. It tends to sting humans only in self-defense.[40]

Centruroides exilicauda venom contains at least five neurotoxins, which through several mechanisms affect the function of membrane sodium channels. The resulting derangement of sodium flow causes spontaneous, repetitive, and prolonged axonal action potentials throughout the nervous system.[8]

Presentation. The sting site itself may be difficult to identify, as the punctum, edema, and erythema are trivial in most cases. A positive "tap test" can prove diagnostic in uncertain cases: sharp percussion of the suspected site may elicit relatively severe tenderness for the degree of inflammation otherwise apparent.[33]

Systemic effects result from aberrant nerve conduction within the sympathetic, parasympathetic, and neuromotor systems. Sympathomimetic effects include tachycardia, hypertension, hyperthermia, mydriasis, and diaphoresis. Parasympathomimetic effects include salivation, lacrimation, bradycardia, urination, and vomiting; in rare cases there may also be clinically significant pulmonary edema. Neuromotor effects include muscle fasciculations, opisthotonos, roving eye movements, nystagmus, and generalized hyperactivity. Lethargy, confusion, and occasionally seizures occur; these may be a result of direct central nervous system toxicity, hypoxia, or both.[4,17,18,28,44]

Young children are particularly prone to develop the more serious cardio-respiratory and neuromotor manifestations of scorpion envenomation. Whereas 80% of those under age 2 years stung by bark scorpions show these signs, only 5% of adults have significant neuromuscular involvement.[18]

Management. Immediate local treatment of scorpion sting is best limited to routine wound care. The site should be cleaned, and an ice cube may be briefly applied to minimize pain. All children under the age of 5 years, and adults with significant systemic symptoms, should be evaluated by a physician.

Pain in the majority of cases can be managed effectively with brief local applications of ice and simple analgesics such as acetaminophen; in the majority of cases involving adults, no further intervention is necessary. Caution is urged in the use of opiates, as these may exacerbate neurologic symptoms and hypoventilation.

Respiratory compromise is generally the most significant risk following a serious envenomation, and it is most common in infants. Although this usually results from neuromotor paralysis of incoordination, pulmonary edema may be a complicating factor. Judicious use of benzodiazepines may improve the motor defect, but increased respiratory depression is a potentially serious drawback to this method. Atropine may be useful for treatment of edema. Specific antivenom treatment should be considered in cases of respiratory compromise.

Cardiovascular effects are usually transient, and specific intervention is rarely necessary. The parasympathetic effects of *C. exilicauda* envenomation are usually brief as well, and atropine is seldom required. Tachyarrhythmias, when they occur, may be managed with beta blockers. Severe hypertension is rare; but this may in theory be treated with nitroprusside, diazoxide, or hydralazine.

The area of greatest controversy in treatment of bark scorpion sting surrounds the issue of neuromuscular manifestations. Respiratory depression is risked with all of the common pharmaceutical interventions, and it should be kept in mind that the outcome of envenomation with intensive care observation alone is unlikely to involve serious long-term morbidity. In the past, large doses of barbiturates and narcotics may have contributed to high mortality, particularly in children.[28,41] Nevertheless, some form of symptomatic treatment is often strongly desired; and in settings where careful monitoring is possible, this may be undertaken with relative safety. Benzodiazepines in conservative doses may prove helpful in reducing neuromotor hyperactivity; phenobarbital in moderate doses (5 to 10 mg/kg IV) may be administered for what is commonly minimal therapeutic benefit. Narcotics, in general, should be avoided.

An antivenin specific to *C. exilicauda* has been developed but is not approved by the Food and Drug Administration; it is available only within the state of Arizona. It has been used with efficacy and minimal incidence of severe side-effects, and it may find more general application once clinical trials have been completed. At this time, however, its use remains controversial due to allergy and serum-sickness that may follow serum administration, and it should be considered an experimental treatment.[38]

Patients with systemic symptoms should be observed for a minimum of 4 hours, as should all children under the age of 5 years. Vital signs should be checked frequently during this time. Those with respiratory compromise, severe tachycardia, or hypertension—or pain or neurologic symptoms requiring ongoing pharmaceutical use—should be admitted to the hospital for medical management and intensive monitoring. In most cases, clinical signs will begin to abate by 6 to 12 hours post-envenomation and will reach a tolerably minimal level by 16 to 24 hours; very mild symptoms may be noted by the patient for several additional days. Hospital discharge is appropriate when neurologic and cardiorespiratory stability status have returned to normal and when drug treatment is no longer necessary; this is usually possible by 24 hours after admission.

Other Scorpions

Other scorpions commonly implicated in envenomations in the U.S. include species of *Vejovis* (devil scorpions), *Hadrurus,* and *Androctonus.* Although many of these species appear outwardly more threatening than do bark scorpions (e.g., *H. arizonensis,* the giant hairy scorpion of the American Southwest), their stings rarely produce symptoms of serious medical importance. Likewise, stings of the non-*exilicauda Centruroides* species of the southeastern United States produce only local pain.

The effects of these stings often resemble those of a bee or wasp. There may be local swelling, erythema, and pain, but systemic signs and symptoms are rare and generally occur only in the presence of hypersensitivity. Medical management consists of cleaning, tetanus prophylaxis if needed, analgesia, and perhaps local application of ice to reduce inflammation. Hospital admission is rarely necessary.[3,4,33]

Centipedes

Centipedes are long, multisegmented arthropods possessing one pair of legs for each segment (millipedes have two pairs per segment). They use venom, injected via a pair of hollow fangs, to kill invertebrate and small vertebrate prey. The largest centipede species exceed 25 cm in length, but most are considerably smaller.[40]

Although any species with large enough fangs may to some extent envenomate humans, the only U.S. species of particular medical significance is the giant desert centipede, *Scolopendra heros*. Centipede venom contains a variety of enzymes, including acid and alkaline phosphatase and amino acid naphthylamidase, lipoproteins, histamine, and serotonin.

Burning pain, edema, erythema, lymphangitis, and lymphadenopathy are common after centipede bite. Reports of systemic toxicity are rare. Following the initial presentation, envenomation by *Scolopendra* species may be very slow to evolve, with local pain, tense edema, erythema, and lymphangitis persisting for 1 to 3 weeks. During this phase it is sometimes impossible to distinguish uncomplicated envenomation from cellulitis, and antibiotics may be administered. Careful observation of tightly swollen extremities should include repeated examination for potential compartment syndrome; intracompartmental pressure monitoring may be indicated. Laboratory evaluation is not necessary in cases of mild envenomation but should include urinalysis, complete blood count, and electrolyte and renal function testing in more serious cases.

Medical management is restricted to routine wound care; local infiltration with lidocaine may be used for immediate pain relief. There is not an antivenin available, and systemic care is primarily supportive; antihistamines and steroids have been suggested for more severe reactions.[6,23]

EDUCATION AND PREVENTION

Diverse popular lore and changing medical recommendations have been the source of much confusion regarding bites and stings. Despite improved understanding of envenomation in recent decades, first aid and early medical management commonly make use of outdated measures that are futile at best and harmful at worst. Education is clearly essential if farm workers and rural physicians are to minimize injury associated with envenomation. Resources for treatment and for development of educational programs are suggested in Table 4.

Farmers likely to encounter venomous creatures should above all be made aware of their local type and habitat, as avoidance of direct contact is certainly the best preventive measure. Sturdy boots, gloves, and full-length pants and sleeves should be worn when appropriate. Worksite first aid kits should be checked for the presence of potentially injurious snakebite-treatment implements, such as blades and electric voltage delivery devices. Suction extractors and restricting bands, when these are present, should be accompanied by clear written instructions to prevent misuse. Region-specific details should be available from biologists and poison information specialists at the nearest university or Poison Control Center.

When a bite or sting occurs on the farm, the second priority of those involved (after ensuring the safety and proper care of the victim) is often removal of the

TABLE 4.   Available Resources

Core references:	Russell FE: *Snake Venom Poisoning*[32]
	Klauber LM: *Rattlesnakes: Their Habits, Life Histories & Influence on Mankind*[16]
	Tu AT: *Rattlesnake Venoms: Their Action and Treatment*[43]
	Auerbach PS, Geehr EC: *Management of Wilderness and Environmental Emergencies*[4,23,27]
Clinical Consultants:	Regional Poison Control Center
	Clinical Toxicologist at University or Poison Center
Animal Identificaiton:	Herpetologist at local university or zoo
	Entomologist at local university or zoo
Antivenin:	Wyeth crotalid polyvalent for all North American pit vipers
	Merck, Sharp and Dohme *Latrodectus* for widow spiders
	Regional Poison Control Center for local antivenin availability

offending animal. When identification is in doubt, arthropods may be contained or killed and held for possible entomological examination. Venomous snakes, even dead ones, should be considered an envenomation hazard at all times; these should be captured or dispatched only when this can be done safely *and* when doing so is necessary for the safety of other workers. In many communities, fire department or animal-control personnel are trained to remove snakes safely; ideally, their availability should be known to farm supervisors in advance of any acute crisis.

REFERENCES

1. Alario A, Price G, Stahl R, Bancroft P: Cutaneous necrosis following a spider bite: A case report and review. Pediatrics 79:618–621, 1987.
2. Babcock JL, Marner DJ, Steele RW: Immunotoxicology of brown recluse spider *(Loxosceles reclusa)* venom. Toxicon 24:783–790, 1986.
3. Banner W: Bites and stings in the pediatric patient. Curr Probl Pediatr 8–69, 1988.
4. Banner W: Scorpion envenomation. In Auerbach PS, Geehr EC: Management of Wilderness and Environmental Emergencies, 2nd ed. St. Louis, C.V. Mosby, 1989, pp 603–616.
5. Binder LS: Acute arthropod envenomation: Incidence, clinical features and management. Med Toxicol Adverse Drug Exp 4:163–173, 1989.
6. Burnett JW, Calton GJ, Morgan RJ: Centipedes. Cutis 37:241, 1986.
7. Butz WC: Envenomation by the brown recluse spider (Aranae, Scytodidae) and related species. A public health problem in the United States. Clin Toxicol 4:515–524, 1971.
8. Curry SC, Vance MV, Ryan PJ, et al: Envenomation by the scorpion *Centruroides sculpturatus.* J Toxicol Clin Toxicol 21:417–449, 1984.
9. Denny WF, Dillaha CJ, Morgan PN: Hemotoxic effect of *Loxosceles reclusa* venom: *In vivo* and *in vitro* studies. J Lab Clin Med 64:291–298, 1964.
10. Ginsburg CM, Weinberg AG: Hemolytic anemia and multiorgan failure associated with localized cutaneous lesion. J Pediatr 112:496–499, 1988.
11. Horen WP: Arachnidism in the United States. JAMA 185:839–843, 1963.
12. Iserson KV: Methemoglobinemia from dapsone therapy for a suspected brown spider bite. J Emerg Med 3:285–288, 1985.
13. Key GF: A comparison of calcium gluconate and methocarbamol (Robaxin) in the treatment of lactrodectism (black widow spider envenomation). Am J Trop Med Hyg 30:273–277, 1981.
14. Kitchens CS: Envenomation by the Eastern coral snake: A study of 39 victims. JAMA 258:1615–1618, 1987.
15. King LE, Rees RS: Dapsone treatment of a brown recluse bite. JAMA 250:648, 1983.
16. Klauber LM: Rattlesnakes: Their Habits, Life Histories, & Influence on Mankind, abridged edition. Berkeley, CA, University of California Press, 1982.
17. La Grange RG: Elevation of blood pressure and plasma renin levels by venom from scorpions, *Centruroides sculpturatus* and *Leiurus quinquestriatus.* Toxicon 15:429–433, 1977.
18. Likes K, Banner WJ, Chavez M: *Centruroides exilicauda* envenomation in Arizona. West J Med 141:634–637, 1984.

19. Lowe CH, Schwalbe CR, Johnson TB: The Venomous Reptiles of Arizona. Tucson, AZ, Arizona Game and Fish Department, 1986.
20. Maretic Z: Epidemiology of envenomation, symptomatology, pathology and treatment. In Bettini S: Arthropod Venoms. New York, Springer-Verlag, 1978, pp 185–212.
21. Maretic Z, Lebez D: Araneism. Belgrade, Nolit Publishing, 1979.
22. Maretic Z: Lactrodectism: Variations in clinical manifestations provoked by *Latrodectus* species of spiders. Toxicon 21:457–466, 1983.
23. Minton SA, Bechtel HB: Arthropod envenomation and parasitism. In Auerbach PS, Geehr EC: Management of Wilderness and Environmental Emergencies, 2nd ed. St. Louis, C.V. Mosby, 1989, pp 513–541.
24. Pennell TC: The management of snake and spider bite in the southeastern United States. Am Surgeon 53:198–204, 1987.
25. Rachesky IJ, Banner WJ, Dansky J, et al: Treatments for *Centruroides exilicauda* envenomation. AJDC 138:1136–1139, 1984.
26. Rees RS, O'Leary JP, King LE: The pathogenesis of systemic loxoscelism following brown recluse spider bites. J Surg Res 35:1–10, 1983.
27. Rees RS, Campbell DS: Spider bites. In Auerbach PS, Geehr EC: Management of Wilderness and Environmental Emergencies, 2nd ed. St. Louis, C.V. Mosby, 1989, pp 543–561.
28. Rimza ME, Zimmerman DR, Bergeson PS: Scorpion envenomation. Pediatrics 66:298–302, 1980.
29. Russell FE: Muscle relaxants in black widow spider *(Latrodectus mactans)* poisoning. Am J Med Sci 243:81–83, 1962.
30. Russell FE, Waldron WG, Madon MB: Bites by the brown spiders *Loxosceles unicolor* and *Loxosceles arizonica* in California and Arizona. Toxicon 7:109–117, 1969.
31. Russell FE, Marcus P, Streng JA: Black widow spider envenomation during pregnancy: Report of a case. Toxicon 7:188–189, 1979.
32. Russell FE: Snake Venom Poisoning. New York, Scholium International, 1983.
33. Russell FE: Venomous arthropods. In Schachner LA, Hansen R: Pediatric Dermatology. New York, Churchill Livingstone, 1988, pp 1600–1618.
34. Russell FE, Banner W: Snake venom poisoning. In Rakel RE: Conn's Current Therapy. Philadelphia, W.B. Saunders, 1988, pp 1002–1005.
35. Ryan PJ: Preliminary report: Experience with the use of dantrolene sodium in the treatment of bites by the black widow spider *Latrodectus hesperus*. J Toxicol Clin Toxicol 21:487–489, 1983.
36. Schenone H, Suarez G: Venoms of scytodidae: Genus *Loxosceles*. In Bettini S: Handbook of Experimental Pharmacology, Vol 48. New York, Springer-Verlag, 1978, pp 247–275.
37. Shaw CE, Campbell S: Snakes of the American West. New York, Alfred A. Knopf, 1974.
38. Schnur L, Schnur P: A case of allergy to scorpion antivenin. Ariz Med 413–415, 1968.
39. Sissom WDL: Systematics, biogeography, and paleontology. In Polis GA (ed): The Biology of Scorpions. Palo Alto, CA, Stanford University Press, 1990, pp 64–160.
40. Smith RL: Venomous Animals of Arizona. Tucson, AZ, University of Arizona, 1986.
41. Stahnke HL: The genus *Centruroides* (Buthidae) and its venom. In Bettini S: Arthropod Venoms. New York, Springer-Verlag, 1978, pp 277–307.
42. Stewart RM, et al: Antivenin and fasciotomy/debridement in the treatment of the severe rattlesnake bite. Am J Surgery 158:543–547, 1989.
43. Tu AT: Rattlesnake Venoms: Their Action and Treatment. New York, Marcel Dekker, 1982.
44. Wang GK, Strichartz GR: Purification and physiological characterization of neurotoxins from venoms of the scorpions *Centruroides sculpturatus* and *Leiurus quinquestriatus*. Molecular Pharmacol 23:519–533, 1982.
45. Wasserman GS, Anderson PC: Loxoscelism and necrotic arachnidism. J Toxicol Clin Toxicol 21:451–472, 1983.
46. Wingert WA, Chan L: Rattlesnake bites in Southern California and rationale for recommended treatment. West J Med 148:37–44, 1988.

KENNETH ABRAMS, MD
DANIEL J. HOGAN, MD
HOWARD I. MAIBACH, MD

PESTICIDE-RELATED DERMATOSES IN AGRICULTURAL WORKERS

From the Department of
   Dermatology (KA, HIM)
University of California, San
   Francisco, School of Medicine
San Francisco, California, and
Department of Dermatology (DJH)
University of Miami School
   of Medicine
Miami, Florida

Reprint requests to:
Kenneth Abrams, MD
Department of Dermatology
University of California, San
   Francisco, School of Medicine
Box 0989, Surge 110
San Francisco, CA 94143-0989

AGRICULTURAL CHEMICALS

The health hazards of working in the agricultural industry are both occupational and a consequence of rural living. Besides the many infectious diseases and traumatic injuries farmers risk on a regular basis, pesticide exposure, often daily and in concentrated form, presents a unique hazard.[79a] It can lead to problems ranging from acute illness—such as acute toxicity, irritant contact dermatitis, or bronchitis—to carcinogenesis. Approximately 60% of all pesticides used in the United States are applied in the agriculture industry.

In 1988 the average employment for the agriculture, forestry, and fishing industry reported by the U.S. Department of Labor Statistics was over 1.3 million people earning over 17.9 billion dollars. Hired workers on the farms are not counted with great accuracy. It is estimated that between 100,000 to 300,000 hired hands work on farms in California (CA), the largest agricultural state. However, they usually work at jobs for less than 25 days a year with different exposures and with different inherent health risks. Besides mixing, diluting, and spraying the crops with pesticides, farmers and their workers fertilize and harvest them. They contact numerous other chemical irritants and potential allergens doing other farm-related activities, such as mixing animal feed, grooming and tending to animals, and using building materials such as cement and petroleum products.

Farmers are not the only people exposed to agrichemicals. Forty percent of these chemicals are used outside the agricultural industry. Home gardeners use fertilizers and weedkillers. Household pest-control agents contain some of the same pesticides used on farms. Chemical workers, professional exterminators, animal feed mill workers, and some food handlers are other workers who may make contact with these compounds on a daily basis.

Pesticides

A pesticide is defined as any toxic chemical used to control unwanted insects, fungi, viruses, weeds, and rodents. Insecticides, herbicides, fungicides, fumigants, and rodenticides are all pesticides. Their names denote the type of pest to which the chemicals are directed. More than 13,000 pesticide products are registered for use in CA alone. It is one of the few states keeping reasonable statistics of pesticide use and resultant illness. These products contain more than 800 active ingredients and more than 1,000 inert ingredients. They are formulated in different ways, such as liquids, wettable powders, dusts, and fumigants. Approximately 100 million pounds of active ingredients in over 550 million pounds of pesticide products purchased in CA alone were used in 1989.[26,97]

Pesticide Usage

Assessing the extent and consequences of pesticide exposure is difficult and stems from the complexity of the subject. Nationally, pesticide use by the agriculture industry is monitored by the Department of Agriculture, the Environmental Protection Agency (EPA), and the Department of Health and Human Services. Several state organizations and labor unions also monitor their use, but none of these organizations keeps the detailed annual statistics needed to properly assess the extent of use. The states follow and control pesticide use through various regulatory agencies. In CA, which ranks first in 36 of 60 major crops grown in the U.S., the most detailed annual statistics of pesticide use and exposure-related illnesses are kept. The state regulatory activities are the most comprehensive in the U.S. and include enforcement, registration, information services, medical toxicology, environmental monitoring, and worker health and safety. These services are all done within the state Department of Food and Agriculture (DFA) through the Divisions of Pest Management, Environmental Protection, and Worker Health and Safety.

Despite this concerted effort, it is still not known exactly how much pesticide has been used on what specific crops in CA. Before 1991 farmers were required only to register their pesticide purchases. They are now additionally required to report their intended pesticide usage (e.g., for storage, for mixing with other pesticides, etc.) and exactly how much is used on which specific crops, how it is applied, and the amount of acreage exposed. These new requirements should give the CA DFA more accurate statistics of actual pesticide use. Large quantities of pesticides are used in nonagricultural settings. Institutional, industrial, and structural pest control uses accounted for an average of 34% of the pesticides used in CA; 15% of pesticides sold were used in homes and gardens.

In CA, approximately one-third of reported illnesses and injuries due to pesticides involve the skin.[44]

HEALTH RISKS OF PESTICIDE USAGE

The medical consequences from exposure to these compounds vary according to numerous factors such as type of exposure (e.g., inhalation vs. cutaneous vs. ingestion), concentration of chemical, exposure time, physical state of the compound (e.g., liquid vs. solid), site of exposure (e.g., hand vs. scalp), repeated vs. single exposure, potential chemical combinations or routes of exposure, body temperature, and numerous environmental influences, such as ambient temperature, relative humidity, wind direction, and speed. Above all, there are numerous human variables such as wearing the same clothing day after day, not bathing after exposure, and eating food without washing hands, as well as interactions between chemicals and personal medications, which can change the relative risk of exposure. The adverse reactions to pesticides, especially fatal reactions, are more common in third world countries.[87] In CA, the agriculture industry ranked fourth in death rate among industries from 1980–1985. There were 16 deaths per 100,000 workers compared to the statewide industry average of 7.1 deaths per 100,000. This disparity can be explained by a higher rate of traumatic injuries and not from pesticide exposure. Occupational fatalities attributed to pesticide use averaged one per year from 1977-1987. The prevalence of pesticide-related illnesses has remained almost the same since 1950, even as the pesticide use has increased four-fold (Table 1).[108] This may reflect reduced toxicity of modern pesticides rather than safer application and pesticide use.

TABLE 1. Occupational Illness/injury Cases Associated with Exposure to Pesticides Reported by Physicians in California Summarized by Work Activity and Illness/injury Type in 1987*[†]

| Work activity | Illness/injury type | | | | |
	Systemic	Eye	Skin	Eye/skin	Total
Applicator, aerial	0	2	0	0	2
Applicator, ground	53	46	48	3	150
Applicator, hand-held equipment	30	48	16	2	96
Applicator, other	44	72	32	5	153
Coincidental exposure	124	37	15	3	179
Emergency response personnel	13	2	5	0	20
Exposed to concentrate (nonuse)	30	13	4	1	48
Exposed to residue, agricultural field	137	18	190	27	372
Exposed to residue, commodity	7	20	14	1	42
Exposed to residue, nonagricultural	230	15	7	2	254
Flagger	8	1	0	0	9
Fumigator, chamber	16	1	2	0	19
Fumigator, field	9	5	5	0	19
Fumigator, tarp	8	1	1	0	10
Manufacture/formulation plant worker	4	5	2	0	11
Mixer/loader, aerial application	11	3	4	0	18
Mixer/loader, ground application	18	66	14	4	102
Mixer/loader, unknown application type	2	1	0	0	3
Total	744	356	359	48	1507

Total cases received (all potential pesticide-related cases) 2897
Total cases determined to be related to pesticide exposure 1754
Total occupational illnesses/injuries 1507
Total nonoccupational illnesses/injuries 247
Cases "unlikely" to be related to pesticides 100
Cases without sufficient data to determine an exposure to illness/injury relationship 339
Cases determined to be "unrelated" to pesticide exposure 704

* From Maddy KT, et al: Illness, Injuries, and Deaths from Pesticide Exposures in California 1949–1988. Reviews of Environmental Contamination and Toxicology 114:57–123, 1990, with permission.
[†] This table includes those cases with a relationship of definite, probable, or possible.

CUTANEOUS EXPOSURE TO PESTICIDES

The majority of reports on adverse cutaneous reactions to pesticides originate from North America and Europe. It has been stated that contact dermatitis due to pesticides is rare considering the extent of their use,[149] but it is possible that pesticides cause more contact dermatitis than is reported.[38,174] In CA between 1978 and 1983, 2,722 claims were filed for lost work time from the agricultural industry attributed to skin conditions (Table 2).[134] Many cases were attributed to allergic contact dermatitis from plants, but these workers were also exposed to pesticides protecting the crops. Only through patch testing could one distinguish irritant from allergic dermatitis and allergy to plants versus allergy to pesticides. Experimentally certain pesticides are strong sensitizers, even though proven cases

TABLE 2. Distribution of Pesticide-related Skin Disease in California Agriculture from 1978–1983*

SIC group[b]	Total employed[c]	Pesticide-related dermatitis Cases	Pesticide-related dermatitis Rate[d]	Systemic pesticide illness Cases	Systemic pesticide illness Rate[d]	Plant-related dermatitis Cases
018 Horticulture	125,826	64	5.1	150	11.9	200
072 Crop services	177,246	84	4.7	252	14.2	34
025 Poultry/eggs	41,670	16	3.8	38	9.1	6
016 Vegetables/melons	258,492	72	2.8	308	11.9	96
019 General crop farms	290,856	74	2.5	172	5.9	98
071 Soil prep services	8,046	2	2.5	16	19.9	0
017 Fruits/trees/nuts	603,615	138	2.3	226	3.7	354
076 Farm labor services	354,669	60	1.7	82	2.3	144
013 Nongrain cash crop	135,401	22	1.6	80	5.9	22
024 Dairy farms	61,669	8	1.3	38	6.2	6
021 Nondairy livestock	34,877	4	1.1	24	6.9	14
011 Cash grains	26,538	2	0.8	40	15.1	8
075 Nonvet animal services	24,309	2	0.8	12	4.9	2
078 Landscaping services	127,655	8	0.6	60	4.7	394
082 Forest nurseries	37	0	0.0	0	0.0	2
091 Commercial fishings	11,862	0	0.0	0	0.0	0
029 General livestock	10,375	0	0.0	2	1.9	10
074 Veterinary services	48,931	0	0.0	4	0.8	0
084 Gathering forest products	76	0	0.0	0	0.0	0
085 Forestry services	2,026	0	0.0	0	0.0	12
081 Timber tracts	478	0	0.0	0	0.0	0
027 Animal specialties	10,571	0	0.0	0	5.7	8
092 Fish hatcheries	481	0	0.0	0	0.0	0
097 Hunting and trapping	66	0	0.0	0	0.0	0
Total	2,355,802	556	2.4	1,150	6.4	1,418

* From O'Malley MA, Mathias CGT, Coye MJ: Epidemiology of pesticide-related skin disease in California agriculture. In Dosman J, Cockcroft D (eds): Principles of Health and Safety in Agriculture. Boca Raton, FL, CRC Press, 1989, p 302, with permission.

a Based on cases reported to the U.S. BLSs (for 1978, 1979, 1980, 1981, and 1983) by the California Department of Internal Relations from tabulations of Employers' First Reports of Occupational Injury or Illness. All cases involved one or more lost days.

b SICs used in SIC Manual, 1972; with 1977 supplement; the Statistical Policy Division, Office of Management and Executive Office of the President: U.S. Government Printing Office.

c Employment figures are derived from unemployment insurance records by the California Department of Employment Development. Reported figures are the sum of mid-third quarter employment (peak agricultural employment) for the study period, 1978, 1979, 1980, 1981, and 1983).

d Rates are reported as number of cases/10,000 workers employed.

of allergic contact dermatitis to pesticides are infrequently reported.[81,96,120] It has been suggested that the dilution of pesticides prior to their use in the field minimizes their capacity to sensitize exposed workers, because induction of sensitization requires a minimal concentration of an allergen.[96] Once individuals are sensitized to pesticides, they may react on patch-testing to dilutions of the pesticide in acetone as low as 1 in 1,000,000.[81,120]

Within the agricultural industry, pesticide handlers have the greatest potential exposure to these chemicals. They participate in mixing, loading and applying, and cleaning and maintaining the equipment. Their potential dermal exposure (PDE), the amount of pesticide found daily on the outermost garment, can sometimes be measured in grams/person. Protective outer clothing and enclosed cabs are important barriers that effectively reduce the PDE by 90% and thus lower the absorbed daily dose.[97] It is estimated that < 1%–30% of daily dermal exposure (DDE) is absorbed percutaneously based on animal studies.

Contact dermatitis may be the main adverse health effect of certain pesticides in man. In CA, where physicians are required by law to report all cases of illness or injury that may have resulted from exposure to pesticides, there have been reports of epidemics of contact dermatitis due to pesticides.[152]

The precise prevalence and incidence of skin diseases in agriculture is unknown. Illness reports from workers' compensation boards are inadequate to assess the incidence of occupational skin disease, because self-employed farmers are excluded from workers' compensation laws in most jurisdictions. In certain jurisdictions voluntary coverage by workers' compensation boards is available for self-employed farmers, but most farmers do not elect this coverage. Many transient agricultural workers may not report occupational diseases, or do not know how to enter the health care system. Most centers for occupational medicine are located in urban areas and may not emphasize occupational disorders in agriculture. Despite these difficulties, the agricultural sector was noted to have the highest rate of occupational skin disease of any industry in CA.[114] Risk of occupational skin disease was four times higher in agriculture than the all-industry average risk. The rate of occupational skin disease in agriculture was twice as high as the rate in the manufacturing sector. Occupational skin disease usually accounts for 40% of all occupational disease, but occupational skin disease accounted for approximately 70% of all occupational disease in agriculture in CA. The risk of occupational skin disease and the types of occupational skin disease vary with the crops, livestock, farming practices, and climate of an area. In CA, pesticides were second to poison oak as reported causes of occupational skin disease in agriculture.

Irritant contact dermatitis as a reaction to pesticides is more frequent than allergic contact dermatitis. The chief cutaneous irritants among the pesticides are inorganic compounds such as copper sulfate. Insecticides such as carbamates have been the most frequently reported causes of allergic contact dermatitis due to pesticides.[104]

Field Conditions

Under field conditions the skin is the organ most exposed to pesticides.[185] Farmers and agricultural workers are exposed to pesticides while mixing, loading, and spraying pesticide formulations as well as while cleaning spray equipment and disposing of pesticide containers.[188] Skin exposure to pesticides is maximal on the hands while mixing and loading pesticides and while spraying pesticides from tractor-powered sprayers. The use of protective gloves markedly decreases cutaneous exposure to pesticides. A knapsack sprayer with a boom helps minimize the exposure of the hands to pesticides.[1] However, the use of knapsack spraying equipment results in the legs, especially the lower legs, being the site most exposed to pesticides.

There is usually no certification program to ensure that farmers and other agricultural workers are competent to use pesticides and agricultural chemicals safely. Most farmers and agricultural workers do not always employ adequate skin protection when using pesticides. Surveys in Saskatchewan confirm that only a minority of farmers always use skin protection while handling pesticides (data on file, Sections of Dermatology and Respirology, Department of Medicine, University of Saskatchewan). Lack of adequate skin protection when using pesticides is most likely to occur in hot weather or during very busy work periods. In a 1985 study field workers in CA vineyards were most likely to develop rashes after thinning vines and during hot days.[184] Pesticides in general and propargite in particular did not appear to be a major cause of skin rashes, though outbreaks of rashes in grape field workers have been attributed to propargite and/or sulfur exposure in CA.

Adequate washing facilities are frequently absent in the fields where the pesticides are being applied and most farmers believe they cannot afford expensive safety equipment. Barrier creams are not proven to be effective in protecting the skin from pesticides. Pesticides may persist on the skin for long periods. Chlordane and dieldrin have been claimed to persist on skin for up to 2 years.[92] Ordinary laundering is not a very effective way of removing pesticide residues from clothing. The degree of contamination of the worker's skin and clothing by pesticides also varies with the skill and attitude of the applicator, the type of pesticide spray (low volume concentrate, conventional spray, etc.), type of crop (i.e., orchard or row crop), wind, and quality of spray equipment.[188]

Certain highly toxic pesticides such as the organophosphate parathion are rapidly absorbed through the skin without producing any dermatitis. Severe neurologic symptoms or death have followed percutaneous absorption of certain organophosphate pesticides.[172] Experimentally percutaneous absorption is five times greater in some individuals than others and is greater through inflamed skin than normal skin. Feldmann and Maibach[52] studied the percutaneous absorption of 12 pesticides. The least absorbed of these was diquat and the most absorbed was carbaryl.

The EPA recommends that workers not be allowed into fields that have been treated with pesticides until an adequate time interval has elapsed. For organo-phosphate and n-methyl carbamate pesticides having acute dermal toxicity, a 48-hour interval is proposed. The EPA proposals recommend rubber of chemical-resistant gloves for exposed workers. Mixers and loaders would be required to wear resistant aprons to reduce exposure from splashes and spills from handling bulk pesticides. Other protective equipment includes headgear, face shields, and chemical-resistant footwear for high toxicity compounds. The EPA draft proposals also require that water, soap, and single-use towels be available for decontamination, and that these must be located near the workers. Provisions would also require that handlers and mixers of pesticides receive training. Workers using organophos-phate compounds for 3 consecutive days should have their serum cholinesterase level determined. Chemical manufacturers would also be required to update warning instructions on pesticide labels. The rules would extend existing require-ments to cover workers in forests, nurseries, greenhouses, and all other handlers of pesticides. Enforcement would be up to state agencies responsible for agricultural programs.[73]

Pesticide sprays contain emulsifiers, adjutants, carrier liquids, and surfactants. To prove that a case of allergic contact dermatitis is due to a particular pesticide, it is necessary to perform patch testing to a nonirritating concentration of analytic-grade pesticide in an appropriate vehicle. Contaminants may be the main allergen in pesticide formulations. For example, diethyl fumarate was found to be the sensitizer in technical grade malathion.[120] Predictive tests to assess a pesticide's capacity of inducing allergic contact dermatitis is now required prior to registration of a pesticide for sale.[143]

PESTICIDE TYPES

Pesticides Derived from Plants

Pyrethrum. Pyrethrum is comprised of the dried flowers of *Chrysanthemum cinerariaefolium* containing not less than 1% pyrethrins. Pyrethrin esters constitute a powerful degradable contact insecticide. They have a low order of systemic toxicity to man and produce no harmful residues on food crops. The flowers and extracts for pyrethrum are imported from Kenya and Ecuador into the U.S. The active principals are pyrethrins I and II, cinerins I and II, and jasmolin I and II, collectively known as pyrethrins. Pyrethrins are used extensively in stock sprays, pet sprays, household sprays, aerosols, and food protection in warehouses. Pyrethrins are stable for long periods of time in water-based aerosols where modern emulsifiers are used. Dermatitis from natural pyrethrins usually occurs on parts of the body exposed to the spray. The substance is a moderately potent allergic sensitizer. Cross-reactions occur among pyrethrum, chrysanthemum, shasta daisy, and ragweed oleo resin.[54,121] Asthma and urticaria have also been reported as reactions to natural pyrethrin.[50,69] In 1972 Mitchell et al. found that a sesquiterpene lactone, pyrethrosin, was the chief allergen in pyrethrin.[122] Contact dermatitis due to pyrethrum is usually mild, but bullous reactions have been reported.[75] In Denmark positive patch test reactions to pyrethrum were obtained in 1–2% of dermatitis patients.[109]

Pyrethroids. Pyrethroids are synthetic compounds produced to duplicate the biologic activity of the active principals of pyrethrum. Pyrethroids have a longer duration of activity against insects than pyrethrum and are not teratogenic or mutagenic. These compounds include: allethrin, alphametrin, barthrin, bioresmethrin, biopermethrin, cismethrin, cyclethrin, cyfluthrin, cypermethrin, decamethrin, deltamethrin, dimethrin, fenothrin, fenpropanate, fenvalerate, flucythrinate, fluvalinate, furethrin, indothrin, permethrin, phthalthrin, resmethrin, and tetramethrin. Allergic contact dermatitis due to pyrethroids has not been reported. Temporary paresthesias manifested by numbness, itching, burning, tingling, and warmth have been reported following cutaneous exposure to the synthetic pyrethroid fenvalerate. Fenvalerate, produced in the U.S., produces more paresthesias following topical exposure than pyrethrin and other pyrethroids. It has been suggested that topical vitamin E acetate is highly effective in treating paresthesias induced by pyrethroids.[61]

Nicotine. Little or no nicotine is now produced in the U.S. for use as an insecticide, because organophosphate insecticides have largely replaced it. Limited supplies are imported from India. Nicotine may be absorbed through the skin of people harvesting tobacco leaves. Vero and Genovese[180] patch-tested a number of workers with dermatitis who made cigars from various tobacco leaves; no positive reactions were found. Exposed workers may develop nausea, vomiting, dizziness, prostration, and weakness. Abrasions on the skin occur during the harvesting of tobacco leaves, and abrasions increase the percutaneous absorption of nicotine. The use of work gloves significantly decreases nicotine absorption in workers.[71]

Rotenone. Rotenone is a selective contact insecticide with some acaricidal properties. Cubé is now the only commercial source in the U.S. of rotenone for insecticide production, although derris, timbo, and other related rotenone-containing plants have been utilized. Peru is the main source of the cubé root. The root may be ground as a dust or extracted to provide concentrate. Rotenone has been long used as dust for garden insects, lice, and ticks on animals. Rotenone may also be used in combination with pyrethrin and piperonyl butoxide (a synergist) for control of a wide variety of insects on food crops. Skin irritation from rotenone has been reported among workers in rotenone-processing plants in South America. Skin inflammation was most notable in intertriginous areas or where the powder had been trapped by perspiration on the skin.[75] A similar outbreak was reported among workers in France, but improved ventilation and dust masks diminished the occurrence of dermatitis in these workers.[75]

Inorganic and Organo-metal Pesticides

Arsenic. The earliest insecticides against chewing insects were the arsenicals, chiefly copper acetoarsenite (Paris green), lead arsenate, and calcium arsenate. Sodium arsenite has been used as a sterilant herbicide and a potato-vine killer. Inorganic arsenic is both a cutaneous irritant and sensitizer.[38] Hyperkeratosis, hyperhidrosis, and melanosis are considered evidence of chronic systemic exposure. The hyperpigmentation is most marked on surfaces exposed to light; it does not extend to mucous membranes. There may be a speckled depigmentation of pigmented areas, giving a "raindrop" appearance. Compounds similar or identical with those used as pesticides have caused skin cancer in man.[75] Agricultural workers are also exposed to chronic ultraviolet light, and Emmett believes that ultraviolet light exposure was a more significant factor for these workers than their exposure to inorganic arsenic.[48]

Inorganic arsenicals have been superseded because of their hazard to man and animals. Sodium arsenate was formerly the toxicant in many ant syrups for household use, but this application also has been discontinued. Organic arsenicals are at present of the most interest because of their value as selective herbicides.

Sulphur. Sulphur is a commonly used fungicide and acaricide. It is compatible with most other insecticides and fungicides. Insoluble in water but soluble in organic solvents, wettable sulphur is prepared by adding wetting and dispersing agents to finely ground sulphur. Micronized wettable sulphur is made by a special manufacturing process to ensure an extremely fine particle size. Grapes and peanuts are examples of crops requiring fungicides such as sulphur. Many cases of irritant dermatitis are attributed to sulphur in CA,[44] but there are few reports of allergic dermatitis.[183]

Triphenyltin Hydroxide. Triphenyltin hydroxide is a fungicide used on a variety of crops. Irritant patch-test reactions are frequent if patients are patch-tested to 1% triphenyltin (phentin hydroxide).[104]

Tributyltin oxide is a severe skin irritant but not a sensitizer.[68]

Copper Sulphate.   Copper sulphate is a fungicide and algicide. Lisi et al. in 1987 reported positive patch test reactions to 1% copper sulphate in agricultural workers.[104] Additional normal controls and use of provocative tests should help clarify whether these responses are irritant or allergic.

Phenylmercury Nitrate.   Phenylmercuric salts were previously widely used as herbicides and agricultural fungicides. Phenylmercury nitrate is still used for tree wound dressings. Contact dermatitis to phenylmercury nitrate used as a herbicide has been reported.[123] Patch-testing with organic mercuric salts presents technical challenges. Patch-test concentrations currently used may be marginal irritants. Until far more is known about current concentration dose and vehicle, provocative tests provide a convenient method to help confirm the presence of allergy.

Solvents

Kerosene.   Kerosene, first used in 1877, was apparently the first petroleum oil to be used for insect control. Presently it is widely used as a solvent for household and industrial pesticide sprays. The kerosene may be sulfonated to provide an odorless oil or deodorants may be added. Kerosene is a cutaneous irritant. Barnes and Wilkinson described an eruption similar to that of toxic epidermal necrolysis, "irritant pseudo-toxic epidermal necrolysis," in a boy whose clothing became contaminated with kerosene.[10]

Fumigants

A fumigant is a substance or a mixture of substances that produces gas, vapor, fume, or smoke intended to destroy insects, bacteria, or rodents. Fumigants may be volatile liquids and solids, as well as substances already gaseous. They may be used to disinfect the interiors of buildings or objects and materials that can be enclosed so as to contain the fumigant.[53]

Ethylene Oxide.   Ethylene oxide or epoxy ethane is used as a fumigant and a sterilant. Severe irritant dermatitis and chemical burns have been reported from direct skin contact with ethylene oxide.[75] Ethylene oxide, first used as an agricultural fumigant in 1928,[168] is effective against all microorganisms. It is a potent skin irritant and may produce immediate and possibly delayed contact hypersensitivity. Because the chemical is a potent irritant, it requires careful testing to ascertain if dermatitis is irritant or allergic. Epidemiologic studies strongly suggest that ethylene oxide is carcinogenic in man.[11]

Methyl Bromide.   Methyl bromide is a fumigant used for insect control in grain elevators, mills, ships, and greenhouses. The gas is a soil fumigant as well. It is also used for termite control, agricultural fumigation, and rodent control. Direct skin contact with methyl bromide produces chemical burns.

Acrylonitrile.   Toxic epidermal necrolysis was reported in four patients 11 to 21 days after their homes were fumigated with a 2:1 mixture of acrylonitrile and carbon tetrachloride.[139] Three of the four cases died. It is not clear if these cases represented true toxic epidermal necrolysis or a "pseudo-toxic epidermal necrolysis" due to irritation. This fumigant has subsequently been discontinued.

Metam-sodium.   Metam-sodium, a broad spectrum soil fumigant, is a fungicide, insecticide, nematocide, and herbicide. Richter[142] states that allergic contact dermatitis to metam-sodium (methyl isothiocyanate) may be significant among exposed persons. In his opinion metam-sodium is a potent sensitizer. He also attributed hepatitis in one patient to exposure to metam-sodium.

DD.   DD is a highly toxic mixture of 1,3-dichloropropene, 1,2-dichloro-propane, epichlorhydrin, and related compounds and is a cutaneous irritant. It is used as a soil fumigant. Nater and Gooskens obtained positive patch-tests to 1% DD in acetone.[125] They concluded that occasionally DD could provoke allergic contact dermatitis.

Dazomet.   Dazomet is used as a nematocide, soil fumigant, herbicide, and algicide. Dazomet hydrolizes to formalin. Contact dermatitis, probably irritant, has been reported to dazomet.[14]

Chlorinated Hydrocarbon Insecticides

DDT (Dichloro-diphenyl-trichloroethane).   Since January 1, 1973, DDT has been banned in the U.S. for all except emergency public health measures. Allergic contact dermatitis due to DDT has not been convincingly reported.[43,102,131,164] Positive patch test reactions to 3% DDT was reported in cotton workers with dermatitis of exposed areas. No positive patch test reactions to 1% DDT were obtained among 665 routine eczematous patients patch-tested by the International Contact Dermatitis Research Group (I.C.D.R.G.).[38]

Lindane.   Lindane is used for seed treatments for control of wireworms and seed corn maggots on various crops. It is also used to protect tobacco transplants from cutworms and wireworms and as soil treatment, application to foliage on fruit and nut trees, vegetables, ornamentals, timber, and wood protection. It is a skin irritant but allergic contact dermatitis is rare. No positive patch reactions to 1% lindane were obtained in 665 routine eczematous patients patch tested by the I.C.D.R.G.[38]

Dieldrin.   Dieldrin is an insecticide. In the U.S. it is only used for termite control. Dieldrin probably caused dermatitis of the lower legs in 200 of 1209 police recruits exercised to sweating who wore socks mothproofed with dieldrin.[145]

Organophosphate Pesticides

Parathion and Methyl Parathion.   Organophosphate pesticides became widely used following the banning of DDT. Parathion is an insecticide that is extremely toxic to man and animals. It is a restricted use pesticide in the U.S., and exposed workers must wear rubber gloves, protective clothing, goggles, and a respirator. The mask or respirator must be approved by the U.S. Bureau of Mines for parathion protection. Parathion was found on the skin of the hands of one worker 2 months after his last known contact.[92]

Parathion is an experimental contact sensitizer.[104] Allergic contact dermatitis to parathion has been reported in a German vintner.[137] A gardener cut his finger and used a concentrated spray containing parathion and emulsifiers on begonias. The cut finger became swollen and bluish-red a day later. The finger was cool and painless. The author believed the patient had an unusual reaction to parathion. The patient was treated with penicillin.[166]

Erythema multiforme has been reported in a woman who inhaled methyl parathion.[13] Experimental re-exposure reproduced her lesions.

Malathion.   Malathion is an insecticide used to control a wide variety of insects. Milby and Epstein[120] found that nearly half of 87 volunteers developed contact sensitization following a single exposure to 10% malathion and that many of them reacted to dilutions as low as 1 ppm. Similar results were reported by Kligman.[96] However, it was found as part of the first study that only about 3% of people with occupational exposure to malathion had a positive patch test reaction to 1% malathion, and no worker had to change work because of malathion allergy. Only one positive patch test reaction to 0.5% malathion was obtained in 455 routine eczematous patients patch tested by the I.C.D.R.G.[38] This one reaction was of unknown relevance. In practice, malathion appears to be a weak allergic contact sensitizer. Kligman has suggested that the usage concentration of malathion is too low to provoke sensitization. Milby and Epstein determined that the sensitizer in malathion is diethyl fumarate, which is used in the manufacture of malathion. Diethyl fumarate was present at a 3% concentration in technical grade malathion.[96] Diethyl fumarate can produce nonimmunologic contact urticaria.[98]

DDVP. DDVP (dichlorvos) is an insecticide used in sprays, wettable powder, aerosols, resin strips, and flea collars. It is also formulated as an anthelmintic for swine, horses, and dogs. It has an acute dermal LD 50 of 75 mg/kg for rats. Strong positive reactions to flea collars were reported in two patients who had dermatitis attributed to contact with dogs wearing DDVP impregnated flea collars.[53] Cronce and Alden[37] reported primary irritant contact dermatitis to DDVP flea collars in four patients. Patch-testing produced bullous primary irritant reactions in four patients and five controls. Mathias[115] noted negative patch tests to 1% and 0.1% DDVP in petrolatum in a truck driver who developed prolonged contact dermatitis to DDVP. This man also had systemic symptoms of organophosphate toxicity following his exposure to DDVP from a spill of this chemical in his truck. Mathias emphasized that individuals who develop dermatitis from skin contact with pesticides should be carefully questioned about general symptoms. This is particularly important for organophosphate insecticides.

Tetmosol. Tetmosol is used to treat parasitic infestations in dogs and cats and is used as a scabicide and a fungicide. Cronin[38] has reported a 58-year-old woman with chronic eczema whose dermatitis flared after treating her cat with Tetmosol and when she wore rubber gloves. She had positive patch tests to Tetmosol solution and both to 1% tetramethylthiuramdisulphide and 1% tetramethylthiuramdisulphide in petrolatum.

Naled. Naled is an insecticide-acaricide. It is intermediate in toxicity between malathion and parathion. Allergic contact dermatitis to naled has been reported in a few workers.[45] Naled is broken down by hydrolysis within a few hours. Patients allergic to naled may work with plants sprayed with naled once a suitable interval has elapsed.

Thiometon. Thiometon is a systemic insecticide used to control aphids, thrips, and mites. A case of contact dermatitis has been attributed to thiometon.[75]

Rodannitrobenzene. Rodannitrobenzene has been used in insecticide sprays for home use. Fregert has reported a case of severe contact dermatitis due to rodannitrobenzene.[64]

Carbamate Insecticides

Promecarb. Promecarb is a contact insecticide. Contact dermatitis to promecarb has been reported in two workers.[75]

Carbaryl. Carbaryl is a broad-spectrum insecticide used on more than 120 different crops. A case of contact dermatitis to carbaryl spray was reported.[75]

Nitro-compounds and Related Phenolic Pesticides

Chlorinated phenols are effective fungicides but because of their toxicity are used only for fabrics and woods.

Pentachlorophenol (PCP).   PCP has been used a molluscide, insecticide, herbicide, fungicide, bactericide, anti-mildew agent, and preservative, particularly for wood. Lumber impregnated with PCP is relatively resistant to bacteria, fungi, and termites. The wood retains its natural appearance.[186]

Vaguely defined rashes and skin irritation, possible chloracne, and susceptibility to skin infections have been attributed to chronic exposure to pentachlorophenol. Lambert et al.[100] associated pemphigus vulgaris in a 41-year-old man and a 28-year-old woman and chronic urticaria in a 35-year-old man to chronic exposure to pentachlorophenol.

Pentachlorophenate.   Kentor has reported a patient who developed urticaria and angioedema from contact with pentachlorophenate.[93] This patient was felt to have immunologically mediated contact urticaria. He developed urticaria and angioedema at sites distant from his hands, which were the site of skin contact with pentachlorophenate.

Chlorocresol and MCPA (Chloromethylphenoxyacetic Acid).   A positive patch-test reaction to 0.1% chlorocresol in alcohol was reported by Fregert in a man who developed dermatitis on two occasions after using MCPA (chloromethylphenoxyacetic acid) spray.[66] Patch-testing to 1% MCPA was negative. Chlorocresol is used in the manufacture of MCPA.

DNOC (4,6,dinitro-o-cresol).   DNOC is an insecticide, fungicide, herbicide, and defoliant used in North America as a dormant spray for killing insect eggs and to control apple scab. Nail dystrophy has been reported following fingernail contact with 5% dinitro-orthocresol.[9]

Dinocap.   Dinocap is a foliage fungicide and acaricide. One case of allergic contact dermatitis has been described to dinocap.[75]

Tecnazene.   Tecnazene is a fungicide and growth regulator. Cotterill reported a farmer who developed an acute dermatitis while throwing tecnazene granules onto a conveyor belt carrying potatoes.[35] Patch-testing to tecnazene was negative, but this farmer had a strong positive patch-test reaction to 0.01% dinitrochlorobenzene (DNCB). Cotterill attributed his patient's contact dermatitis to DNCB contaminating the tecnazene granules. DNCB could have been formed during the production of tecnazene.

Phenothiazine.   Phenothiazine, an oral insecticide and anthelmintic, introduced in 1925, was the earliest organic insecticide. It is fed in salt or mineral supplements to control fly larvae and certain internal parasites.

Workers spraying apple orchards with phenothiazine in the state of Washington developed severe phototoxic reactions.[41] Phototoxic reactions have also occurred in workers preparing the raw materials. The reactions resembled sunburn and in hair became a pinkish red and the fingernails brown.[136]

Rodenticides

Warfarin.   Warfarin is a rodenticide that is highly effective in controlling Norway rats and house mice. A positive past reaction to 0.05% warfarin in an agricultural worker has been reported by Lisi and colleagues.[104]

ANTU (Naphthylthiourea).   ANTU is a rodenticide for adult Norway rats. A case of occupational contact dermatitis to ANTU has been reported.[75]

Herbicides

Herbicides are now frequently used in place of hand labor or machine cultivation to control unwanted plants.

Glyphosphate. Glyphosphate is a nonselective, postemergence herbicide. In 1986, contact dermatitis attributed to glyphosphate was reported in 33 workers mixing or loading this herbicide in California.[44] Maibach extensively investigated glyphosphate and has found it to be a nonsensitizer in the Draze Repeat Insult Patch Test and less irritating to the skin than baby shampoo.[111] A phototoxic reaction to benzisothiazolone, a preservative present in glyphosphate, has been reported. Phototoxicity to glyphosphate itself was not demonstrated.[77]

Paraquat. Paraquat is a contact herbicide and desiccant. Irritant contact dermatitis has been reported to paraquat. Workers in factories where paraquat is manufactured have an increased risk of occupationally induced keratoses, Bowen's disease, and squamous cell carcinoma of the skin.[16,182] Paraquat itself is probably not the etiologic agent for these premalignant and malignant skin lesions. Discoloration of the fingernail, nail deformity, onycholysis, and loss of the nail have been reported in workers whose fingernails came into contact with paraquat sprays and concentrates.[9,76]

A case with periungual eczematous dermatitis with striking nail lesions due to paraquat was reported by Botella et al.[15] Patch-testing to paraquat 0.001% and 0.01% in water was negative. A necrotic ulcer of the scrotum following direct contact with paraquat solution was reported by Sharvill.[157] Deaths arising from percutaneous absorption of paraquat have also been reported.[130]

Nitralin. Allergic contact dermatitis to nitralin and its precursor 4-chloro-3,5-dinitrophenylmethyl sulfone was reported in a man working in a factory producing this herbicide. He also showed cross-sensitivity to DNCB.[132] The manufacture of nitralin in the U.S. has been subsequently discontinued.

Amitrole. Amitrole (aminotriazole) is a systemic herbicide used to control nonselective grasses, broadleaf weeds, cattails, poison ivy, and certain aquatic weeds. One case of allergic contact dermatitis to aminotriazole has been reported in a contract weed control operator.[49]

Chloridazon. Chloridazon (pyrazon), a herbicide used to protect beets, persists in the soil for several months. Allergic contact dermatitis to chloridazon spray has been reported in a farmer by Bruze and Fregert.[20]

Phenmedipham. Phenmedipham is a postemergence herbicide. Severe allergic dermatitis to phenmedipham has been reported in two farmers.[127]

Dichlobenil. Dichlobenil is a herbicide. Six men engaged in mixing or bagging dichlobenil developed dermatitis within 1 week to 5 months after first exposure. Although the condition involved comedones and was spoken of as chloracne, no cysts were observed, and judging from the description and one photograph, the dermatitis was not severe. The possibility that this mild condition may have been associated with a contaminant may not have been explored.[75]

Atrazine. Atrazine is a selective herbicide. Severe contact dermatitis to atrazine has been reported in a farmer with a history of dermatitis caused by propachlor. This patient had a positive patch-test reaction to 1:1000 dilution of a commercial atrazine formulation.[75]

Propazine. Propazine and simazine are selective herbicides. Many cases of contact dermatitis have been reported among workers manufacturing propazine and simazine.[75]

Oxydiazol. Chloracne has been reported in workers manufacturing oxydiazol (methazole). This resulted from exposure to 3,4,3',4'tetrachloroazoxybenzene (TCAB), an extraneous intermediate produced during the manufacture of the herbicide.[167]

Alachlor. Alachlor is a pre-emergence herbicide. Iden and Schroeter reported five individuals with positive allergic patch-test reactions to alachlor.[86] They found that 3 of the 21 patients patch-tested to alachlor reacted to both alachlor (Lasso) and propachlor (Ramro). Further studies may help clarify whether these were irritant or allergic patch-test reactions.

Trichlorobenzyl. Trichlorobenzyl chloride is a herbicide used in pre-emergence application only in combination with allidochlor (Randox). Skin irritation was also reported to this chemical by Spencer.[161]

2,4-D (2,4,Dichlorophenoxyacetic Acid). 2,4-D is a selective herbicide used for weed control, water hyacinth control, and various other uses. Several companies manufacture 2,4-D. 2,4,5-T, salts, and esters are used widely to control woody plants on industrial sites and rangeland. Amine formulations are used extensively for weed control on rice. the action and properties of these compounds are similar to those of 4,5-T preparations.

2,4-D–2,4,5-T mixtures are used in combination for the destruction of mixed growth of woody plants and herbaceous weeds. Severe contact dermatitis has been reported to a mixture of 2,4-D and 2,4,5-T.[75] A major epidemiologic study found an association between the use of 2,4-D and non-Hodgkin's lymphoma in Kansas. The greater the use of 2,4-D, the greater the incidence of non-Hodgkin's lymphoma among exposed farmers.[78] This study did not confirm previously reported associations between 2,4-D use and soft-tissue sarcoma or Hodgkin's disease.[21,23,33,84,89,93,124]

Barban. Barban (barbamate, barbane, chlorinate) is a selective herbicide of low systemic toxicity. Allergic contact dermatitis to barban has been documented.[17,81] Marked sensitivity to barban may develop when only minute concentrations of barban are sufficient to produce strongly positive patch-test reactions. Hypopigmentation was noted following one case of allergic contact dermatitis to barban.[17] It is a potent experimental sensitizer.

Dazomet. Dazomet is a herbicide, fungicide, slimicide, and nematocide. Black in 1973 reported a tomato grower using dazomet as a soil fumigant.[14] A 0.5% concentration in water resulted in a positive reaction on patch-testing, and a significant reaction also occurred at 96 hours following open testing. Black described dazomet as a strong sensitizer, a primary irritant, and possibly a vesicant.

Fungicides

Benomyl. Benomyl is a systemic fungicide widely used for the control of a broad range of diseases of fruits, nuts, vegetables, field crops, and ornamentals. Allergic contact dermatitis in areas exposed to benomyl was reported in seven Japanese women working in a hot, humid greenhouse where benomyl was being sprayed on carnations. Ten Hispanic co-workers were unaffected. Undiluted benomyl and benomyl diluted 1:5 in olive oil produced negative patch tests in three controls, but a Japanese medical assistant developed a 2+ reaction when these patch test sites were exposed to 30 seconds of ultraviolet light. The seven Japanese workers had positive patch-test reactions to benomyl 1:10 in olive oil.[153] Fregert reported one case with a positive patch-test reaction to benomyl 0.1% in water.[67] He wondered whether most cases of dermatitis due to benomyl were transient. Van Ketel reported a begonia grower with contact dermatitis due to this fungicide.[176] The dermatitis was caused not by spraying but by picking the leaves. Patch-testing with 1% in petrolatum was positive. Van Joost, Naafs, and van Ketel state that picking plants containing residues of benomyl is an important source of sensitization to benomyl.[174]

Hexachlorobenzene.   Hexachlorobenzene is a seed protectant used on wheat. Contact may cause slight skin irritation. Hexachlorobenzene produced an epidemic of sever porphyria cutanea tarda in Turkey from 1955–1959. The disease occurred almost exclusively in persons who admitted eating wheat distributed for seed not for food. This wheat had been treated with hexachlorobenzene. Many infants died from exposure to hexachlorobenzene in this epidemic.[36]

Thiophanatemethyl.   Thiophanatemethyl is a systemic fungicide with a broad spectrum of activity for plant disease. Many cases of apparent irritant contact dermatitis but few cases of allergic contact dermatitis to thiophanatemethyl have been reported.[75]

Captafol.   Captafol is used to prevent blight on potatoes and on fruit and farm crops. Camarasa reported severe pruritus, morbiliform urticarial eruptions, and asthma among 7 out of 41 workers in a company that packed captafol (Difolatan).[29] Four of these patients had strong patch-test reactions to captafol. The sudden appearance of vesiculation and edema of the face and hands of a welder associated with wheezing was attributed to contact with bags of captafol. Subsequent re-exposure led to recurrences.[75] Irritant contact dermatitis has been associated with the use of captafol by farmers in Japanese tangerine orchards; 25–30% of workers were affected.[38] Some of these reactions were severe.[75] Captafol was the pesticide accounting for the greatest number of cases of contact dermatitis in Japanese regions.[117]

Stoke states that at least one-third of exposed workers will develop dermatitis to captafol if adequate precautions are not taken.[163] Up to 65% of exposed workers have been reported to develop captafol dermatitis. The risk of dermatitis from captafol can be minimized by appropriate worker training and industrial hygiene. The manufacturers of captafol regard it as a potent sensitizer.[34] Cottel also reported two farmers with dermatitis of exposed areas who had positive patch tests to 0.1% captafol in water.

Captan.   Captan is a widely used protectant-eradicant fungicide. Agricultural workers may be heavily exposed to captan during and after spraying operations. One California vineyard applied it 75 times in one season. The EPA reviewed the chemical because bacterial and rodent studies suggested that captan is mutagenic and carcinogenic. Urticaria due to captan has been documented in a gardener who reacted to captan and to captan-treated plants.[75] Fregert reported a fruit farmer who developed dermatitis of his hands and face after 3 weeks exposure to captan.[65] Patch-testing with captan and the related folpet (Phaltan), 1% in petrolatum, gave positive reactions. Marzulli and Maibach demonstrated that captan in a concentration of 1% is a significant contact allergic sensitizer.[113] Out of 205 human test subjects, 9 were sensitized. The International and North American Contact Dermatitis Groups later found captan in a 1% concentration to be irritant on patch-testing; 0.25% in petrolatum is now preferred for patch-testing. Relevant allergic reactions to captan appear to be rare.[38]

Captan had been reported as a successful topical treatment for tinea versicolor.[75,83]

Folpet.   Folpet is a protective fungicide used as a 50% wettable powder and in various dusts on fruits, berries, vegetables, flowers, and ornamentals. Six agricultural workers had positive patch-test reactions to 0.1% folpet but irritant reactions were seen in some controls.[104]

The International Contact Dermatitis Research Group patch-tested 509 patients with suspected contact dermatitis to folpet. Fifty patients had positive patch-test reactions but only one was relevant. One hundred and seven patients were patch-tested to 0.1% folpet. Three patients had positive reactions but no positive patch-test reactions were deemed clinically relevant.[38]

DNCB (Dinitritochlorobenzene).   Occupational allergic contact dermatitis has been reported to DNCB used as an algicide.[112,190] Adams, Zimmerman et al. emphasized that this potent sensitizer should be only used in completely enclosed systems not allowing skin contact with DNCB.[190]

PCNB (Pentachloronitrobenzene).   PCNB is used as a soil fungicide and seed-treatment chemical. It is especially useful for Brussel sprouts, broccoli, and artichokes.

Cronin described a 46-year-old man packing pesticide powders who developed dermatitis of his arms, legs, forehead, trunk, and scrotum.[38] Patch-testing to PCNB, 1% in petrolatum, was positive. The patient's shoes were heavily contaminated with PCNB dust. DCNA (2,6 dichloro-4-nitroaniline) is a related compound.

Ditalmifos.   Ditalmifos (marketed only in Europe) is a contact fungicide used for the control of powdery mildews and scab of apples and pears. Allergic contact dermatitis to ditalmifos used as a rose spray was reported by van Ketel.[175]

Plondrel.   Plondrel is sprayed on roses to protect them from mildew. It is left on as a deposit on roses; therefore, both sprayers and florists are exposed. Four patients with occupational allergic contact dermatitis to plondrel were reported by van Ketel.[175] Cronin reported a case of occupational contact dermatitis due to plondrel.[38]

Maneb and Zineb.   Maneb and zineb are used to treat many plant diseases. Maneb may be used in combination with other pesticides including lindane, hexachlorobenzene, captan, and zineb. Zineb may be combined with other pesticides including thiram and sulfur. Maneb and zineb are related to the carbamate class of rubber accelerators and are of relatively low systemic toxicity; however, they are important allergic sensitizers.

Matsushita et al., using the guinea pig maximization test, demonstrated the strong sensitization potential of maneb and zineb.[117] Six patients with dermatitis from zineb were reported by Scepa and Ippolito in 1959.[38] Cases of allergic contact dermatitis in workers spraying tobacco were reported by Laborie.[97a] Nater et al. described three cases of allergic contact sensitization due to maneb.[128] Two of the patients worked in rooms heavily decorated with plants, and the third was a florist. Patch-testing was done at 1%, 2%, and 5%, but studies of cross-reactions to zineb and other dithiocarbamates were not done. Cronin reported a rose gardener who had a strong patch-test reaction to maneb rose spray and zineb 1%.[38] Adams and Manchester reported a case of allergic contact dermatitis to maneb in the wife of a residential gardener.[2] Several severe episodes of dermatitis occurred before the cause was discovered. The patient's husband had stored a large bag of maneb next to the washing machine in the garage. Patch test to maneb 1% and thiram 1% in petrolatum were strongly positive, whereas testing with zineb was negative.

Members of the International Contact Dermatitis Research Group tested 655 eczematous patients with zineb 1% and maneb 1% in petrolatum. Three patients had positive reactions to zineb but none was thought clinically relevant; 35 patients had positive reactions to maneb but only one was thought to be relevant.

Allergic contact dermatitis to ethylenediamine used in the manufacture of zineb has been reported.[171]

Ziram. Ziram, a fungicide used extensively on almonds and peaches, is the most stable of the metallic dithiocarbamates. A positive patch-test reaction to ziram in an agricultural worker has been reported by Lisi and colleagues.[104]

Mancozeb. Mancozeb (manzeb), a fungicide related to both maneb and zineb, combines the benefits of these two earlier fungicides into a distinctive chemical used on a wide range of crops. It has an acute dermal LD 50 of >15,000 mg/kg in rats. Burry reported allergic contact dermatitis from mancozeb in South Australia in a worker treating barley and wheat seeds and in a farmer planting the seeds.[25] Patch-testing was performed at 0.5% concentration; 10 controls were negative. Testing for cross-reactivity to thiram was not done. Allergic contact dermatitis due to mancozeb in an agricultural worker has also been reported by Lisi and Carfinni.[105] This patient was also allergic to maneb.

Thiram. The chemical name is bis(dimethylthiocarbamoyl) disulfide, or tetramethylthiruram disulfide. Thiram, thirame, and TMTD are common names for this fungicide, seed protectant, and animal repellent.

It was first reported as a cause of dermatitis by Shulz and Hermann in five dock laborers unloading bananas treated with the fungicide.[156] Shelley described dermatitis from its use as a fungicide on a golf course.[158] Cronin related dermatitis in a man who had applied thiram to his garden.[38] Thiram (TMTD) has been reported to cause allergic contact dermatitis in a Polish flower vendor. She was in contact with flowers treated with the Polish fungicide Sadoplon, which contains 75% TMTD.[147] Fisher lists fungicides and animal repellents that may contain thiuram.[58]

Chlorothalonil. Chlorothalonil is a broad-spectrum fungicide approved for use on vegetables, fruits, flowers, and trees. Chlorothalonil 0.1% in acetone is a moderate cutaneous irritant; 0.1% chlorothalonil in petrolatum is much less irritating, and 0.1% chlorothalonil in saline is nonirritating to the skin of New Zealand white rabbits.[61] Stable on exposure to ultraviolet light, it has a half-life of about 2 months. Contact dermatitis has been reported in vegetable growers, woodworkers, and in flower growers.[19] Patch-testing is performed with 0.01% chlorothalonil in petrolatum. This is a marginally irritant concentration of chlorothalonil. Chlorothalonil is a strong cutaneous irritant at the concentrations used in spraying.

Chlorothalonil is used as a wood preservative in Northern Europe. Johnsson has reported an epidemic of contact dermatitis in a Norwegian woodenware factory;[90] 14 out of the 20 workers had work-related skin complaints, and 7 workers had contact dermatitis. Bach and Pederson reported contact dermatitis to tetrachloroisophthalonitrile in a cabinet maker.[7] Spindeldreier and Deitchmann have also reported three cases of contact dermatitis to tetrachloroisophthalonitrile.

Fatal toxic epidermal necrolysis (TEN) has been attributed to chlorothalonil. A 30-year-old navy pilot had played 81 holes of golf in the week prior to developing toxic epidermal necrolysis. The golf course had been sprayed with chlorothalonil. The authors state that special photographic techniques using ultraviolet light demonstrated chlorothalonil on the deceased's golf clubs, balls, and shoes.[106] It is not known if this case represented the TEN syndrome or an irritant variant. Chlorothalonil has produced severe immunologic contact urticaria with systemic signs, including an anaphylactoid reaction (Danmaker C, Maibach H, in preparation).

Dithianone. Dithianone is a broad-spectrum fungicide. Calnan reported dermatitis in a female horticulturalist working in a fruit orchard who became sensitive to dithianone.[28] Contact occurred from the sprayed trees while pruning and also from cleaning the spraying machines. Patch-testing was positive with 1% dithianone in petrolatum.

Dinobuton. Dinobuton is a fungicide and acaricide used to control the mites of deciduous fruits, citrus, cotton, cucumbers, and other vegetables. It is also valuable for controlling powdery mildew on apples, cucumbers, hops, and other crops.

In 1974 Wahlberg reported yellow staining of the hair and nails in workers with allergic contact dermatitis from dinobuton who were manufacturing dinobuton in a factory in northern Sweden.[181] Wahlberg noted that dinobuton did not appear to be a strong primary irritant; patch-testing with 40% dinobuton caused spontaneous flare reactions (sensitization) in two workers 9–10 days after application. The chemical relationship to picric acid was considered significant.

Octhilinone. Octhilinone is a biocide used in cooling water plants, cutting oils, cosmetics, shampoos, and as a leather preservative. Two cases of occupational allergic contact dermatitis to octhilinone used as a fungicide for surface paint of roof sheets were reported by Thormann.[170] Both workers had severe allergic contact dermatitis. Allergic reactions to other chemically related preservatives have been reported (1,2 benzisothiazolin-3-1 and 3-ethyl amino-1,2 benzisothiazolin hydrochloride [etisazol]).[8,39] Etisazol is a veterinary antifungal agent.

Slimicides

Slimicides are used in paper manufacture. If the wood pulp slurry becomes contaminated with slime molds, blemishes appear in the paper that is produced. Slime molds are not true fungi, though they possess characteristics resembling fungi. Slimicides are chemical treatments added to wood pulp slurry to prevent the growth of slime molds. Rycroft and Calnan reported irritant contact dermatitis to slimicides in a paper mill.[148] The active constituents in the slimicides include bis-1,4-bromoacetoxy-2 butene and 2,3-dichloro-4-bromo-tetrahydrothiophene-1,1-dioxide.

Antibiotics

Streptomycin is used to control bacterial plant diseases such as fireblight. It may be used in combination with oxytetracycline and tetracycline. It has been reported to cause allergic contact dermatitis among agricultural workers.[62]

Miticides

Propargite. Irritant contact dermatitis to propargite has been reported.[38] Propargite is the active ingredient in Omite-30W, a miticide widely used on grapes in California. Propargite is also the active ingredient of Omite-CR for use on citrus.

An outbreak of dermatitis among 114 of 198 orange pickers exposed to Omite-CR has been reported. The dermatitis occurred predominantly on exposed areas of the neck and chest. The prolonged residual action of propargite in Omite-CR was suggested as the cause of this outbreak of dermatitis.[152]

Dienochlor. Dienochlor is a miticide of low toxicity that has been in use for 20 years. The Farm Chemical handbook[53a] stated that dienochlor was neither a primary irritant nor a sensitizer, but a positive patch-test reaction to dienochlor has been reported in a florist with hand dermatitis by van Joost.[174]

Plant-growth Inhibitors

Choline Chloride. Choline chloride is a growth inhibitor used in agriculture. Fischer has reported a case of contact dermatitis to choline chloride.[59]

Insect Repellents

Deet (Diethyltoluamide). Deet was first synthesized in 1954 and came into use as an insect repellent in 1957. Poorly soluble in water, it is soluble in ethanol and propylene glycol. Diethyltoluamide, considered the best all-purpose insect repellent,[141] is especially effective against mosquitos. It remains effective for several hours post-application. The concentration of deet present in sprays, liquids, or sticks for application to skin or clothes varies from 1% to 100%.

Antecubital erythema progressing to hemorrhagic bullae was reported in 10 young soldiers by Reuveni and Yagupsky.[141] The antecubital area was the area involved in two patients who had permanent scarring. In Vietnam, some American soldiers developed bullae followed by scarring from deet.[99] Deet has been reported to exacerbate seborrhea and acne vulgaris as well as to produce contact dermatitis.[75]

Immunologic contact urticaria to deet was documented in a patient reported by Maibach and Johnson and subsequently verified by several other groups.[110] Toxic encephalopathy and death have been rarely reported in children from skin contact with deet.

LIVESTOCK

Dairy farmers may develop irritant contact dermatitis from extended wet work. Disinfectants that may cause irritant or allergic contact dermatitis are often used to clean the udders prior to milking.[62] Equipment is cleaned with sodium hydroxide and nitric acid. Dairy farmers are also exposed to hypochlorite, iodine, phenolic compounds, quaternary ammonium compounds, and hairs and secretions of cows. Dairy farmers may also develop allergic contact dermatitis to rubber compounds such as IPPD.[177]

Contact dermatitis due to cow saliva has been documented in a farm worker by Camarasa.[30] Contact urticaria due to horse saliva was reported by van der Mark.[173] Itching and flaring of eczema is not uncommon among veterinarian surgeons doing obstetric work. Veterinarians may be allergic to cowhair and dander or the obstetric fluid of cows.[138]

Farmers may develop irritant contact dermatitis to animal feeds. Medicaments mixed in the feeds may be primary irritants as well as sensitizers. Farmers sometimes neglect to wear protective gloves while mixing drugs to be administered to animals. Antimicrobial agents, including antibiotics, are used in feed not only for the treatment of disease but also to promote growth of animals. Contact dermatitis due to ethylenediamenedihydroiodine, as a source of iodine, furazolidone (a synthetic derivative of nitrofurazone), the antioxidant hydroquinone, and halquinol as an antibacterial agent have been reported from animal feed ingredients.[24,187]

Allergic contact dermatitis to the antioxidant, ethoxyquin, present in animal feed has been reported in farmers as well as feed mill workers. Ethoxyquin was also used to control scald in fruit. It was reported to cause allergic contact dermatitis in apple pickers.[24,187]

Quindoxin was used as a growth-promoting factor in animal feeds. Photocontact dermatitis due to quindoxin in animal feed has been reported. Quindoxin photosensitivity with a persistent light reaction has been reported in pig farmers.[88] Quindoxin is not registered for use in the U.S. and Canada.

Severe contact eczema due to quinoxaline present in animal feeds was reported by Dawson and Scott.[40] Quinoxaline is also an acaricide.

Olaquindox is a derivative of quinoxaline used as a feed additive to prevent bacterial enteritis in pigs. Both allergic contact and photocontact dermatitis due to olaquindox have been reported in Italy.[12,63] Photoallergic contact dermatitis has been reported to farmers who used chlorpromazine to tranquilize pigs.[95]

Piperazine, phenothiazine, and levamisole are anthelmintics that may cause allergic contact dermatitis. Allergic contact dermatitis to nitrofurazone has been reported. This anticoccidian is used in cattle feed. Formaldehyde is the allergen in nitrofurazone. Allergic contact dermatitis to 3,5 dinitro-o-toluamide, an anticoccidian used in chicken feeds, has been reported.[62]

Neomycin, ethylenediamine, and thiabendazole have also been used as feed additives. Sulfacetamide, sulfamethazine, chlortetracycline, oxytetracycline, and bacitracin have been used as growth promoters for livestock.[129] Farmers have become allergic to both nitrofurazone and tylosin in animal feed, particularly feed for hogs. Spiramycin and tylosin were the most common sensitizers among antibiotics used by farmers in Denmark.

Tylosin is a macrolide antibiotic used to combat swine dysentery in pigs and respiratory infections in poultry in the U.K. Tylosin can produce both irritant and allergic contact dermatitis.[179] Cases of occupational allergic contact dermatitis due to the macrolide spiramycin and tylosin have been reported in hog farmers and veterinarians.[82,178]

Allergic contact dermatitis to virginiamycin, a food additive for pigs and poultry, has also been reported.[169] Veien patch-tested 180 farmers to 5% virginiamycin in petrolatum but obtained no positive reactions.[177]

Approximately one-half of veterinarians surveyed in Scandinavia have occupational contact dermatitis, predominantly irritant contact dermatitis. Occasionally occupational dermatoses force veterinarians to abandon general veterinary practice.[52]

Penethamate has been reported as a common sensitizer in veterinarians. Penethamate is a strongly sensitizing penicillin derivative used in Europe for local treatment of mastitis in cows.[52,82]

MILK TESTERS

Chromate has been used as a preservative for milk that is to be analyzed for quality control purposes. Several reports document chromate allergy in milk testers and in milk analysis laboratories.[85,144,146]

Milk preservative solutions in the U.K. now contain 8% bronopol and 20% methyl-chloroisothiazoline and methylisothiazoline (KathonR CG). Allergic contact dermatitis to bronopol and KathonR CG was reported in three milk recorders by Grattan, Harman and Tan.[72] Bronopol has also been used as a seed treatment and foliar spray in some countries.

PATCH-TESTING

Agricultural workers may have the greatest exposure rate to the aforementioned compounds, but one must remember that these chemicals can reside on clothing that is brought back into the household and are found in many household exterminator preparations and garden products. Accumulation of these compounds in the skin after repeated exposures sometimes creates "reservoirs" of pesticide in the stratum corneum that effectively increase their concentration and their irritant capacity, as well as potential toxic effects. A good investigative history will usually help verify a relationship between possible pesticide exposure and dermatitis.

It is easy to see just how complicated evaluation can become of a patient with a history of possible pesticide exposure. Separation of those patients in need of a complete diagnostic work-up to isolate the offending compound from those who should be empirically treated for an irritant contact dermatitis with topical corticosteroids and emoliants may be relatively easy.

The well-established and accepted diagnostic test for allergic contact dermatitis is the patch-test. All agricultural workers suspected of suffering from chronic dermatitis (>1 month) or any patient requiring more than one course of oral prednisone deserves further diagnostic testing and should be patch-tested to all plants they are in contact with, as well as to the pesticides they use or are exposed to. It is simple, relatively inexpensive, and under optimal conditions has a high sensitivity and specificity. The Finn Chamber with paper adhesive tape is recommended. Patch-testing should be on the upper back, 48 hours in duration, and observations made at 48 and 96 hours. Erythema, vesicles, papules, and edema at the patch-test site suggest contact allergy. Pesticides may be generally patch-tested at 1% dilution.[174] A dilution of 0.1% is also suggested to avoid false-positive patch-test reactions. A minority of pesticides are commercially available in proper vehicles and concentrations for patch-testing. False-negative reactions occur in patch-testing for insecticides.[83] Fear of systemic toxicity may deter one from patch-testing with adequate concentrations of organophosphous insecticides, such as parathion. Some pesticides are sometimes dissolved in primary irritants, necessitating extreme dilutions for patch-testing. Using 15 microliters of a 0.1% to 1% solution for patch-testing excludes few concentrations because of acute toxicity. Pesticide manufacturers have some information on file regarding cutaneous irritation and allergenicity of their products.

Access to these antigens by dermatologists for patch-testing is limited and difficult. Few dermatologists demand these chemcials for testing. Manufacturers have little incentive to provide them, and there is no political motivation through governmental regulations. Improving the credibility of the current science is necessary. If the government required manufacturers to make their compounds available for diagnostic testing by responsible dermatologists and research groups, the minimal irritant concentration and proper vehicle could be determined before the compound came to market. Their irritant potential to skin should be tested at low- and high-level exposures to simulate actual farming situations.

RECOMMENDATIONS FOR IMPROVING THE CURRENT STATE OF PESTICIDE-INDUCED DERMATOSES

Improvement in the current state of science as it stands today is necessary. Anecdotal case reports in the literature only create misinterpretation, disorganization, and nonstandardization when assigning a pesticide an allergic- or irritant-potential. There needs to be a more scientific approach to determine the true nonirritant concentration of pesticides through patch-testing, by using appropriate controls, vehicles, and numbers of subjects. This would ultimately create a listing of chemicals as to their irritant potential, their vehicle's irritant potential, and at what specific concentration the skin irritation takes place.

The value of provocative use tests (PUT) via repeat open application test (ROAT) should be incorporated into the investigation of pesticide allergic/irritant dermatitis. Occasionally patch-testing will not give a definitive answer, and the ROAT may clarify the issue. Careful interpretation of the literature regarding the validity of the diagnosis made in case reports without scientific proof (i.e., a positive patch-test, or a positive ROAT) regarding irritant versus allergy must be made. The so-called excited skin syndrome may alter the validity of patch-testing, and repeat testing on normal skin will confirm a true allergy. The contact urticaria syndrome needs to be explored. Photo-allergy patch-testing is a valuable diagnostic test when the dermatitis is on the sun-exposed areas, as is common in field workers. Preexisting dermatitis may speed percutaneous absorptions of some pesticides, especially the organic phosphorus compounds. Dermatologists need to remember to search for unusual systemic toxic effects in all explored patients.

ZOONOTIC INFECTIONS

There are numerous dermatologic consequences of farming besides pesticide-induced dermatoses. Interaction with livestock presents a unique situation for zoonotic skin diseases. These dermatophyte, viral, and bacterial infectious diseases are transmitted from direct exposure to an infected animal, an asymptomatic carrier, or sometimes from contact with an inanimate object such as a bush, saddle, or comb.

Dermatophytosis (Tinea, Ringworm)

Among the three etiologic groups of dermatophytoses, only the zoophilic group will be discussed, because it is far more common in the farming community. Common dermatophytes in farm animals and pets derive from *Trichophyton* and *Microsporum* species. They are: *T. mentagrophytes, T. verrucosum, T. equinum,* and *M. canis.*

The hosts are cattle, dogs, and horses, but can include sheep, pigs and wildlife. A pustular folliculitis with loss of hair, usually over the exposed areas of the body, is generally more severe when in man than in nonhumans. Diagnosis is made microscopically and through culture. Hyphae can remain viable on inanimate objects for years if kept in a dry, cool environment, which makes direct contact with an infected animal nonessential.

Infectious disease controls include treatment of all infected animals with anti-fungal agents, initial isolation, and cleaning of the infected animals' environment, use of gloved hands when in contact with the animals, and good personal hygiene such as washing hands with antifungal soaps and a change of clothes when needed.

Viral Infections

The major infectious agents are from the pox viruses. These infect cattle, causing pseudocowpox, and sheep, causing contagious ecthyma (sore mouth). These viruses will produce milkers' nodule and orf virus disease in man. Both diseases are transmitted via direct contact with infected animals or contaminated inanimate objects. The virus can withstand drying and is viable at room temperature for years.

The lesions seen in humans are indistinguishable for both orf virus and milker's nodule. They begin as a small red or reddish blue papule that enlarges to form a flat-topped hemorrhagic pustule, often crusted in its umbilicated center. Diagnosis is made by clinical observation and by complement-fixation test, tissue culture, or electron microscopy.

Infection control is essentially the same as dermatophytic infections. Vaccination of noninfected animals for milker's nodule protection is recommended after isolation and treatment of infected animals are complete. Using rubber gloves when handling infected animals usually will prevent human infection.

Bacterial Infections

Tularemia, erysipelas, anthrax, brucellosis, salmonella dermatitis, and staphylococcal folliculitis and cellulitis can all be transmitted to humans from farm and wild animals. Diagnosis is made through bacterial cultures taken from clinically suspected infected individuals. Transmission requires direct contact, often after animal bites. Appropriate antibiotics are given and vaccination programs work well to lower the incidence of erysipelas in pigs and turkeys and anthrax in all animals. The best prevention from all bacterial infections includes using protective gloves and good personal hygiene, especially after minor skin injuries.

Anthrax, caused by *Bacillus anthracis*, is a spore-forming, gram-positive rod that produces a lethal endotoxin. An effective vaccine was discovered by Pasteur in 1881. In the U.S., almost all human infections are cutaneous and limited to workers handling imported goat hair, wool, and hides from endemic regions with poor infectious disease controls.

Direct inoculation from a puncture wound or abrasion can cause cutaneous infection. A small papule forms and enlarges to a purplish red, sharply marginated mass topped with a hemorrhagic vesicle or bulla. Necrosis of the bulla ensues and satellite vesicles appear. Diagnosis is made by culture, and treatment is with penicillin and tetracycline.

Brucellosis is caused by three different gram-negative rods: *Brucella suis* from pigs, *B. abortus* from cattle, and *B. melitensis* from sheep and goats. Infection is from handling infected animals or ingesting contaminated unpasteurized milk or cheese. The skin manifestations can include maculopapular lesions, petechiae, a chronic ulcer at the site of inoculation, and a urticarial eruption with subsequent vesiculopustules. Treatment is oral tetracycline plus streptomycin intramuscularly. Prevention of brucellosis in humans is based on elimination of animal brucellosis. Immunization of animals is done with a live attenuated *Brucella* vaccine.

Tularemia is a disease found in many wild animals in North America, but 90% of human cases are after contact with cottontail rabbits. The pleomorphic gram-negative coccobacillus causes an ulcer at the inoculation site, with massive regional lymphadenopathy and constitutional symptoms. The ulcer becomes necrotic and a black eschar forms. Treatment includes streptomycin, tetracycline, or chloramphenicol.

Salmonella dermatitis, caused by *S. dublin*, produces a erythematous rash followed by a papular, pustular eruption. These pustules are contagious and infected humans can spread the disease.

SKIN CANCER

Because the most common cause of nonmelanoma skin cancers (squamous and basal cell carcinomas) is ultraviolet light, it is not surprising to find a slightly increased rate of skin cancers in outdoor workers compared to indoor workers.[51] Agricultural workers with light skin, light eye coloring, and light hair who sunburn easily and tan poorly, or of Celtic descent, are even more susceptible. Women tend to have slightly lower rates secondary to sun protection from increased sun screen and cosmetic use.[51] It is therefore recommended that all persons working outdoors wear sun protection at work.

SUMMARY

We need to improve education of farm workers and their families to the potential hazards of exposure to the chemicals and other agents that they are in contact with on a daily basis. Simple measures such as showers in the fields and a change of clothes after work might lower the cutaneous reactions to these chemicals significantly. To that end, physicians can better educate themselves to highlight this area more intensely to residents in training, to offer lectures on the subject at dermatology conferences, and to foster better communication between our public health agencies and the pesticide industry itself. Companies are often cooperative when made aware of the benefits of irritant- and allergic-potential testing. Pesticide registration should require from the companies patch-testing before the product comes to market to determine the threshold irritant concentration and irritant potential of the vehicle.

REFERENCES

1. Abbott IM, Bonsall JL, Chester G, et al: Worker exposure to a herbicide applied with ground sprayers in the United Kingdom. Am Ind Hyg Assoc J 48:167–175, 1987.
2. Adams RM, Manchester RD: Allergic contact dermatitis to maneb in a housewife. Contact Dermatitis 8:271, 1982.
3. Adams RM, Zimmerman MC, Bartlett JB, Preston JR: 1-Chloro-2,4-dinitrobenzene as an algicide: Report of four cases of contact dermatitis. Arch Dermatol 103:191–193, 1971.
4. Adams RM (ed): Occupational Skin Diseases, 2nd ed. Philadelphia, W.B. Saunders, 1990.
5. Alexander JO: Arthropods and Human Skin. Suffolk, William Clowes, 1984, pp 1–9.
6. Ancona AA: Biologic causes. In Adams RM (ed): Occupational Skin Disease, 2nd ed. Philadelphia, W.B. Saunders, 1990, pp 89–112.
7. Bach B, Pedersen NB: Contact dermatitis from a wood preservative containing tetrachlorisophthalonitrile. Contact Dermatitis 6:142, 1980.
8. Bang Pedersen N: Occupational allergy from 1,2-benzisothiazolin-3-one and other preservatives in plastic emulsions. Contact Dermatitis 2:340–342, 1976.
9. Baran RL: Nail damage caused by weed killers and insecticides. Arch Dermatol 110:467, 1974.
10. Barnes RL, Wilkinson DS: Epidermal necrolysis from clothing impregnated with paraffin. Br Med J 4:466–467, 1973.
11. Becker CE: Recognizing the health hazards of ethylene oxide. West J Med 148:75, 1988.
12. Bedello PG, Goitre M, Cane D, Roncarolo G: Allergic contact dermatitis to Bayo-N-OX-1. Contact Dermatitis 12:284, 1985.
13. Bhargava RK, Singh V, Soni V: Erythema multiforme resulting from insecticide spray. Arch Dermatol 113:686–687, 1977.
14. Black H: Dazomet and chloropicrin. Contact Dermatitis Newsletter 14:410–411, 1973.
15. Botella R, Sastre A, Castells A: Contact dermatitis to paraquat. Contact Dermatitis 13:123–124, 1985.
16. Bowra GT, Duffield DP, Osborn AJ, Purchase FH: Premalignant and neoplastic skin lesions associated with occupational exposure to "tarry" byproducts during manufacture of 4,4'-bipyridyl. Br J Ind Med 39:76–81, 1982.
17. Brancaccio RR, Chamales MH: Contact dermatitis and depigmentation produced by the herbicide Carbyne. Contact Dermatitis 3:108–109, 1977.
18. Bruecker G, Hofs W: Kobalthaliges Futtermittel fur Wiederkauer als berufliches Ekzematogen. Derm Wochenschr 152:528–530, 1966.
19. Bruynzeel DP, van Ketel WG: Contact dermatitis due to chlorothalonil in floriculture. Contact Dermatitis 14:67–68, 1986.
20. Bruze M, Fregert S: Allergic contact dermatitis to chloridazon. Contact Dermatitis 8:427, 1982.
21. Buesching DP, Wollstadt L: Cancer mortality among farmers. J Nat Cancer Inst 72:503, 1984.
22. Budavari S (ed): The Merck Index. Merck & Co, 1989.

23. Burmeister LF, Everett GD, Van Lier SF, et al: Selected cancer mortality and farm practices in Iowa. Am J Epidemiol 118:72–77, 1983.
24. Burrows D: Contact dermatitis in animal feed mill workers. Br J Dermatol 92:167–170, 1975.
25. Burry JN: Contact dermatitis from agricultural fungicide in South Australia. Contact Dermatitis 2:288–296, 1976.
26. California Department of Food and Agriculture, Division of Pest Management and Pesticides Enforcement Branch: Report of pesticides sold in California for 1989 by pounds of active ingredients. Sacramento, CA, 1990, pp 1–17.
27. California Department of Food and Agriculture, California Agriculture Statistical Review, 1989. Sacramento, CA, 1990.
28. Calnan CD: Dithianone sensitivity. Contact Dermatitis Newsletter 6:119, 1969.
29. Camarasa JG: Difolatan dermatitis. Contact Dermatitis 1:127, 1975.
30. Camarasa JG: Contact eczema from cow saliva. Contact Dermatitis 15:117, 1986.
31. Cantor KP: Farming and mortality from non-Hodgkin's lymphoma: A case-control study. Int J Cancer 29:239–247, 1982.
32. Cohen ML, Moll MB, Maley PW: Statistical description of agricultural injuries in the United States. In Dosman JA, Cockcroft D (eds): Occupational Health and Safety in Agriculture. Boca Raton, FL, CRC Press, 1989.
33. Cook RR: Dioxin, chloracne, and soft-tissue sarcoma. Lancet i:618–619, 1981.
34. Cottel WI: Difolatan. Contact Dermatitis Newsletter 11:252, 1972.
35. Cotterill JA: Contact dermatitis following exposure to tetrachloronitrobenzene. Contact Dermatitis 7:353, 1981.
36. Cripps DJ, Gocmen A, Peter HA: Porphyria turica. Twenty years after hexachlorobenzene intoxication. Arch Dermatol 116:46–50, 1980.
37. Cronce PC, Alden HS: Flea collar dermatitis. JAMA 206:1563–1564, 1968.
38. Cronin E: Pesticides. In Cronin E: Contact Dermatitis. Edinburgh, Churchill Livingstone, 1980, pp 393–413.
39. Dahlquist I: Contact allergy to 3-ethylamino-1,2-benzisothiazole hydrochloride, a veterinary fungicide. Contact Dermatitis 3:277, 1977.
40. Dawson TJA, Scott KW: Contact eczema in agricultural workers. Br Med J 3:469–470, 1972.
41. De Eds F, Wilson RH, Thomas JO: Photosensitization by phenothiazine. JAMA 114:2095–2097, 1940.
42. Dosman JA, Cockcroft DW: Principles of Health and Safety in Agriculture. Boca Raton, FL, CRC Press, 1989.
43. Dunn JE, Dunn RC, Smith BS: Skin-sensitizing properties of DDT for the guinea pig. Public Health Rep 61:1614, 1946.
44. Edmiston S, Maddy KT: Summary of illnesses and injuries reported in California by physicians in 1986 as potentially related to pesticides. Vet Hum Toxicol 29:391–397, 1987.
45. Edmundson WF, Davies JE: Occupational dermatitis from naled: A clinical report. Arch Environ Health 15:89, 1967.
46. Elliott GF: Compensation programs for farmers. In Dosman JA, Cockcroft D (eds): Boca Raton, FL, CRC Press, 1989.
47. Emil M, Darby W, et al: Report of the Secretary's Commission on Pesticides and Their Relationship to Environmental Health. Washington, D.C., U.S. Department of Health, Education, and Welfare, December 1969.
48. Emmett EA: Occupational skin cancer. A review. J Occup Med 17:44–49, 1976.
49. English JSC, Rycroft RJG, Calnan CD: Allergic contact dermatitis from aminotriazole. Contact Dermatitis 14:255–256, 1986.
50. Epstein E: Urticaria due to an insecticide (pyrethrum). Urol Rev 48:829, 1938.
51. Epstein JH, Ormsby A, Adams RM: Occupational skin cancer. In Adams RM (ed): Occupational Skin Diseases, 2nd ed. Philadelphia, W.B. Saunders, 1990, pp 136–159.
52. Falk ES, Hektoen H, Thune PO: Skin and respiratory tract symptoms in veterinary surgeons. Contact Dermatitis 12:274–278, 1985.
53. Farber GA, Burks JW: Flea-collar dermatitis. CUTIS 9:809–812, 1972.
53a. Farm Chemical Handbook. Willoughby, Ohio, Meister Publishing Co., 1986.
54. Feinberg SM: Pyrethrum sensitization: Its importance and relation to pollen allergy. JAMA 102:1557–1558, 1934.
55. Feinstein A, Kahana M, Schewach-Millet M, Levy A: Idiopathic calcinosis and vitiligo of the scrotum. J Am Acad Dermatol 11:519–520, 1984.
56. Feldmann RJ, Maibach HI: Percutaneous penetration of some pesticides and herbicides in man. Toxicol Applied Pharmacol 28:126–132, 1974.

57. Fisher AA: Occupational dermatitis from pesticides: Patch testing procedures. CUTIS 31:483–492, 1983.
58. Fisher AA: Contact Dermatitis, 3rd ed. Philadelphia, Lea & Febiger, 1986.
59. Fischer T: Contact allergy to choline chloride. Contact Dermatitis 10:316–317, 1984.
60. Flannigan SA, Tucker SB, Key MM, et al: Synthetic pyrethroid insecticides: A dermatological evaluation. Br J Ind Med 42:363–372, 1985.
61. Flannigan SA, Tucker SB: Influence of the vehicle on irritant contact dermatitis. Contact Dermatitis 3:177, 1985.
62. Foussereau J, Benezra C, Maibach HI, Hjorth N: Agricultural occupations. In Foussereau J, et al (eds): Occupational Contact Dermatitis. Copenhagen, Munksgaard, 1982, pp 90–107.
63. Francalanci S, Giola M, Georgini S, et al: Occupational photocontact dermatitis from Olaquindox. Contact Dermatitis 15:112–114, 1986.
64. Fregert S: Allergic contact dermatitis from the pesticide rodannitrobenzene. Contact Dermatitis Newsletter 2:4, 1967.
65. Fregert S: Allergic contact dermatitis from the pesticides captan and phaltan. Contact Dermatitis Newsletter 2:28, 1967.
66. Fregert S: Allergic contact dermatitis from p-chloro-o-cresol in a pesticide. Contact Dermatitis Newsletter 3:46, 1968.
67. Fregert S: Allergic contact dermatitis from two pesticides. Contact Dermatitis Newsletter 13:367, 1973.
68. Gammeltoft M: Tributyltinoxide is not allergenic. Contact Dermatitis 4:238, 1978.
69. Garratt JR, Bigger JW: Asthma due to insect powder. Br Med J 2:764, 1923.
70. Garcia-Perez A, Garcia-Bravo B, Beneit SV: Standard patch tests in agricultural workers. Contact Dermatitis 151–156, 1984.
71. Ghosh SK, Gokani VN, Parikh JR, et al: Protection against "green symptoms" from tobacco in Indian harvesters: A preliminary intervention study. Arch Environ Health 42:141–144, 1987.
72. Grattan CEH, Harman RRM, Tan RSH: Milk recorder dermatitis. Contact Dermatitis 14:217–220, 1986.
73. Hanson D: EPA proposes expanded rules to protect pesticides workers. Chemical & Engineering News 4:14–15, 1988.
74. Haverstock LM: Farm stress: Research considerations. In Dosman JA, Cockcroft D (eds): Occupational Health and Safety in Agriculture. Boca Raton, FL, CRC Press, 1989, pp 427–430.
75. Hayes WJ: Pesticides Studied in Man. Baltimore, Williams & Wilkins, 1982.
76. Hearn CED, Keir W: Nail damage in spray operators exposed to paraquat. Br J Ind Med 28:399–403, 1971.
77. Hindson PC, Diffey BL: Phototoxicity of a weed killer: A correction. Contact Dermatitis 11:260, 1984.
78. Hoar SK, Blair A, Holmes FF, et al: Agricultural herbicide use and risk of lymphoma and soft-tissue sarcoma. JAMA 256:1141–1147, 1986.
79. Hoffman MS: Farms—Number and acreage by States. In Hoffman MS (ed): The World Almanac Book of Facts 1988. New York, Pharos Books, 1988, p 119.
79a. Hogan DJ: Pesticides and other agricultural chemicals. In Adams RM (ed): Occupational Skin Disease, 2nd ed. Philadelphia, W.B. Saunders, 1990, 546–577.
80. Hogan DJ, Lane PR: Dermatologic disorders in agriculture. Occup Med State Art Rev 1:285–300, 1986.
81. Hogan DJ, Lane PR: Allergic contact dermatitis due to a herbicide (barban). Can Med Assoc J 132:387–389, 1985.
82. Hjorth N, Weismann K: Occupational dermatitis among veterinary surgeons caused by Spiramycin, Tylosin, and Penethamate. Acta Dermatovener 53:229–232, 1973.
83. Hjorth N, Wilkinson DS: Contact dermatitis. II. Sensitization to pesticides. Br J Dermatol 80:272–274, 1968.
84. Honchar PA, Halperin WA: 2,4,5-T, trichlorophenol, and soft-tissue sarcoma. Lancet i:268–269, 1981.
85. Huriez C, Martin P, Lefebre M: Sensitivity to dichromate in a milk analysis laboratory. Contact Dermatitis 1:247, 1975.
86. Iden DL, Schroeter AL: Allergic contact dermatitis to herbecides. Arch Dermatol 113:983, 1977.
87. Jeyaratnam J, de Alwis Seneviratne RS, Copplestone JF: Survey of pesticide poisoning in Sri Lanka. Bull WHO 60(4):615–619, 1982.

88. Johnson BE, Zaynoun S, Gardiner JM, Frain-Bell W: A study of persistent light reactions in quindoxin and quinine photosensitivity. Br J Dermatol 93(Suppl 11):21–22, 1975.

89. Johnson FE, Kugler MA, Brown SM: Soft-tissue sarcomas and chlorinated phenols. Lancet ii:40, 1981.

90. Johnsson M, Buhagen M, Leira HL, Solvang S: Fungicide-induced contact dermatitis. Contact Dermatitis 9:285–288, 1983.

91. Jung HD, Rothe A, Heise H: Zur Epikutantestung mit Pflanzenschutz und Scha "dlingsbeka" mpfungsmitteln (Pestiziden). Dermatosen 35:43–51, 1987.

92. Kazen C, Bloomer A, Welch R, et al: Persistence of pesticides on the hands of some occupationally exposed people. Arch Environ Health 29:315–319, 1974.

93. Kentor PM: Urticaria from contact with pentachlorphenate. JAMA 256:3350, 1986.

94. Kleibl K, Rackova M: Cutaneous allergic reactions to dithiocarbamates. Contact Dermatitis 6:348–349, 1980.

95. Klein HM, Schwanitz HJ: Photocontact allergy to chlorpromazine in farmers. In Abstracts of 17th World Congress of Dermatology Part II. CMD-Scientific Secretariat (ed). G Braum Druckerei und Verlage. Karlsruhe, Germany, 1987, p 346.

96. Kligman AM: The identification of contact allergens by human assay. III. The maximization test: A procedure for screening and rating contact sensitizers. J Invest Dermatol 47:393–409, 1966.

97. Krieger R, et al: Gauging pesticide exposure of handlers (mixer/loaders/applicators) and harvesters in California agriculture. Proceedings of the Pesticide Workshop, Milan, 1990.

97a. Laborie F, Laborie R, Dedieu EH: Allergie aux fongicides de la gamme du menebe et du zinebe. Arch Mal Prof Med Tavail Securite Soc 25:419–424, 1964.

98. Lahti A, Maibach HI: Contact urticaria from diethyl fumarate. Contact Dermatitis 12:139–140, 1985.

99. Lamberg SI, Mulrennan JA Jr: Bullous reaction to diethyl toluamide (deet) resembling a blistering insect eruption. Arch Dermatol 100:582–586, 1969.

100. Lambert J, Schepens P, Janssens J, Dockx P: Skin lesions as a sign of subacute pentachlorophenol intoxication. Acta Derm Venereol 66:170–172, 1986.

101. Lane HU: Hired farmworkers: Workers and earnings 1970 to 1983. In Lane HU (ed): The World Almanac Book of Facts 1986. New York, Scripps Howard, 1985, p 162.

102. Leider M: Allergic eczematous contact-type dermatitis caused by DDT. J Invest Dermatol 8:125–126, 1947.

103. Lisi P, Carafinni S, Assalve D: A test series for pesticide dermatitis. Contact Dermatitis 15:266–269, 1986.

104. Lisi P, Carafinni S, Assalve D: Irritation and sensitization potential of pesticides. Contact Dermatitis 17:212–218, 1987.

105. Lisi P, Carafinni S: Pellagroid dermatitis from mancozeb with vitiligo. Contact Dermatitis 13:124–125, 1985.

106. Lord JT, Moats R, Jones J: Too much golf. J Forensic Sci Soc 24:359, 1984.

107. MacCaulay JC: Occupational high-pressure injection injury. Br J Dermatol 115:379–381, 1986.

108. Maddy KT, Edmiston S, Richmond D: Illness, injuries, and deaths from pesticides exposures in California 1949–1988. Reviews of Environmental Contamination and Toxicology 114:57–123, 1990.

109. Magnusson B, Blohm S-V, Fregert S, et al: Routine patch testing IV. Acta Dermato-venereologica 48:110–116, 1968.

110. Maibach HI, Johnson HL: Contact urticaria syndrome. Arch Dermatol 111:726–730, 1975.

111. Maibach HI: Irritation, sensitization, photoirritation and photosensitization assays with a glyphosate herbicide. Contact Dermatitis 15:152–155, 1986.

112. Malten KE: DNCB in cooling water. Contact Dermatitis Newsletter 15:466, 1974.

113. Marzulli FN, Maibach HI: Antimicrobials: Experimental contact sensitization in man. J Soc Cosmet Chemists 24:399–421, 1973.

114. Mathias CGT: Epidemiological aspects of occupational skin disease in agriculture. In Dosman JR, Cockcroft D (eds): Occupational Health and Safety in Agriculture. Boca Raton, FL, CRC Press, 1989.

115. Mathias CGT: Persistent contact dermatitis from the insecticide dichlorvos. Contact Dermatitis 9:217–218, 1983.

116. Matsushita T, Nomura S, Wakatsuki T: Epidemiology of contact dermatitis from pesticides in Japan. Contact Dermatitis 6:255–259, 1980.

117. Matsushita T, Arimatsu Y, Nomura S: Experimental study on contact dermatitis caused by dithiocarbamates maneb, mancozeb, zineb, and their related compounds. Int Arch Occup Environ Health 37:169–178, 1976.

118. Mehler L, Edmiston S, Richmond D, et al: Summary of illnesses and injuries reported by California physicians as potentially related to pesticides. HS-1541 Worker Health and Safety Branch, 1990.
119. Merck Index: An Encyclopedia of Chemicals, Drugs, and Biologicals. Windholz M (ed). Rahway, NJ, Merck & Co., 1983.
120. Milby TH, Epstein WL: Allergic contact sensitivity to malathion. Arch Environ Health 9:434–437, 1964.
121. Mitchell JC: Allergic contact dermatitis from Compositae. Trans St. John's Hosp Derm Soc 55:174–183, 1969.
122. Mitchell JC, Dupuis G, Towers GHN: Allergic contact dermatitis from pyrethrum. Br J Dermatol 86:568–573, 1972.
123. Morris GE: Dermatoses from phenylmercuric salts. Arch Environ Health 1:53–55, 1966.
124. Moses M, Selikoff IJ: Soft-tissue sarcomas, phenoxy herbicides, and chlorinated phenols. Lancet i:1370, 1981.
125. Nasution D, Klokke AH, Nater JP: A survey of occupational dermatoses in Indonesia. Berufsdermatosen 21:215–222, 1973.
126. Nater JP, Gooskens VH: Occupational dermatosis due to a soil fumigant. Contact Dermatitis 2:227–229, 1976.
127. Nater JP, Grosfeld JCM: Allergic contact dermatitis from Betanol (phenmedipham). Contact Dermatitis 5:59–60, 1979.
128. Nater JP, Terpsta H, Bleumink E: Allergic contact sensitization to the fungicide maneb. Contact Dermatitis 5:24–26, 1979.
129. Nelder KH: Contact dermatitis from animal feed additives. Arch Derm 106:722–723, 1972.
130. Newhouse M, McEvoy D, Rosenthal D: Percutaneous paraquat absorption. Arch Dermatol 114:1516–1519, 1978.
131. Niedelman ML: Contact dermatitis due to DDT. Occup Med 1:391–395, 1946.
132. Nishioka K, Asagami C, Kurata M, Fujita H: Sensitivity to the weed killer DNA-nitralin and cross-sensitivity to dinitrochlorobenzene. Arch Dermatol 119:304–306, 1983.
133. O'Malley MO, Mathias CGT, Coye MJ: Skin injury associated with pesticide exposure in California 1974 to 1983. In Dosman JA, Cockcroft D (eds): Principles of Health and Safety in Agriculture. Boca Raton, FL, CRC Press, 1989, pp 335–338.
134. O'Malley MO, Mathias CGT: Distribution of lost-work-time claims for skin disease in California agriculture: 1978–1983. Am J Ind Med 14:715–720, 1988.
135. Peachey RDG: Skin hazards in farming. Br J Dermatol 105(Suppl 21):45–50, 1981.
136. Pennsylvania Dept of Health, Division of Occupational Health: Occupational Health News and Views. Winter, 1969.
137. Pevny I: Pesticide allergy: Allergic contact eczema of a vintner. Derm Beruf Umwelt 28:186–189, 1980.
138. Prahl P, Roed-Petersen J: Type 1 allergy from cows in veterinary surgeons. Contact Dermatitis 5:33–38, 1979.
139. Radimer GF, David JH, Ackerman AB: Fumigant-induced toxic epidermal necrolysis. Arch Dermatol 110:103–104, 1974.
140. Rasmussen JE: Lindane. Arch Dermatol 123:1008–1010, 1987.
141. Reuveni H, Yagupsky P: Diethyltoluamide-containing insect repellent: Adverse effects in worldwide use. Arch Dermatol 118:582–583, 1982.
142. Richter G: Allergic contact dermatitis from methyisothiocyanate in soil disinfectants. Contact Dermatitis 6:183–186, 1980.
143. Ritter L: Assessment of pesticide toxicity: Regulatory viewpoints. In Dosman JA, Cockcroft D (eds): Principles of Health and Safety in Agriculture. Boca Raton, FL, CRC Press, 1989, pp 237–239.
144. Rogers S, Burrows D: Contact dermatitis to chrome in milk testers. Contact Dermatitis 1:387, 1975.
145. Ross CM: Sock dermatitis from dieldrin. Br J Dermatol 76:494–495, 1964.
146. Rudski E, Czerwinska-Dihnz I: Sensitivity to dichromate in milk testers. Contact Dermatitis 3:107–108, 1977.
147. Rudzki E, Napiorkowska T: Dermatitis caused by the Polish fungicide Sadoplon 75. Contact Dermatitis 6:300–301, 1980.
148. Rycroft RJG, Calnan CD: Dermatitis from slimicides in a paper mill. Contact Dermatitis 6:435–439, 1980.
149. Rycroft RJG, Wilkinson JD: The principal irritants and sensitizers. In Rook A, Wilkinson DS, et al (eds): Textbook of Dermatology. Oxford, Blackwell Scientific Publications, 1986, p 551.

150. Samitz MH, Mori P, Long CF: Dermatological hazards in the cigar industry. Ind Med Surg 18:434–439, 1949.
151. Samman PD, Johnston ENM: Nail damage associated with handling of paraquat and diquat. Br Med J 1:818–819, 1969.
152. Saunders LD, Ames RG, Knaack JB, et al: Outbreak of Omite-CR induced dermatitis among orange pickers in Tulare County, California. J Occup Med 29:409–413, 1987.
153. Savitt LE: Contact dermatitis due to benomyl insecticide. Arch Dermatol 105:926–927, 1972.
154. Schuman SH, Dobson RL, Fingar JR: Dyrene dermatitis. Lancet ii:1252, 1980.
155. Scott KW, Dawson TAJ: Photo-contact dermatitis arising from the presence of quindoxin in animal feeding stuffs. Br J Dermatol 90:5436, 1974.
156. Schultz KH, Hermann WP: Tetramethylthiuramdisulphide, ein Thioharnstoffderivat also Ekzemnoxe bei Hafenarbeiten. Berufsdermatosen 6:130–135, 1958.
157. Sharvill DE: Reaction to paraquat. Contact Dermatitis Newsletter 9:210, 1971.
158. Shelley WB: Golf course dermatitis due to thiram fungicide. JAMA 188:415–417, 1964.
159. Smith JG: Paraquat poisoning by skin absorption: A review. J Hum Toxicol 7:15–19, 1988.
160. Solomons B: Sensitization to Nitrofen. Contact Dermatitis Newsletter 12:336, 1972.
161. Spencer MC: Herbicide dermatitis. JAMA 198:169–170, 1966.
162. Spindeldreier A, Deichmann B: Contact dermatitis against a wood preservative with a new fungicidal agent. Derm Beruf Umwelt 28(3):88–90, 1980.
163. Stoke JCJ: Captafol dermatitis in the timber industry. Contact Dermatitis 5:284–292, 1979.
164. Stryker GV, Godfrey B: Dermatitis resulting from exposure to DDT. J Missouri Med Assoc 43:384, 1946.
165. Sulzberger MB: Studies in tobacco hypersensitivity. I. A comparison between reactions to nicotine and to denicotinized tobacco extract. J Immunol 24:85–91, 1933.
166. Svindland HB: Subacute parathion poisoning with erysipeloid-like lesion. Contact Dermatitis 7:177–179, 1981.
167. Taylor JS, Wuthrich RC, Lloyd KM, Poland A: Chloracne from manufacture of a new herbicide. Arch Dermatol 113:616–619, 1977.
168. Taylor JS: Dermatologic hazards from ethylene oxide. Cutis 19:189–191, 1977.
169. Tennstedt D, Dumont-Fruytier M, Lachapelle JM: Occupational allergic contact dermatitis to virginiamycin, an antibiotic used as a food additive for pigs and poultry. Contact Dermatitis 4:133–134, 1978.
170. Thormann J: Contact dermatitis to a new fungicide, 2-n-octyl-4-isothiazolin-3-one. Contact Dermatitis 8:204–221, 1982.
171. Tsyrkunov LP: Toksiko-allergicheskii dermatit ot vozdeistviia etilendiamina v proizvodstve gerbitsida tsineba. Gig Tr Prof Zabol 8:45–46, 1987.
172. Upholt WM, Kearney PC: Pesticides. N Engl J Med 275:1419–1426, 1966.
173. van der Mark S: Contact urticaria from horse saliva. Contact Dermatitis 9:145, 1983.
174. van Joost TH, Naafs B, van Ketel WG: Sensitization to benomyl and related pesticides. Contact Dermatitis 9:153–154, 1983.
175. van Ketel WG: Allergic dermatitis from a new pesticide. Contact Dermatitis 1:297–300, 1975.
176. van Ketel WG: Sensitivity to the pesticide benomyl. Contact Dermatitis 2:290–291, 1976.
177. Veien NK: Occupational dermatoses in farmers. In Maibach HI (ed): Occupational and Industrial Dermatology. Chicago, Year Book, 1987, pp 436–446.
178. Veien K, Hattel T, Justesen O, Norholm A: Occupational contact dermatitis due to spiramycin and/or tylosin among farmers. Contact Dermatitis 6:410–413, 1980.
179. Verbov J: Tylosin dermatitis. Contact Dermatitis 9:325–326, 1983.
180. Vero F, Genovese S: Occupational dermatitis in cigar makers due to contact with tobacco leaves. Arch Dermatol 43:257–263, 1941.
181. Wahlberg JE: Yellow staining of hair and nails and contact sensitivity to dinobuton. Contact Dermatitis Newsletter 16:481, 1974.
182. Wang JD, Li WE, Hu FC, Hu KH: Occupational risk and the development of premalignant skin lesions among paraquat manufacturers. Br J Ind Med 44:196–200, 1987.
183. Wilkinson DS: Sulphur sensitivity. Contact Dermatitis 1:58, 1975.
184. Winter CK, Kurtz PH: Factors influencing grape worker susceptibility to skin rashes. Bull Environ Contam Toxicol 35(3):418–426, 1985.
185. Wolfe HR, Armstrong JF, et al: Pesticide exposure from concentrate spraying. Arch Environ Health 13:340–344, 1966.
186. Wood S, Rom WN, White GL, Logan DC: Pentachlorophenol poisoning. J Occup Med 25:527–529, 1983.

187. Wood WS, Fulton R: Allergic contact dermatitis from ethoxyquin in apple packers. Contact Dermatitis Newsletter 11:295–296, 1972.
188. Yoshida K: Cutaneous exposure of pesticide spray applicators. In Dosman JA, Cockcroft D (eds): Principles of Health and Safety in Agriculture. Boca Raton, FL, CRC Press, 1989, pp 331–334.
189. Zaynoun S, Johnson BE, Frain-Bell W: The investigation of quindoxin photosensitivity. Contact Dermatitis 2:343–352, 1976.
190. Zimmerman MC: Dinitrochlorobenzene in water systems. Contact Dermatitis Newsletter 7:165, 1970.

JENNIFER LOWE ELLIS, MD
PAUL R. GORDON, MD

FARM FAMILY MENTAL HEALTH ISSUES

From the Department of Family
and Community Medicine
University of Arizona College of
Medicine
Tucson, Arizona

Reprint requests to:
Jennifer Lowe Ellis, MD
Preventive Medicine Resident
Family and Community Medicine
University of Arizona
Tucson, AZ 85724

For a variety of reasons health care has historically been less available to rural Americans compared to their metropolitan counterparts. Mental health services, which are variably accessible to metropolitan populations, continue to be even less available to rural Americans. The purpose of this chapter is to address this issue, that is, behavioral and mental health problems as manifested in rural farm families and the availability of care. Suggestions are made for health care providers to address and manage these problems in conjunction with the rural community itself. Limitations and possible directions for policy, practice, and research are discussed.

DESCRIPTION OF THE POPULATION

According to the U.S. Bureau of Census, a "rural" population refers to individuals living in towns or specified areas with fewer than 2,500 persons.[31] The farm population is defined by the manual of *Agricultural Statistics* as all persons living in rural places with $1000 or more of agricultural sales per farm in the reporting year.[1] The farm population in the United States declined from 2.9% of the total population in 1978 to 2.0% of the population in 1988.[1] When examined on a larger scale, approximately 60% of the rural population was living on farms in 1920, as compared to less than 10% of the rural population living on farms in 1984.[35] Total farm employment has declined from 3.0% of the total population employed on the farm in 1975 to 1.8% in 1988.[32]

Poverty continues to be highest and median income is lowest among rural farm families, regardless of race.[5] However, in contrast to the increase in services available to growing urban populations, rural and farming communities still suffer a much lower availability of public services and lag significantly behind the urban communities with respect to educational levels and housing quality.[34] Reasons for the disparity in health care services are many. Geographic isolation is a deterrent both for the farmers, who must endure long commutes to receive care, and for the health care facility, which must provide comprehensive services to a sparsely populated region. Transportation can be a problem, due to high fuel prices and lack of public transit. Fewer resources are available to rural communities for use in establishing mental health services because of their lower socioeconomic level and lower tax base, and because of the general scarcity of funds available for program development in mental health and in rural areas in general. Health professionals are less attracted to rural locations; there is difficulty recruiting and keeping qualified personnel in isolated areas.

STRESS IN THE FARMING ENVIRONMENT

In sharp contrast to the widely accepted belief that life on the arm is idyllic, wholesome, and stress-free, farming has been described as one of America's most stressful occupations.[26] The agricultural crisis of the 1980s has served only to intensify pre-existing stress and create a whole new set of stressors in the farming community.

Stress experienced by farmers and their families is largely a product of the occupation itself and of the environment in which the farmer operates. Farming is physically taxing and often dangerous. Physical injury is an ever-present threat, especially when large machinery and animal handling are involved. Exposure to chemical insecticides and inhalation of dusts may lead to a number of illnesses in the farmer and his or her family, and they are additional causes for worry. Farmers recognize that theirs is a hazardous occupation and admit to experiencing anxiety over health and safety issues.[29] Long hours and inflexible schedules leave little or no time for vacation, and stress is compounded if the farmer is stricken with illness, injury, or other disability, as there is rarely someone who can fill in. Postponing or rescheduling is not an option on the farm.

Environmental factors play a large part in the daily life of the farmer. Adverse weather conditions are by definition unpredictable and can be devastating to the farmer, as can insect infestations, crop disease, and erosion. Geographical isolation creates hardship in obtaining needed services. "Cabin fever" in winter months along with geographic isolation can bring on fear of being caught away from home or being unable to respond to an emergency.[18] Escalating fuel prices are another source of anxiety and ultimately another cause of increased isolation. Isolation may interfere with the farmer's ability to utilize available resources because of loneliness, depression, feelings of helplessness, and loss of interpersonal skills.[18]

Farmers may experience emotional conflict in responding to the pressure to produce to keep profits up, many having to adopt less humane conditions for livestock and less environmentally sound agricultural methods. Health and safety issues often have an emotional component. For instance, pesticide and chemical use, although economically essential, carry environmental and occupational hazards in their application and disposal.[24]

Stress is intensified by the fact that many of the forces at play that create stress are largely beyond the farmer's sphere of influence. Unlike other self-employed workers, farmers have very little control over the price of their products and, hence, their ultimate profit margin. All of the environmental variables are part of the competition, and the value and cost of the farmer's products change constantly. This is true both locally and worldwide.[8]

This lack of control over environmental events can lead to a "learned helplessness" that may come about in the face of experiencing adversity in circumstances out of one's control.[25] In many cases, one's motivation to respond in the face of increasing distress wanes, and self-esteem is increasingly disturbed. In the end, depression and anxiety predominate.[25] The economic vulnerability of the agricultural industry and the physical vulnerability of the farm itself when subjected to severe weather conditions are examples of such uncontrollable but regularly occurring events that may lead to depression and anxiety.[18]

CONSEQUENCES OF CHANGE

The changing rural environment in America during the 20th century has had important consequences for the mental health of farmers and their families. Before discussing these changes, it is important to mention certain general characteristics of traditional farming families and rural communities in an effort to understand how this changing environment has affected their mental health.

Rural residents hold more traditional values and are more resistant to change than urban residents.[10] "Traditional values" include emphasis on hard work and mastery of the physical environment, emphasis on the importance of family and community ties, orientation toward traditional moral standards, conformity to group norms, and fatalism.[18] When comparing rural and urban populations, it has been generally found that rural people are less accepting of divorce, of premarital sex, and of making contraception more widely available to teenagers. They are more likely to increase restrictions on the sale of pornography and decrease restrictions on the sale of alcohol. Rural persons tend to be more politically conservative, and greater numbers consider themselves to be "very religious," with a day-to-day dependence on religious faith in dealing with modern life and its problems.[20] The present-day rural community is quite diverse, however, and one must consider carefully any generalizations concerning rural attitudes and values.[9]

The introduction of the consequences of rapid change in the 20th century to the traditional farm environment has brought with it certain stresses. Advances in technology have often been accompanied by a breakdown of traditional support systems and a shift to dependence on the world community as represented in the media. The mass media, movies, and cable TV have introduced urban value systems that often conflict with the traditional farmer's values. Conflict may be a source of discord, especially between children and adolescents and the parents of the farm family. As a result, migration of the younger generations to urban environments is occurring in greater numbers.

Urban migration has affected the mental health of rural inhabitants.[19] A shift in values occurs in which the old ways are abandoned in favor of the more modern and appealing city ways. This results in the gradual deterioration of a lifestyle that had sustained rural people—a progressive breakdown of the culture and social environment—that adversely affects the mental health of the people involved.[15] When a family is in crisis, isolation and powerlessness may be exacerbated, because there are fewer natural resources available for help in these modern times. This is in contrast to the past, when "support groups" rallied around the farmer and his family in times of adversity, providing tangible assistance and tempering the rural tendency to be fatalistic and accepting. With the increasing isolation experienced by rural people comes an increasing vulnerability to powerlessness when faced with crisis.[22]

Since the turn of the century, mechanization has improved the lives and the productivity of farmers and their land. Mechanization has also caused labor displacement and an increase in rural and urban poverty rates.[34] Technological advances have increased productivity but have also created problems, namely, a shift away from the focus on the farm family's contribution to the community towards a larger, depersonalized, organizational framework. For the farmer, this shift may lead to a devalued sense of importance.[18]

Outside pressure to increase productivity and to adopt more scientific methods began in the 1950s. Further reduction in labor requirements resulted in increasing isolation for the farmers who were left in the profession, which in turn exacerbated the dissolution of local support systems and the breakup of extended rural families.[22] All of these changes served only to lessen the farmer's psychological readiness for the hard times to come.

Farmers who were left prospered through the early 1970s as their property values skyrocketed. They responded by increasing their debts with the purchase of more land and expensive machinery in hope that this abnormal prosperity would become the norm in years to come. In the words of one farmer, the accumulation of such debt among farmers did not "leave much room for things to go wrong."[8]

But yet things did go wrong. A combination of changes in policy, a strong U.S. currency overseas, and worldwide overproduction led to the agricultural crisis of the 1980s, which many have claimed has brought about a level of economic deprivation equal to that of the Great Depression. As a result, many farmers left the agricultural profession altogether, and those who remained faced countless new stresses in addition to existing ones.

Thus, the lifestyle of the farming family has been pushed to conform to a set of circumstances that are much more threatening than the seasonal fluctuations with which they routinely have dealt. The 1980s ushered in major changes in the lives of American farm families on the tail of the agricultural crisis. This significant disruption of the farming community continues to be felt and is reflected in a variety of mental health consequences.

MANIFESTATIONS OF FARM STRESS OF THE 1980s

Farmers and their families may respond in different ways to their environment and its inherent stresses. The Career Hotline for farmers in crisis, established by the University of Missouri, reported several psychological themes emerging from their telephone interviews with farm men and women. They describe a "wishing and hoping syndrome" among farmers, or the desire of farmers to close their eyes to the present and move on to better times. Another frequent illusion was a belief that a new farm bill or legislation would come along to "rescue" them from financial crisis. Cynicism and frustration were common, as was fear brought on by "a lack of past experience with life transitions." A grieving process similar to that described by Kubler-Ross over the loss of the farm and the personal identity associated with the farming lifestyle was commonly reported.[13]

The farmer may feel that he has betrayed his expanded family by losing the farm, which may have been handed down for generations.[15] Traditional support systems may not hold up under crisis. Friends may come to represent the farmer's failures, blame may be placed on community members, and the church may become a place where the farmer's family believe they must "maintain appearances." Farmers, when faced with career and lifestyle changes, may become indecisive, anxious, and depressed. The family—each member of which is lost in his or her own set of issues and blame—may pull away from each other instead of displaying mutual support.[13] Children in the farm family may blame themselves in some way for the family's troubles, because they are much less cognizant of the precipitating factors.[15]

The Farm Family Survey of 1989 revealed that farmers report their major concerns to be stress, trauma, and respiratory problems.[29] Nearly 50% of farm illness in the last 10 years in Iowa has been stress-related, with stress being induced or exacerbated by environmental conditions, weather, exposure to occupational hazards, financial strain, and other similar factors. A variety of mental health problems may evolve as a consequence of stress, including anxiety, depression, substance abuse, and violent behavior. Somatic and physical symptoms are also commonly associated with chronic stress, as revealed by a survey of self-reported stress symptoms in farmers. The farmers report complaints of chronic fatigue, forgetfulness, loss of temper, concentration difficulties, back pain, and sleep disruptions.[33] Although seemingly obvious, many farmers do not associate their symptoms with stress and instead ascribe them to yet another force in their lives that is mysterious and out of their realm of control. Their frustration may lead to alcohol abuse, family violence, or other manifestations of disintegration.[15]

A study focusing on new referrals to a rural mental health clinic over a 5-year period during the agricultural crisis showed a steady increase in this group and, of these new referrals, an increasing percentage each year were farmers.[16] The most frequent diagnosis for the entire group of new referrals was alcohol abuse or dependence. A considerable increase in the percentage of farmers with an alcoholic diagnosis was noted during the study period. This is in contrast to the nonfarm group, in which the incidence of alcohol-related diagnoses remained stable. These findings suggest a relationship between increased stress on the farm and maladaptive coping behaviors.[16] Yet when farmers were asked to rate the importance of farm-related health care services, mental health counseling and/or stress workshops were ranked eighth of nine services (the most important services being the availability of water testing for chemicals, health screening for pesticide exposure, and a telephone hotline addressing occupational exposure issues).[26] It is suggested by these findings that either stress and mental illness are not legitimate "health" concerns in the eyes of the farmers, or the farmers do not believe that stress and mental illness can be alleviated by the health care system. It is also possible that farmers may repress any desire to seek help because of the stigma of mental illness.

Rural Elderly. The elderly represent an ever-increasing percentage of the rural farm population. The rural elderly, when compared to their urban counterparts, are often more independent yet less healthy, and have fewer community resources on which to depend.[28] The 1980 National Census found that 43% of those 65 years and older live in rural areas.[30] When surveyed, the rural elderly identify their major concerns to be (1) financial strain, (2) loneliness, (3) not feeling needed, (4) fear of crime, (5) poor health, (6) not enough to do to keep busy, and (7) not enough friends. The rural elderly are more likely to be socially isolated and disengaged, and may be prone to low self-esteem and suicide.[28] Behavioral and mental health consequences implied by these needs are obvious.

Rural Women. Stress experienced by women in rural areas may be distinguished from the typical non-rural woman's stress, according to several studies. The farm wife must integrate her role on the farm with her role in the home, and these multiple simultaneous roles produce stress. One study of farmers' wives written during the agricultural crisis of the 1980s is particularly revealing. It examines role overload, role conflict, and perceived financial situation, and their relationships to mental health complaints (anxiety, irritation, and depressive mood), physical health complaints (including psychosomatic complaints), and self-esteem. The study showed that, despite complaints of role overload with increased farm work, the wife's self-esteem increased with increased participation in work on the farm, and that role overload in this situation had no significant effect on health outcomes.[3] The study also found that the more husband support involved, the higher the woman's self-esteem.

In contrast, the feeling of role overload was greatly influenced by the woman's perceived financial situation. In this case, the more severe the financial situation, the more role overload occurred and the more health-related complaints (mental and physical) were experienced.

Another study of rural women found that anxiety, hostility, and depression were increased in younger women, in families with two or more children under age 14, and in women whose husbands had less than a high school education.[12] Women who attended church more than once a month, who visited their friends more than once a month, and who were involved in decision-making roles in the family were less likely to experience anxiety, hostility, and depression.[14] This may be partly explained by the observation that increased contact with friends and the social support system of the church lessen the sense of isolation often experienced by rural women.

Adolescents. Adolescents whose families have been affected by the agricultural crisis have suffered in different ways. School phobia and chronic truancy in this adolescent population may be manifestations of fear and uncertainty with lifestyle changes and the parent's career transition.[23] A study of the relationship between family economic hardship and adolescent distress among secondary school students in a small Midwestern community revealed that family economic hardship was indeed associated with a significant amount of increased distress in adolescents.[21] The study hypothesizes that depression in these adolescents results from the feeling of events being out of control (with respect to family conditions), with consequent feeling of uncertainty about the future, worthlessness, and helplessness. Loneliness in this group is exacerbated by the decrease in parental nurturing that often occurs in such families during economic hard times. Delinquent and drug-using behaviors in this population are more commonly associated with increases in inconsistent parental discipline brought on by economic hardship.[21] Marital discord induced by financial stress may contribute to decreased parental nurturance and increased inconsistent parental discipline. Likewise parent-child conflicts induced by economic strain may intensify marital discord.[21]

LIMITATIONS IN PROVIDING CARE

As outlined above, mental and behavioral health problems in rural America are varied and multifactorial. Services in general are less available and less accessible to rural persons. This situation is complicated by the observation that rural residents are less willing to participate in outpatient health care and are typically opposed to institutionalization.[4] The farmer may regard help-seeking as a weakness. His independence, self-reliance, and simple, direct coping methods, essential to functioning well on the farm, may also prevent him from seeking services in times of need.[13] Other limitations to improvement of rural mental health care include the "brain drain" of younger rural inhabitants to the cities, the difficulty in recruiting qualified personnel to rural and often isolated areas, and the fact that in most cases, farmers who are forced to sell their farms are not eligible for unemployment benefits, because they had previously been self-employed.

IMPLEMENTATION OF MENTAL HEALTH SERVICES

All practitioners, regardless of specialization, should develop an awareness of mental health problems and their manifestations, and should be able to recognize their signs and symptoms. However, just as not all practitioners care regularly for patients with diabetes or fractures, not all practitioners possess the skills needed to treat mental illness. There will be a subset of practitioners who are more comfortable with psychological and behavioral issues. Some of these practitioners may choose to engage their patients in short-term psychotherapy, whereas others may be trained in and practice family therapy.

Practitioners who are less comfortable with the above interventions may still play an active role in the care of the mentally ill member of the farm family. In addition to being familiar with available referral sources, they may act as advocates for specific services and may serve as facilitators for certain groups and activities as discussed below.

The practitioner should remember that a focus on the family as a unit is helpful, because isolation of family members during crisis often leads to a decreased awareness and appreciation of the strengths of the family and contributions of its individual members.[15] The farmer and his family should be reassured that indecisiveness is caused by stress and as such "should be seen as a natural and understandable response to a highly ambiguous situation."[15] When formulating strategies to make farm communities more cohesive and thus less vulnerable to isolation and depression, practitioners should consider the importance of extra-familial sources of support (i.e., friends, schools, community groups, and churches).[21] These groups "enhance the sense of community, and attendance at one of these gatherings does not identify the farmer as a person at risk."[15] An additional advantage in working with groups that already have the farmers' trust exists in this approach as well.

Hotline staffers have noted that in many cases, women are the first to use their services. Practitioners could advocate self-help groups targeted at these women as the initial contact with the family. Another group that is strategic to reaching displaced farmers is other displaced farmers.[8] Leadership and empowerment are other important issues and should encompass the community and beyond as farmers seek to influence farm policy nationally. Marketing support services is extremely important. The Farm Family Survey reveals that farmers commonly turn to farm family magazines and the Cooperative Extension Service for health information.[29] Polling of callers by the Career Hotline indicated that local newspapers were also frequently used sources.[13]

Support programs that have been successful include the University of Missouri's Career Hotline for Farmers in Transition, the Cooperative Extension Service of Iowa State University's program "Family Stress: Dealing with Blame," which is targeted to farmers' current concerns and sold as a packaged seminar, and the publication "The Family Farm; Can It Be Saved?" published by Brethren Press, a study guide of the current farm issues and a listing of available resources.[8]

The economic situation in rural America will certainly not improve suddenly and will most likely get worse before it gets better. The fragile rural economy is vulnerable to economic disruption, and "the social fabric and networks of a community can be torn apart overnight."[7] Mental health services and research related to their delivery should be prioritized and should be considered as important as medical services in the rural community.[7] Needed mental health services include counselors/workshops dealing with coping skills, family management, stress management, and alcohol/drug use and dependency treatment. Career counseling should be available for farmers and their families, who frequently are burdened with self-doubt in approaching the job market, despite many talents and skills that could be applied to potential new employment.[23] Programs should also be available in schools, with education and the influence of the media working together to eliminate the stigma associated with mental health issues. Practitioners are important players in advocating these services in the community.

In addition to implementation and improvement of programs for the farmworkers, training opportunities for the practitioners themselves should be considered. Area Health Education Centers (AHECs) have been established with government assistance in different areas in the United States for the purpose of training medical students and residents in rural health issues.[11] AHECs operate through university-based linkages to underserved communities, addressing the training needs for health professionals there. The relationship between the community and the academic health science center translates into training opportunities for health care students, with the goal of improved recruitment and retention of providers in shortage areas, and improvement of the quality of services and providers in underserved areas.

Successful programs developed through AHECs or modeled after its example include rural public health and border health rotations for University of Arizona students and residents,[6] special curriculums addressing the underserved at Meharry Medical School[2] and the University of New Mexico,[17] and Commitment to Underserved People (CUP) at the University of Arizona,[27] which provides medical students with educational and service activities on a longitudinal basis. These concepts could certainly be expanded to include mental health care issues in farmworkers.

CONCLUSION

Increasing the amount of mental health services available to rural Americans is only part of the solution. We practitioners are not likely to see an improvement in the mental and behavioral health status of rural Americans until we educate members of the rural community about mental and behavioral health issues relevant to them, shaping positive attitudes toward available community-based services, and thus legitimizing mental health problems and reducing the stigma associated with them.

REFERENCES

1. Agricultural Statistics. Washington, DC, US Government Printing Office, 1989.
2. Arradondo JE: Family Medicine Division at Meharry uses special strategies to meet priority for the underserved. Public Health Rep 95:29–31, 1980.
3. Berkowitz AD, Perkins HW: Stress among farm women: Work and family as interacting systems. J Marriage and the Family February:161–166, 1984.

4. Blazer D, George LK, Landerman R, et al: Psychiatric disorders: A rural/urban comparison. Arch Gen Psychiatry 42:651–656, 1985.
5. Chadwick B, Bahr H: Rural poverty. In Ford T (ed): Rural USA: Persistence and Change. Ames, IA, Iowa State University Press, 1978.
6. Cordes DH, Rea DF: Resident training in rural and border areas: Prevention in cross-cultural settings. Tucson, AZ, Department of Family and Community Medicine, University of Arizona (unpublished report).
7. Cordes SM: The changing rural environment and the relationship between health services and rural development. Health Services Research 2:757–784, 1989.
8. Ferguson SB, Engels DW: American farmers: Workers in transition. The Career Development Quarterly 37:240–248, 1989.
9. Flax JW, Wagenfeld MO, Ivens RE, Weiss RJ: Mental Health and Rural America: An Overview and Annotated Bibliography. National Institute of Mental Health, DHEW Publication No. (ADM) 78-753, Washington, DC, US Government Printing Office, 1979.
10. Ford T: Contemporary rural America: Persistence and change. In Ford T (ed): Rural USA: Persistence and Change. Ames, IA, Iowa State University Press, 1978.
11. Gessert CE, Smith DR: The National AHEC Program: Review of its progress and considerations for the 1980s. Public Health Rep 96:116–120, 1981.
12. Giesen D, Maas A, Vriens M: Stress among farm women: A structural model approach. Behavioral Medicine, Summer:53–62, 1989.
13. Heppner MJ, Johnston JA, Brinkhoff J: Creating a career hotline for rural residents. J Counseling and Development 66:340–341, 1988.
14. Hertsgaard D, Light H: Anxiety, depression, and hostility in rural women. Psychological Reports 55:673–674, 1984.
15. Hook MPV: Harvest of despair: Using the ABCX Model for farm families in crisis. Social Casework: The J of Contemp Social Work. May:273–278, 1987.
16. Hsieh HH, Khan MH, Cheng SC, et al: Increased drinking and the farm crisis: A preliminary report. Hospital and Community Psychiatry 39:315–316, 1988.
17. Kaufman A, Obenshain SS, Voorhees JD, et al: The New Mexico Plan: Primary care curriculum. Public Health Rep 95:25–28, 1980.
18. Keller PA, Murray JD: Rural mental health: An overview of the issues. In Keller PA, Murray JD (eds): Handbook of Rural Community Mental Health. New York, Human Sciences Press, 1982, pp 3–19.
19. Kennedy R: Dr. Kennedy speaks to Dr. Srole's findings. Rural Community Mental Health Newsletter 5(1):19–20, 1978.
20. Larson O: Values and beliefs of rural people. In Ford T (ed): Rural USA: Persistence and Change. Ames, IA, Iowa State University Press, 1978.
21. Lempers JD, Clark-Lempers D, Simons RL: Economic hardship, parenting, and distress in adolescence. Child Development 60:25–39, 1989.
22. Murray JD, Kupinsky S: The influence of powerlessness and national support systems on mental health in the rural community. In Keller PA, Murray JD (eds): Handbook of Rural Community Mental Health. New York, Human Sciences Press, 1982, pp 62–73.
23. Peeks B: School-based intervention for farm families in transition. Elementary School Guidance & Counseling 24:128–134, 1989.
24. Sandfort D: Reaching the difficult audience: An experiment to provide occupational health services to farmers and ranchers in Colorado, USA. Am J Indust Med 18:395–403, 1990.
25. Seligman M: Helplessness: On Depression, Development and Death. San Francisco, Freeman, 1975.
26. Smith M, Cullingan M, Hurrel J: A review of National Institute for Occupational Safety and Health and stress research. In Walker JL, Walker LJS (eds): Self-reported Stress in Farmers. J Clin Psychology 44(1):10–16, 1988.
27. Spencer SS, Outcalt D: Commitment to Underserved People (C.U.P.) Program at the University of Arizona. Public Health Rep 95:26–28, 1980.
28. Talbot DM: Assessing the needs of the rural elderly. J Gerontol Nursing 11:39–43, 1985.
29. Thu K, Donham KJ, Yoder D, Ogilvie L: The farm family perception of occupational health: A multistate survey of knowledge, attitudes, behavior, and ideas. Am J Indust Med 18:427–431, 1990.
30. US Bureau of Census: Demographic aspects of aging and the older population in the United States. In Sourcebook on Aging, 2nd ed. Chicago, Marquis Academic Media, 1979, p 225.
31. US Department of Commerce, Bureau of the Census: County and City Data Book. Washington, DC, US Government Printing Office, 1989.

32. US Department of Commerce, Bureau of the Census: Statistical Abstract of the United States. National Data Book and Guide to Sources. Washington, DC, US Government Printing Office, 1990.
33. Walker JL, Walker LJS: Self-reported stress symptoms in farmers. J Clin Psychology 44:10–16, 1988.
34. Wilkinson K: Changing rural communities. In Keller PA, Murray JD (eds): Handbook of Rural Community Health. New York, Human Services Press, 1982, pp 20–28.
35. Wimberly RC: Agricultural and rural transition. In New Dimensions in Rural Policy Building upon Our Heritage. US Congress Joint Economic Committee, Subcommittee on Agriculture and Transportation. Washington, DC, US Government Printing Office, 1986, pp 39–45.

JOEL S. MEISTER, PhD

THE HEALTH OF MIGRANT FARM WORKERS

From the Southwest Border Rural
  Health Research Center
Department of Family and
  Community Medicine
University of Arizona College
  of Medicine
Tucson, Arizona

Reprint requests to:
Joel S. Meister, PhD
Southwest Border Rural Health
  Research Center
Department of Family and
  Community Medicine
Community Medicine Section
University of Arizona College
  of Medicine
Tucson, AZ 85724

Of the many articles in this issue, only this one focuses on a specific group of farm workers. The others are devoted to a particular health hazard or type of risk or to the regulatory and preventive environment of health in agriculture. Why are migrant farm workers special? Are they not, in fact, at risk of experiencing the same kinds of illnesses and injuries and disabilities as other farm workers?[5] The simplest and probably most accurate answer is that they are, but more so. The "more so" is explained partly by the specific conditions encountered while migrating and partly by other factors associated with migration, such as ethnicity and socioeconomic status. This article will describe the special characteristics of the migrant population and how they are related to health hazards, health status, and health-seeking behavior. It will examine some of the more prominent health issues of this population while attempting to avoid repeating information provided by other authors. And it will address the potential for appropriate actions on the part of the health professions.

It should be acknowledged at the outset that this discussion is hindered by ignorance. We believe that migrant farm workers deserve special attention to their health needs, and anyone who has worked with them or in the vicinity of the fields and orchards and labor camps where they work and live knows that this is so. But most of the "hard facts" are yet to be gathered. Available data are often sparse, incomplete, or inconclusive. This condition of ignorance is itself a consequence of the migrant situation, which will be addressed later in this article.

DEMOGRAPHICS

To begin with, no one really knows how many migrant farm workers there are, and how many family members there are, either nationally or regionally or by state. Different federal agencies even define "migrant" differently. For the purposes of this chapter, we use the Office of Migrant Health's definition: a migrant farm worker is "an individual whose principal employment is in agriculture on a seasonal basis, who has been so employed within the last 24 months and who establishes for the purpose of such employment a temporary abode."[20] A seasonal farm worker, on the other hand, also works cyclically but does not migrate. The federal Office of Migrant Health estimates that there are 3,000,000 migrant and seasonal farm workers and dependents in the U.S.,[30] of whom about 1,000,000 are migrants. Depending on which agency is doing the counting, estimates range from 317,000 to 1,500,000 migrants and dependents.[29] This uncertainty is one consequence of migrancy; you can't count people if you can't find them. And if you can't count them, then you can't undertake population-based research with much confidence in your denominator figures. For example, much has been made in the press of the assertion that the life expectancy of migrant farm workers is 49 years. A recent study tracked this statistic to undocumented congressional testimony in the 1960s and concluded, on the basis of indirect and incomplete but suggestive data, that the figure might be closer to 59 years.[16] Such a discrepancy does nothing to lessen concern about the shortness of life but illustrates the demographic problem. The same concerns are raised about other vital statistics, such as infant mortality and early childhood deaths.[3,4,27]

There are three major migrant "streams" in the United States. One includes the east coast, from a home base in Florida to the northern Atlantic states. The second originates in Texas and spreads throughout the plains states, middle west, and parts of the Rocky Mountains. The third, based in California and Arizona, covers the western states. The eastern stream is the most ethnically heterogeneous, including African Americans, Mexican Americans, Mexicans, Puerto Ricans, Haitians, Jamaicans, and others. The other two streams are over 90% Hispanic but also include American Indians and Southeast Asians.[29] Among the Hispanics there are Mexican Americans, Mexicans, and an increasing number of Central Americans. An unknown but large number of these workers are undocumented. Undocumented status has significant implications for health, which are discussed below.

One can see that migrant farm worker populations vary by race and ethnicity, geographic location, type of work performed, and degree of acculturation. From the Jamaican apple harvester in New England to the African American tobacco worker in North Carolina and the Mexican grape picker in California's central valley, migrants constitute a heterogeneous population with different exposures and reactions to health hazards.

THE MIGRANT CONDITION

The very geographic mobility and transience of migrants create health hazards. If motor vehicle accidents, for example, are a hazard to all farm workers, then one would expect the "more so" situation to apply here. But this transience leads to other serious health risks as well. Migration causes social and physical isolation of farm workers and their families, especially of wives who may not be working themselves. Recent interviews[17] of migrant health center staffs in the western stream yielded the following typical picture: a migrant family arrives at a new site and finds employment and housing on or near a farm with a few other migrants—the large migrant labor camp is the exception. There is no ongoing social network to provide emotional, social, or financial support. The husband leaves at dawn to work in the fields, leaving his family with no transportation to use for schools, shopping, or doctors' visits. The wife speaks no English and may be illiterate in Spanish. She may be fearful as well as depressed about her isolation. Access to health care is difficult at best. Continuity of care and adequate medical follow-up of her or her family are problematic. Specific health problems, such as alcoholism and other substance abuse, are associated with social isolation. For male workers migrating alone, the risk of contracting AIDS and other sexually transmitted diseases is increased. Thus, migrancy in itself exacerbates problems of access and may lead to behavioral problems associated with isolation.

Poverty is not unique to migrant farm workers, but, combined with migrancy, results in a degree of substandard living conditions that have been described as "third world."[2,13] The average family income of migrant farm workers from all sources was estimated at $6,194 in 1985.[24] Of that, $3,295 came specifically from farm labor. In 1981, a migrant family's income was estimated at only $3,995 a year.[29] Housing is sometimes provided by the employer but is typically left to the worker to obtain on his own. The regulation of growers' labor camps is haphazard or nonexistent. As recently as May, 1990, Secretary of Labor Dole was "shocked" by what she saw on a surprise visit to a migrant labor camp in Florida.[1] Unfortunately, what she saw was typical of labor camps as well as of privately available migrant housing throughout the country.[1] Such housing is substandard on every count. It lacks insulation; there is often no indoor plumbing, no running water, no heat, and no electricity. Laundry facilities, which are important in reducing pesticide exposure, are nonexistent. For a minority of workers, California's agricultural counties offer an exception to the rule by providing county operated labor camps for up to 5 months of the year.

Yet, in California as elsewhere, one can also find migrant workers living under plastic sheets or in cardboard boxes in the fields and orchards where they work.[1] Whether living in the fields, in camps, or in privately obtained housing, migrant families are likely to eat and sleep in close proximity to the workplace. They are thus at risk of exposure to pesticide drift or direct accidental spraying in addition to any exposures suffered by working members of the family while at work. Because of the lack of adequate sanitation, water, and laundry facilities, the migrant family may have to use irrigation water for drinking, bathing, and washing clothes. This water is likely to be contaminated by both pesticides and fertilizer runoff. In the case of some crops, such as citrus, the irrigation water itself is used as the delivery vehicle for pesticides.

Child labor is a general problem in agriculture, and, again, this is more so for migrant farm workers, because their relative poverty makes them more dependent on the income of their children. Assuming that there is effective enforcement of child labor statutes (an unsafe assumption of a best-case scenario), it would still be possible for children as young as 10 to harvest potatoes and strawberries, and children of 12 may legally work in any crops. Dunbar and Kravitz[10] estimated that 25% of all farm labor in the U.S. is performed by children.

The intermittency of work, fluctuation of wages based on the piece rate system of payment, and overall low level of income of migrant workers lead to long hours in the fields. The piece rate system also provides disincentives to seek health care. Every minute away from work, no matter the reason, is money lost. A clinic visit which, counting travel time, waiting time, and actual encounter, may take several hours, can be a financial disaster to a migrant worker. I have been told by workers that even the quarter mile walk from the field to the portable toilets takes too much time away from work. Piece rate work also increases the pace of work and decreases the number and length of breaks for any reason.

Migrant workers also fear to leave work, even briefly, for health reasons, because they are easily replaceable by others willing to work hard for low wages under poor conditions. Those most willing to work include the undocumented, primarily Mexicans and Central Americans who have crossed the Mexican border illegally for economic or political reasons, or both. If migrant workers are more at risk than other agricultural workers, then the undocumented workers are even more at risk than other migrants. One could say that their greatest health hazard is the risk of being deported, because their legal jeopardy leads them to avoid any contacts that might lead to their apprehension, and this includes contacts with health care providers. They are also the most likely to be living in the fields. Undocumented workers thus live under more stress, in the worst living conditions, and with the least health care of all migrant workers.[29]

Those workers who were once undocumented but are now enrolled in the amnesty program created by the Immigration Reform and Control Act of 1986 (IRCA) may also avoid health care because of the ambiguity of the regulations requiring amnesty participants to be unlikely to become a public charge. One test of the public charge rule is whether the applicant has received public cash assistance. While medical care is not considered to be such assistance, the Immigration and Naturalization Service (INS) refuses to make a blanket exemption, preferring to make decisions on a case by case basis. The effect of this policy, based on interviews in the western stream, has been to discourage workers from applying for Medicaid or any other publicly sponsored health care.[8]

Language and culture are important factors that exacerbate the health hazards to migrant farm workers. Of workers who are Hispanic, a majority of them speak only Spanish or are much more fluent in Spanish than in English. Smaller numbers of workers speak Haitian French, Creole dialects, or Southeast Asian languages. In all cases, a language and/or cultural difference between the worker and the surrounding culture creates barriers to care, increases social and physical isolation, makes health education more difficult, and increases the likelihood that nonmedical or "traditional" forms of care, such as "curanderos" (healers) or "brujas" (witches) will be used where available.[11] Language and cultural differences, coupled with the personal and family ties of many migrants to Mexico, also increase the likelihood that migrant workers will seek health care in Mexico, not in the U.S.[17] Rather than seeking care in a timely manner, workers will wait until they can return to Mexico for care. And while American providers, especially those at migrant health centers, will provide workers with their medical records and interagency referral forms, Mexican providers do not do so.[17] The result is that this major subgroup of migrant workers is very difficult to follow medically.

Lack of unionization, which is typical of farm workers in general and migrants in particular, has been noted as a contributing factor to health problems.[29] Where workers have been unionized, housing is better, field sanitation and water are better, health insurance is provided, and wages are higher. Another way of stating the issue is that migrant farm workers are probably the politically weakest occupational group in this country, the hardest to organize, and the most poorly represented. They have little political clout. As a consequence, the health care provider may find him- or herself acting by default, but by necessity, as the advocate as well as the caregiver for migrant farm workers.

The condition of migrancy, then, affects health in many ways. It leads to increased exposure to unhealthy living and working conditions; to increased exposure to specific health hazards; to poor utilization of health care; to an overemphasis on acute care relative to routine or preventive care; and to lack of awareness, lack of availability, and lack of accessibility of care.

WHAT DO WE NOT KNOW ABOUT MIGRANT HEALTH?

Migrant farm workers suffer from the same leading causes of death as other Americans—heart disease, cancer, and strokes—but we know little or nothing about prevalence, incidence, or risk factors among migrants.[21] We do know something about the most frequent diagnoses made at migrant health centers. Wilk[29] reports the following diagnoses in descending order of frequency, in 1979–80: acute upper respiratory infection, hypertension, obstetrical problems, diabetes mellitus, otitis media, dermatitis, trauma, urinary tract infection, anemia, obesity, gastroenteritis, family planning activities, and heart disease. In a 1986 study of one migrant health center in Arizona, injuries were the most common diagnosis, followed by hypertension, respiratory diseases, diabetes mellitus, digestive diseases (including dental caries), and mental disorders, primarily depression and anxiety.[16] There were also differences in frequency between upstream and downstream (home base) clinics.[29] Among the upstream clinics, skin disorders were the most frequent diagnosis, whereas dermatitis was eighth in frequency at downstream clinics. Parasitic infections, which ranked ninth at upstream clinics, were too infrequent to rank at downstream clinics. These changes in frequency are likely related to changes in working and living conditions when migrant workers are "on the road."

A recent review of the literature summarized questions regarding migrant health "to which we find virtually no answers in the peer-reviewed medical literature."[24] Rust identified 40 distinct areas of ignorance, of which several have been mentioned above. Other major lacunae include the following: perinatal outcome data, including birthweight, congenital anomalies, and maternal morbidity/mortality; adequacy of prenatal care; prevalence of chronic diseases; incidence of cancers; pesticide exposure; injuries; dermatitis; obesity; malnutrition; tobacco and alcohol use; other substance abuse; risk factors for AIDS; suicide, homicide, and family violence; immunization status; ulitlization of cancer screening; delays in diagnosis or treatment, and so on.

Data on chronicity in general are lacking. Questions related to low-level, long-term pesticide exposure, occupationally related cancers, and musculoskeletal diseases or disabilities cannot, therefore, be answered with assurance. Wilk[29] enumerates several probable chronic problems caused by pesticide exposure alone, including dermatitis, fatigue, headaches, sleep disturbances, anxiety, disturbances of memory and concentration, cancer, birth defects, sterility, blood disorders, and abnormal liver and kidney function. Moreover, we cannot document illness due to the workplace environment as distinct from illness due to poverty.

Certainly one cause of our ignorance is the lack of provider training in "agrimedicine." Lack of training results in misdiagnoses as well as missed opportunities to ask the relevant questions of patients as part of the history or during examination. For example, an emergency medical technician (EMT) attending an agrimedicine workshop organized by the author recounted an incident in which his ambulance had been called to a field where a worker had collapsed. It was months later, during the workshop, that the EMT realized that the worker had exhibited all the symptoms of acute pesticide poisoning, which were somewhat similar to those of a myocardial infarction for which the EMT had provided first aid. There had never been any training in the recognition and treatment of pesticide poisoning provided to the emergency medical service crews in this agricultural community, nor had the physicians or nurses at the local migrant health center received any similar training. This issue is addressed further at the end of the chapter.

HAZARDS TO MOTHERS, CHILDREN, AND FETUSES

The field labor characteristically performed by migrant and seasonal farm workers presents a wide range of health hazards. In regard to chemical risk factors, a California study[29] found that children of farm workers were four times as likely to have limb defects as the nonfarm population, if both parents were farm workers. (Little as we know about maternal health effects, we know even less about reproductive effects on the male.) Uterine bleeding may be a response to chemical exposure.[29] Both the active and inert ingredients of pesticides may cross the placental barrier and have mutagenic, teratogenic, carcinogenic, or neurotoxic effects. Dehydration, a common risk for field workers, may decrease the effectiveness of the placental barrier and increase fetal exposure to contaminants. Pesticide-caused anemias may also interfere with a normal pregnancy. The effects of such exposures "may not manifest themselves until later in childhood, in adolescence, or even later."[29]

Physiological changes associated with pregnancy may also increase health hazards. For example, changes in lung function increase the risk of inhalation-related illness. Musculoskeletal changes may increase the risk of falls and therefore of miscarriage and prematurity. Occupational fatigue in general—standing, load carrying, repetitive work—carries the risk of accident and injury. Urinary retention as the result of lack of field toilets may lead to urinary tract infections. Unsanitary work conditions can lead to fecal-oral contaminations and diarrhea, anemias, or malnutrition, and to viral infections that cause miscarriages, stillbirths, or congenital defects. Pregnancy itself, as a physiological stress, may trigger symptoms of previously asymptomatic conditions, such as pneumonitis.[29]

Children are at risk both directly, as laborers themselves, and indirectly, as members of migrant families. Infants, for example, can be exposed to toxic agents in breast milk or by skin contact with the mother's skin or clothes. Children are at high risk of pesticide poisoning because of their low body weight, faster metabolism, and potentially long-term exposures. Elevated rates of brain tumors and leukemia have been noted among some migrant children.[29]

The Department of Labor estimated that approximately 400,000 children, ages 8–15, worked in agriculture in 1981.[29] More recently, Pollack reported that 23,500 children a year suffer from nonfatal trauma in agriculture.[23] The Migrant Clinicians' Network estimated that 300 children a year die from work-related injuries in agriculture.[19] These figures apply to all child farm labor and have not been broken down for migrant or seasonal farm workers.

PESTICIDES

As of 1985, there were more than 1,500 active ingredients used in more than 45,000 registered pesticide products on the U.S. market.[7] In 1989, the Government

Accounting Office (GAO) reported to Congress that the Environmental Protection Agency (EPA) had not completed a final assessment of any of the 45,000 pesticide products sold in the U.S., but that they were close to completing three.[31] In addition to the active ingredients, there are inert ingredients that may be highly toxic to humans, such as benzene, carbon tetrachloride, and others. Those are not listed on the warning label because they do not affect the target pest and are considered trade secrets. Rust concluded that the available epidemiological data on pesticide exposure, while poor, suggest links to limb-reduction birth defects, childhood leukemias and brain tumors, adult lymphomas, and lymphosarcomas.[24] Other health problems not already mentioned include spontaneous abortion, sterility, menstrual dysfunction, immune system abnormalities, and various nervous system effects, including motor coordination, thought processes, anxiety, and depression.[31]

Several difficulties in documenting pesticide exposures should be noted. Lack of training of physicians and other medical personnel is negatively reinforced by the lack of a national reporting system for exposures, by the absence of information among farm workers and/or their inability to read labels on pesticide containers, by farm workers' ignorance of the specific pesticides being used in their vicinity, by the reluctance of farm workers to report pesticide poisonings, and by the use of providers in Mexico when they are accessible. Both California and Arizona requires physicians to report all cases of pesticide poisoning within 24 hours. Compliance is poor and, as of early 1990, this appeared to be due to a combination of ignorance of the requirement and resistance to regulation.[26]

Another difficulty in documenting exposure and the effects of specific pesticides is that many different pesticides may be used on one crop in a short period of time. Apples, for example, are treated with a minimum of 12 to 16 chemicals between blooming and storage.[12] The pesticides being used change from year to year and vary from place to place as well as from crop to crop. There is a sort of "folklore" of pesticides among growers such that one grower may discover a particular pesticide to have been especially effective, and this information will be passed along informally, leading to the adoption of the same pesticide by other growers in the vicinity. The same crop, grown in another area, may be treated with different pesticides, depending on the local folklore, as well as manufacturers' recommendations. Thus, adequate documentation of pesticide exposures, requiring the identification of the specific pesticide, may depend on information that is site-specific, crop-specific, time-specific, and pesticide-distributor-specific.

Migrant farm workers are probably at greater risk than others of pesticide poisoning, both acute and chronic, for several reasons. They live close to—and some live in—the fields and therefore may be exposed outside of as well as during working hours. Poor sanitation and water facilities may lead to the use of contaminated water for washing, drinking, and laundering. Lack of laundry facilities may lead to contamination of all family members by clothing. The labor intensive crops with which migrants work also receive heavy pesticide application. Reentry periods— the time after application during which workers may not return to the field or orchard—vary by state and by federal EPA standards and are the subject of much controversy. For example, the EPA reentry interval for azinphos methyl is 24 hours. In California, the state-mandated interval for the same pesticide is 30 days for citrus, 21 days for grapes, and 14 days for peaches, nectarines, and apples.[29]

Workers are exposed to pesticides in several ways. These include direct spraying, both aerial and ground; drift from aerial spraying or windy conditions on the ground; contact with plants; eating or smoking with contaminated hands; eating the fruits or vegetables being harvested without washing them; drinking water from contaminated utensils; drinking, cooking, or bathing with contaminated water; using contaminated leaves as toilet paper; contaminating the genitals with unwashed hands; and wearing contaminated clothing rather than laundering it immediately upon leaving the fields.

We do not know the true pesticide-related mortality or morbidity among farm workers. For reasons already noted—lack of a population denominator, inaccessibility of the population, confounding variable, difficulty in measuring extent of exposure—it is more difficult to gather these data for migrants than for other categories of workers. Given these difficulties, the potential for prevention represented by EPA testing and regulations is all the more important for reducing the health hazards of pesticides.

CANCER

Another article in this issue contains a complete summary of cancer among farmers (p. 335). However, there are no reliable estimates of cancer mortality among migrant and seasonal farm workers.[7] Case-control studies of stable farm populations reported elevated risks for leukemia, Hodgkin's disease, non-Hodgkin's lymphoma, multiple myeloma, and cancers of the lip, stomach, skin, prostate, testis, brain, and connective tissue. Other studies have linked cancers in children to farming and farm labor.[29] None of these studies focuses specifically on migrant workers.

Carcinogenic exposures may have multiple sources.[25] Chemical exposures could include pesticides, fertilizers, solvents, fuels, oil, and welding fumes. Zoonotic viruses and fungi are biological threats, and sunlight is a physiological source. Most attention has been given to the carcinogenicity of pesticides, but even here the data are skimpy. In 1988, the AMA's Council on Scientific Affairs reviewed 53 agricultural chemicals.[6] It determined that two of the 53, arsenicals and vinyl chloride, were carcinogenic; that 13 were probably carcinogenic; and that 16 were possibly carcinogenic, making of a total of 31 suspect chemicals of the 53 reviewed.

The Council report called attention to the extreme frustration inherent in attempts to measure the effects of low level or prolonged exposure. With a latency of 15 to 30 years for chemically induced tumors, "no adverse effect may be apparent until long after the cancer-causing exposure has occurred."[6] In the face of "only conjectural evidence at best that pesticides may be carcinogenic," the Council calls epidemiological studies in humans the "ideal choice."[6] Again, migrants are at risk both because they are exposed to pesticides and because their exposures are the most difficult to document over time.

OTHER HAZARDS

Accidents, infectious diseases, dermatoses, allergic and respiratory conditions, musculoskeletal conditions, and behavioral health issues are covered elsewhere in this publication. Following the principle of "the same, but more so" regarding migrant farm workers, the reader interested in these hazards should consult the other articles in this issue. A few additional words are in order, however, regarding "stoop labor" and musculoskeletal conditions. The disability rate of migrant and seasonal farm workers may be three times that of the general population, much of it due to arthritis and chronic back injury.[29] Heavy physical labor may cause detectable spinal degeneration that develops up to 10 years prematurely.[28]

The short-handled hoe was for many years the nemesis of the migrant farm worker, requiring the worker to bend low in order to cultivate row crops, allowing him to stand only briefly at the end of one row before beginning to work on the next. To stand at any other place in the field, or for any more than a very short time, made the worker easily spotted by the crew leader or foreman and put him at risk of harassment or firing.

The short-handled hoe is now banned in California, Arizona, Texas, and Washington. There is no national ban. Growers seem to have been convinced that longer hoes are as efficient as the short ones, and there are no recent documented reports of use of the latter. Stoop labor, however, continues to be very much a part of the migrant worker experience. The harvesting and packing of melons, cauliflower, broccoli, lettuce, strawberries, and other low-growing vegetables and fruits require low bending for long periods and lifting heavy loads from ground level onto trucks or conveyor belts. There have been no formal studies of the actual work performed by migrant farm workers; e.g., lifting and carrying heavy loads, emptying these loads into trucks, carrying heavy loads up and down ladders, and bending, all of which are likely to exact a heavy physical toll over time.

THE REGULATION OF MIGRANT LABOR

Farm workers are excluded from most labor laws. Only 30 states provide workers' compensation coverage to farm workers. An analysis of all 544 workers' compensation claims paid to Arizona farm workers in 1985 revealed that not one involved pesticide poisoning, even though the authors had considerable anecdotal evidence of such poisonings.[15] The data did confirm the hazardous conditions of farm work due to the use of machines, knives and other tools, lifting of heavy objects, and working on ladders. The weakness of the workers' compensation program lies partly in worker and physician ignorance of the existence of the program, of how the process is initiated, or of how the injury is documented and reported. Growers with access to Mexico are known to have sent injured workers across the border for treatment in order to avoid reporting the injury.[9]

Farms with fewer than 10 employees are exempted from the requirements of the Occupational Safety and Health Act of 1970. Since 85% of migrant and seasonal farm workers work on just such farms, they are not protected by OSHA regulations. Similarly, the Field Sanitation Standard applies to employers of 11 or more. Current laws applying to employers and workers under the OSHA Hazard Communication Standard do not apply (as of 1990) to pesticide use by agricultural employers. In states whose field sanitation regulations do cover many migrants, standards such as the requirement that toilets be placed within one quarter mile of the work area are not as effective as they should be. Workers paid on a piece rate basis, as noted earlier, will avoid a quarter mile long walk as long as possible, whether it be to use a toilet or to drink potable water.

Since 1970, the EPA has had primary responsibility for overseeing and regulating pesticides. Other federal agencies, such as the Department of Agriculture, the Food and Drug Administration, OSHA, and the Consumer Product Safety Commission, are involved in controlling pesticide exposures. According to the AMA Council on Scientific Affairs, all these agencies are fairly consistent in setting permissible limits.[6] Regulation is likely if a substance is expected to cause an increase of more than four cases per 1,000 persons, and it is highly unlikely if the expected increase is less than 1:1,000,000. However, between these limits, cost-effectiveness rules: regulation is likely if the cost of regulation is less than $2,000,000 per life saved.

Under current federal law, only commercial applicators must keep records of their use of restricted use pesticides. Most growers are not required to keep records of their pesticide usage. Eleven states require private applicators to keep some records. Large food processors and growers cooperatives also require records, e.g., Campbell Soup, Heinz, Gerber, Ocean Spray, Del Monte, Vlasic, and Diamond Fruit Growers. Despite the existence of regulations like these, their effect is weakened or even nullified by lax or nonexistent enforcement.[22]

WHAT IS TO BE DONE?

Occupational and preventive medicine can respond in several ways to the challenges of migrant health. The ritual call for more research is only one of those, although this article should make clear that the need for documentation of migrant health status is genuine and urgent. There are other urgent needs as well. Education is indicated for at least three groups: health professionals, farm workers, and growers. Professional education on an inservice and continuing education basis would probably be more effective than injecting brief units, easily forgotten, into the formal curricula of undergraduate and graduate training institutions.

Most providers working in migrant health centers, for example, are family practitioners, pediatricians, or general internists who were originally assigned there by the National Health Service Corps or who decided to work there late in their formal training. Thus, the opportunities to provide relevant training are limited until the provider is actually on-site. Once on-site, however, the educational opportunities should be plentiful. Some migrant health centers provide a formal orientation to "agrimedicine" to their new providers. Content and length seem to be highly variable. There are many benefits to conducting such training on-site. Learning occurs at the point of need—it is immediately relevant. Different types of providers who actually must work cooperatively can be brought together for training, e.g., physicians, nurses, EMTs, and pharmacists. Local conditions can be incorporated into training: types of crops in the area, which determine the types of hazards; specific pesticides in use at the time; and, specific resources available in the area, such as a poison control center, county extension agents, and local and state health departments.

Between 1987 and 1990, two models of continuing education were tested in Arizona. One was centralized and specialized, offering a 4-hour seminar on pesticides to physicians in two urban locations. The seminar was presented by a toxicologist. Turnout in both locations was meager.[14] The other model was decentralized and general, offering a 3-hour agrimedicine workshop on several aspects of farm worker health, with emphasis on pesticides, to a mixed group of providers at several rural locations. Presenters included a family physician with clinical experience in migrant health, the state pesticide coordinator, and the regional director of an insurance company that provides health insurance for migrant workers. The latter model was effective educationally but required considerable manpower resources to plan and conduct. In 1991, the state pesticide coordinator's office will conduct at least one regional pesticide workshop for health professionals.

Because the physicians who actually treat migrant workers are unlikely to be well trained in occupational health, they would benefit from having an occupationally relevant medical history form to guide them. Such a form, the (Arizona)

Farmworker Health History, was developed in both English and Spanish versions. Designed to be completed by the patient, if possible with assistance from clinic staff, the history attempts to elicit information regarding pesticide exposure and other occupationally related health problems over the previous 5 years. The form is then reviewed by the examining physician, who has the opportunity to followup with questions and a more detailed examination, if indicated (see Appendix I).

Growers, too, could benefit from health education. They are insulated in many ways from their workers. Frequently, the grower is not even the legal employer. Instead, a labor contractor, or *contratista*, is contracted by the grower to hire the field workers, who then become the contractor's employees. Nevertheless, it is the grower who ultimately determines working conditions, pesticide use, wages, and health benefits. Growers may be ignorant, either innocently or willfully, of just how bad the workers' living and working conditions are, or of how these conditions affect workers' health. County extension agents, who work closely with growers, could provide agricultural health education along with the latest information on seeds and fertilizers. Occupational health specialists could provide much needed information and training to the staffs of cooperative extension services in all states with land grant institutions.

Education for farm workers is clearly indicated, and here the challenge is great. Some of the conditions of migrancy that make it difficult to provide health care—transience, physical and social isolation, language and cultural differences— also increase the difficulty of providing effective education. A community-based program, utilizing lay educators, informal teaching, and various forms of outreach, might well succeed. Such a program would recruit farm workers and train them to deliver agricultural and general health education. They in turn would recruit other farm workers to attend short classes just before or just after the work day, or would provide information to workers while in the fields or in buses on the way to the fields. This model—"Su Salud Vale Mucho" (Your Health is Worth a Lot)—is derived from a successful prenatal outreach and education program that also targets farm worker families.[18] Such a program would provide occupational and preventive medicine specialists, as well as other health professionals, the important role of "training the trainers." As uninformed as researchers and health professionals still are about migrant health, they have much skill, knowledge, and experience that could benefit the migrant population. The recommendations made here are intended to make the professional reservoirs of knowledge more accessible and more useful to those who need it the most, the people who live and work in the fields.

APPENDIX I

The Arizona Farmworker Health History

Historial Medico del Trabajador Agricola en Arizona

University of Arizona, Rural Health Office

Please answer all questions as fully as possible. If a question does not apply to you, leave it blank. The information you provide us will be used for medical and research purposes only. Your name will be kept strictly confidential.

1. Mother
   (1) Is your mother living? Yes __ No __
   (2) If she is living, how old is she? _____
   (3) If she is dead, how old was she at death? ___
   (4) What caused her death? _____
   (5) Did she ever work in agriculture? _____
   (6) How long? _____

2. Father
   (1) Is your father living? Yes __ No __
   (2) If he is living, how old is he? _____
   (3) If he is dead, how old was he at death? ___
   (4) What caused his death? _____
   (5) Did he ever work in agriculture? _____
   (6) How long? _____

3. Please answer these questions about your children
   (1) Were there any miscarriages? Yes __ No __   (3) Was any child born prematurely? Yes __ No __
   (2) Was any child born dead? Yes __ No __   (4) Did any child die at birth? Yes __ No __
   (5) Was any child born with a birth defect? Yes __ No __

Explain any yes answer_____

4. Where do you work now? _____

5. How long have you worked there?   Years _____ Months _____

6. If retired, what kind of work did you do before you retired?_____

7. (1) Do you live in a camp provided by your employer? Yes __ No __
   (2) Do you live in an apartment or house? Yes __ No __
   (3) Do you have other housing? Yes __ No __

8. How do you get to and from your work?_____

9. Describe what you do on your job: _____

10. (1) In the past five years, have you been around chemicals or pesticides on your job? Yes __ No __
    (2) Have you had any training on the dangers of pesticides and how to handle them properly?
        Yes __ No __
    (3) Check any protection equipment you use on the job:
        Gloves __   Mask __   Special suit over clothes __
        Goggles __   Rubber boots __   Head covering __
        Hearing protection __
        Other_____
    (4) In the past five years, have you been exposed to any of the following?
        Pesticides __   High noise levels __   Fumes and dust __
        Vibration __   Excess heat or cold __   Emotional stress __
        Other_____

11. (1) In the past five years, have you carried or lifted heavy objects as part of your job? Yes __ No __
    (2) Do you have back problems? Yes __ No __ If yes, explain_____

If you HAVE Worked in Farmwork in the Last Five Years, PLEASE CONTINUE ON: IF NOT, STOP HERE.

12. If you have worked on any of these types of farms in the last five years, check the ones you have
    worked on:
      Vegetable or truck farm __   Fruit orchard __   Cotton farm __
      Grain farm __   Animal or dairy farm __ Poultry __
      Other_____

13. In the past five years, have you used the short-handled hoe?   Yes __ No __
    Do you currently use the short-handled hoe?   Yes __ No __

14. In the past five years, have you had any skin rashes or other skin problems?   Yes __ No __

15. In the past five years, have you had any allergies such as asthma or other respiratory problems?
    Yes __ No __

16. At work, where does the water you use for washing your hands come from? Is it:
    Brought to the fields from home __   From a well in the fields __
    Irrigation water at the fields __   From some other source __
                                                Don't know __

17. At work, where does your drinking water come from? Is it:
    Brought to the fields from home __   From a well in the fields __
    Irrigation water at the fields __   From some other source __
                                                Don't know __

18. Are there toilets near where you work?   Yes __ No __
    If yes, are they close enough for you?   Yes __ No __

19. Is there any particular hazard or part of your job that you think has caused your health problems?
    Yes __ No __
    If yes, explain:_____

20. Have you ever been injured at work?   Yes __ No __
    If yes, explain:_____

21. In the past five years, what different kinds of work have you done? (For example: weeding lettuce,
    packing melons, cutting broccoli.)
    _____
    _____
    _____

22. Add anything else you want to tell us:_____
    _____
    _____

THANK YOU FOR YOUR COOPERATION

```
— FOR OFFICE USE ONLY —          Date: _____        Site ID No.: _____

Patient/Family ID No.: _____

Chief Complaint: 1. _____     Treatment:  1. _____
2. _____           2. _____
3. _____           3. _____

Assessment:  1. _____
2. _____
3. _____
```

HISTORIAL MEDICO DEL TRABAJADOR AGRICOLA EN ARIZONA

Universidad de Arizona, Oficina de Salud Rural

Por favor, conteste las siguientes preguntas tan completo como le sea posible. Si alguna de las preguntas no aplica a usted, deje el espacio en blanco. La información que usted está dando será usada con el único fin de investigación medica y científica. Su nombre sera estrictamente confidencial.

1. Madre
   (1) ¿Vive su madre? Sí __ No __
   (2) ¿Si vive su madre, que edad tiene? _____
   (3) ¿Si esta muerta, a que edad murió? _____
   (4) ¿Cuál fue la causa de su muerte? _____
   (5) ¿Trabajó alguna vez en la agricultura?
       Sí __ No __
   (6) ¿Por cuánto tiempo? _____

2. Padre
   (1) ¿Vive su padre? Sí __ No __
   (2) ¿Si vive su padre, que edad tiene? _____
   (3) ¿Si esta muerto, a que edad murió? _____
   (4) ¿Cuál fue la causa de su muerte? _____
   (5) ¿Trabajó alguna vez en la agricultura?
       Sí __ No __
   (6) ¿Por cuánto tiempo? _____

3. Por favor, conteste las siguientes preguntas sobre sus hijos.
   (1) ¿Hubo algun mal parto (aborto)? Sí __ No __   (4) ¿Murió durante el nacimento algun hijo?
   (2) ¿Nació muerta algun hijo? Sí __ No __   Sí __ No __
   (3) ¿Nació prematuro algun hijo? Sí __ No __   (5) ¿Nació alguno de sus hiijos con un defecto?
                                                                        Sí __ No __

Si es así, explique: _____

4. ¿Actualmente dónde trabaja? _____

5. ¿Cuánto tiempo tiene trabajando alli? Años _____ Meses _____

6. Si esta jubilado, ¿en que trabajaba antes de jubilarse? _____

7. (1) ¿Vive usted en alojamiento del dueño del campo? Sí __ No __
   (2) ¿Vive usted en apartemento o casa? Sí __ No __
   (3) ¿Vive usted en otra clase de vivienda? Sí __ No __

8. ¿Qué medio de transporta usa para ir y venir de su trabajo? _____

9. ¿Qué hace en su trabajo? _____

10. (1) ¿En los últimos cinco años ha tenido contacto con productos químicos o insecticidas en su trabajo? Sí __ No __
    (2) ¿Ha tenido entrenamiento acerca de los peligros y el manejo de los insecticidas? Sí __ No __
    (3) Indique que equipo de seguridad usa en su trabajo:
        Guantes __   Máscara __   Traje especial sobre la ropa __
        Botas de hule __   Cubierta para la cabeza __   Espejuelos/gafas protectoras __
        Protección para los oídos __
        Otro _____
    (4) En los últimos cinco años ha estado expuesto a cualquiera de los siguientes:
        Insecticidas __   Altos niveles de ruido __   Vapores/gases y polvo __
        Vibraciones __   Temperaturas extremamente   Tensión emocional __
                                altos o bajos __
        Otro _____

11. (1) ¿En los últimos cinco años ha levantando o cargado objetos/cosas pesadas en su trabajo?
        Sí __ No __
    (2) ¿Tiene problemas de la espalda? Sí __ No __ Si es así, explique _____

Si usted ha trabajado en el campo en los últimos cinco años favor de continuar; si no, no conteste las siguientes preguntas.

12. Indique si en los últimos cinco años ha trabajado en cualquiera de los siguientes:

    Finca de vegetales/verduras or camiónes __   Huerta de fruta __
    Finca de animales or lechería __   Finca de algodón __
    Finca de grano/cereal __   Finca de aves de corral __
    Otro _____

13. ¿En los últimos cinco años ha usado "el cortito?" Sí __ No __
    ¿Actualmente, usa "el cortito?" Sí __ No __

14. ¿En los últimos años has teenido erupciones en la piel u otros problemas en la piel? Sí __ No __

15. ¿En los últimos cinco años ha tenido problemas alérgicos tales como asma u otra clase de problemas respiratorios? Sí __ No __

16. Cuándo está trabajando, ¿de dónde viene el agua que use para lavarse las manos? Es:

    Traída de los campos desde la casa __   De una noria/pozo en los campos __
    Agua de riego en los campos __   De alguna otra fuente __
                                                     No sabe __

17. Cuándo está trabajando, ¿de dónde viene el agua que tome? Es:

    Traída de los campos desde la casa __   De una noria/pozo en los campos __
    Agua de riego en los campos __   De alguna otra fuente __
                                                     No sabe __

18. Hay baños/excusados cerca de su trabajo? Sí __ No __
    Si es así, estan batante cerca de usted? Sí __ No __

19. Hay algún riesgo o parte de su trabajo que puede ser la causa de sus problemas de salud?
    Sí __ No __
    Si es así, explique _____

20. Se ha lastimado en el trabajo? Sí __ No __
    Si es así, explique _____

21. En los últimos cinco años, que trabajos ha desempeñado? (Por ejemplo: deshierbando lechuga, empacando melones or cortando broculi.)

    _____
    _____
    _____

22. Alguna otra cosa que le gustaría mencionar:

    _____
    _____
    _____

Muchas Gracias Para Su Cooperación

--- FOR OFFICE USE ONLY ---   Date: _____   Site ID No.: _____

Patient/Family ID No.: _____

Chief Complaint: 1. _____   Treatment: 1. _____
2. _____   2. _____
3. _____   3. _____

Assessment: 1. _____
2. _____
3. _____

REFERENCES

1. A Continuing Harvest of Shame: Conditions Facing Migrant Farmworkers in 1990. Washington, DC, Farmworkers Justice Fund, 1990.
2. Abrams HK: The short-handled hoe: Ergonomics comes to the farmworker. Occupational Health and Safety News 2(2):1–4, 1986.
3. Carlson ML, Petersen GR: Mortality of California agricultural workers. J Occup Med 20:30–32, 1978.
4. Chase HP, Kumar V, Dodds JM, et al: Nutritional status of preschool Mexican American migrant farm children. Am J Dis Child 122:316–324, 1971.
5. Cordes DH, Rea DF: Health hazards of farming. Am Fam Phys 38:233–244, 1988.
6. Council on Scientific Affairs: Cancer risk of pesticides in agricultural workers. JAMA 260:959–966, 1988.
7. Coye MJ: The health effects of agricultural production. I. The health of agricultural workers. J Public Health Policy 6:349–370, 1985.
8. de Zapién JG: Personal communication.
9. de Zapién JG, Meister JS, LaBrec PA: Where have all the farmworkers gone? Working paper no. 1. Tucson, AZ, Southwest Border Rural Health Research Center, 1988.
10. Dunbar A, Kravitz L: Hard Traveling: Migrant Farm Workers in America. Cambridge, MA, Ballinger Publishing Company, 1976.
11. Estrada AL, Treviño FM, Ray LA: Health care utilization barriers among Mexican Americans: Evidence from HHANES 1982–84. Am J Public Health 80(suppl):27–31, 1990.
12. Finch G: Farmworkers and pesticide exposure in the apple orchards. Farmworker Justice News 4(2):2–3, 1990.
13. Goldsmith MF: As farmworkers help keep America healthy, illness may be their harvest. JAMA 261:3207–3213, 1989.
14. LaBrec PA: Personal communication.
15. LaBrec PA, Meister JS, de Zapién JG: Arizona farmworkers and workers' compensation. Working Paper No. 3. Tucson, AZ, Southwest Border Rural Health Research Center, 1988.
16. Meister JS, de Zapién JG, LaBrec PA: The Arizona Farmworker Health History and Data Base. Working Paper No. 2. Tucson, AZ, Southwest Border Rural Health Research Center, 1988.
17. Meister JS: Report on site visits to migrant health centers and evaluation of progress on migrant referral network. Tucson, AZ, University of Arizona, 1991 (unpublished).
18. Meister JS, Warrick LH, Wood AH, et al: Using lay workers: Case study of a prenatal outreach, education and advocacy program. J Community Health (in press).
19. Migrant Clinicians Network, Occupational Health Subcommittee: Migrant Health Newsline Clinical Supplement 7(3):1–4, 1990.
20. Migrant Health Program Target Population Estimates. Rockville, MD, U.S. Department of Health and Human Services, 1980.
21. National Center for Health Statistics: Births, marriages, divorces, and deaths for 1988. Monthly Vital Statistics Report 37(12):13–14, 1988.
22. Pesticide Regulation: Report to the Arizona Legislature. Phoenix, AZ, Office of the Auditor General, 1990.
23. Pollack SH: Health hazards of agricultural child labor. Migrant Health Newsline Clinical Supplement 7(3):1–4, 1990.
24. Rust GS: Health status of migrant farmworkers: A literature review and commentary. Am J Public Health 80:1213–1217, 1990.
25. Schenker M: Agricultural occupations and cancer. San Francisco, University of California (unpublished).
26. Selvey D: Personal communication.
27. Slesinger D, Christensen B: Health and mortality of migrant farm children. Soc Sci Med 23(1):65–74, 1986.
28. Wickstrom G: Effect of work on degenerative back disease: A review. Scand J Work Environ Health 4:1–12, 1978.
29. Wilk VA: The Occupational Health of Migrant and Seasonal Farmworkers in the United States, 2nd ed. Washington, DC, Farmworkers Justice Fund, 1986.
30. Wilk VA: Occupational Health of Migrant and Seasonal Farmworkers in the US: Progress Report. Washington, DC, Farmworker Justice Fund, 1988.
31. Wilk VA: Farmworkers and the health risks of pesticides. Farmworker Justice News 4(2):3–4, 1990.

PAUL A. JAMES, MD
RICKY L. LANGLEY, MD, MPH

USING THE COOPERATIVE EXTENSION SERVICE IN AGRICULTURAL HEALTH EDUCATION

From the Department of Preventive
Medicine and Public Health
Policy (RLL) and
Department of Family Medicine
(PAJ)
East Carolina University School
of Medicine
Greenville, North Carolina

Reprint requests to:
Ricky L. Langley, MD, MPH
Department of Preventive Medicine
and Public Health Policy
East Carolina University School
of Medicine
Greenville, NC 27858-4354

Agriculture is one of the oldest yet one of the least studied occupational industries. Agrarian life has been a part of man's existence for several thousand years. Yet, over the last 100 years enormous changes in agricultural production have increased the ability of farmers to feed larger numbers of the population. In 1910, the average farmer could feed little more than his immediate family. However, in the 1990s, American farmers, who are less than 2% of the population, feed not only all of America but export significantly to foreign countries. This highlights the success of enhanced production in agriculture. Science and technology have played a significant role in this success through the use of fertilizers, pesticides, genetic engineering, and technological mechanization.

However, the use of these important advances has caused an increased risk of injuries and chronic illness. Agriculture has one of the highest mortality rates of all occupations.[7] Its morbidity rate is also significant. Attempts at improving the health of agricultural workers have been difficult and have not fit easily into traditional medical models.

The agricultural industry presents multiple barriers to improved health care. These barriers include geographic isolation, poor access to health care services, lower socioeconomic status, diversity of agricultural practices, language barriers, social barriers, cultural barriers, and racial barriers. Agricultural workers have varied educational backgrounds, and the work force is often transient. Finally, no medical specialty considers the problems of agricultural and rural health to be directly within its domain.

The agricultural work force can only experience improved health through the use of preventive medicine. The most important tool in preventive medicine is education. The Cooperative Extension Service (CES) serves an integral role in educating the agricultural and rural population, especially in the use of science and technology to improve agricultural production. In North Carolina, the East Carolina University–North Carolina State University (ECU-NCSU) Agromedicine Program has found the CES to be an integral part of health education in its attempts to improve agricultural health. This chapter will discuss the benefits of using the CES to improve the health education and the health status of the agricultural population.

THE HISTORY OF COOPERATIVE EXTENSION

The CES was established in 1914, with the enactment of the Smith-Lever Act, to develop a nationwide extension network of field educators to work with rural people in their communities, homes, and farms.[10] These educators were to serve as liaisons between the local population and land grant colleges, with support from the United States Department of Agriculture. The initial focus of the CES would be upon improved agricultural production, home economics, the status of youth, and related subjects. Planning and development of these educational programs would be based at the state level rather than the federal level.[12] The CES has traditionally divided responsibilities between agricultural extension and home economics extension.

The CES is a unique educational organization that receives financial support from three levels of government: state, federal, and local. The agricultural extension service has close ties to land grant universities and serves as a bridge between rural citizens and researchers at these universities, as well as scientists at the United States Department of Agriculture. Additionally, the CES receives support from commodity and farm organizations, agribusinesses, foundations, and individuals.

Every county in the United States is served by a local agricultural extension agent who is the link to university specialists. These specialists provide the scientifically based information people require to solve their local problems. Each extension office develops lay leaders who are involved in the Extension Advisory Leadership System. These lay leaders inform university researchers and extension professionals of local concerns and issues, thus placing the extension office in a position to provide two-way communication between local citizens and a university system.

The CES educates local rural citizens through several mechanisms. One-on-one consultations are the most frequent and personal tool. Meetings, workshops, and seminars are useful for larger audiences. Printed brochures and fact sheets are distributed for more mass communication. Finally, the Extension Advisory Leadership System is available to disseminate information within communities.

The success of the CES, especially in production agriculture, can be attributed to two salient features of the system. First is flexibility in adapting to the local needs.[4] The firm belief of the CES in involving its constituents in program planning requires constant reassessment of program objectives. Secondly, the CES provides a delivery system that extends into every county in the nation. This network provides a valuable resource for dissemination of information.

From early in its development, health has been a component of CES outreach. The most visible component early on was through one of the four points of its youth program under 4-H ("head, heart, hands, and health"). In the 1940s, many states placed increasing emphasis on health, especially in the context of rural health and improved access to care. Nebraska and Ohio developed full-time specialists in rural health.[5] These early specialists realized the need for facilitators to network between farm organizations, health departments, and medical societies. However, the conservatism of the 1950s brought a decline in the activities of rural health in the extension service. By the 1960s and 1970s, the CES witnessed increasing interests both from within its structure and from the public to become more active in health. In 1971, the Extension Committee on Organization and Policy began to study the CES's role in health education. Many of the policies drawn up were approved in 1974.[13] The home economics extension arm of the CES has focused more on health issues such as nutrition counseling and health access. More recently, the agricultural extension arm of the CES has shown interest in agricultural health education such as farm safety.

AGROMEDICINE UTILIZES THE COOPERATIVE EXTENSION MODEL

In response to concerns about pesticide management in third-world countries, the National Academy of Sciences recommended the development of an agromedical team as a multidisciplined approach to solving problems.[9] This team was to use and share the expertise not only of agricultural professionals, but of health professionals, epidemiologists, nurses, statisticians, economists, and environmental scientists. To develop solutions to the health-related problems of agriculture, cooperation among divergent disciplines was the key. The agromedicine concept strongly incorporated this tenet into its philosophy of problem-solving in agricultural medicine.

Dr. Stanley Schuman, at the Medical University of South Carolina, initiated the agromedicine concept when forming the South Carolina Agromedicine Program, a cooperative venture with Clemson University. This program first developed agricultural and health care professionals as equal partners. Secondly, the program used an extension model of university outreach to rural and agricultural areas. This was accomplished by encouraging local private physicians to cooperate as volunteers with extension agents in each county as Agromedicine Program Consulting Physicians.

The Cooperative Extension Model served as a useful tool to the medical community as a method for medical university outreach. The CES provided access for health care professionals to isolated groups that often had little trust in the medical profession. Additionally, by working with the CES, health care professionals were more able to deploy state and community resources. The Cooperative Extension Model provided an established agent in each community to assist local physicians in educational outreach.

The CES has access not only to farmers but farm families and wives, who oftentimes control the health practices of their families. Table 1 highlights the different assets and liabilities of involving different organizations in agricultural health education.[2]

THE NORTH CAROLINA EXPERIENCE

Agriculture has a major influence on the economy of North Carolina. In 1987, farmers received over 4.9 billion dollars in cash receipts from farming. The

TABLE 1. Assets and Liabilities of Selected Agencies for the Conduct of Health Education Programs

Organization	Asset	Liability
Official health agencies	1. Legal authority in field 2. Broad knowledge of health problems 3. Ability to consider facts, make decisions, and organize action 4. Built-in base for coordination of variety	1. Political limitations 2. Frequent lack of flexibility 3. Fragmentation of service 4. Frequently viewed as service for indigents
Voluntary health agencies	1. Knowledge of special subject matter 2. Local contacts 3. Speed of response 4. Capacity to influence decision-makers in relation to special subject 5. Network of volunteers for policies and service	1. Uncertainties of funding 2. Narrow specialization
Cooperative Extension Service	1. Capacity to reach all socio-economic levels 2. Facility for outreach, especially to rural persons 3. Continuing local contacts and access to total family 4. Professional-volunteer relationship 5. Primary function of education 6. Access to university resources and ability to bring them to local level	1. Lack of medical knowledge base 2. Lack of staff trained in health 3. Tradition of heavy involvement in non-health educational work
Medical schools	1. Technical knowledge 2. Well-trained manpower	1. Lack of local contacts 2. Frequent lack of ability to work with local community
Churches and civic groups	1. Flexibility 2. Capacity for fundraising	1. Lack of knowledge of health 2. Lack of staff trained in health

From Johnston HL, Crawford C: Potentials for interstate, interagency cooperation. In D'Onofrio C, Wang VL (eds): Cooperative Rural Health Education. Thorofare, NJ, C.B. Slack, 1975, p 41, with permission.

value of agriculture, forestry, and fishery enterprises totaled more than one fourth of North Carolina's gross income.[14] Agriculture in North Carolina is heavily diversified, producing over 60 commodities, which are processed into numerous food and fiber products.

Injuries and illnesses in North Carolina agricultural workers have recently attracted the attention of various agencies within the state. In 1987, the North Carolina Department of Labor reported the incidence of occupational injuries and illnesses in the agriculture, forestry, and fishery industries to be 8.3 per 100 full-time workers. In 1988, the rate of agricultural injury increased by 18% to 9.8 per 100 full-time workers.[11] This compares to an injury and illness rate of 7.8 per 100 full-time workers in all North Carolina industries for 1988.

Recently, a North Carolina Farm and Rural Life Study conducted by North Carolina State University evaluated a random sample of farm operators in North Carolina on health-related issues. Approximately 10% of respondents stated that they or a family member had been injured on the farm seriously enough to miss a day's work or schooling, or to require a visit to a doctor. Eighteen percent of operators reported experiencing a chronic problem that occasionally interfered with work or recreational activities.[6] A study of occupational fatalities in North Carolina from 1984 through 1988 identified 123 individuals accidentally killed performing an agriculturally related activity on the farm. Nearly 20% of the victims had been consuming alcohol. The rate of unintentional occupational fatalities in North Carolina for this period was 41 per 100,000 agricultural workers.[1] This is more than twice the rate of 18 per 100,000 workers reported by the National Traumatic Occupational Fatality Survey for North Carolina for the period 1980 through 1985.[8] Major efforts are currently underway in North Carolina to increase the level of awareness of agricultural injuries and illnesses among farm workers, extension agents, and health personnel. Some of these activities are described.

Health Education

East Carolina University School of Medicine is located in a rural region with a large agricultural work force. A specific mission of the school is to produce primary care physicians to serve in rural counties. The medical school has embarked on a goal of introducing rural and agricultural health early in the medical curriculum.

First-year medical students take, in addition to the traditional basic science courses, a primary care conference series on topics related to clinical medicine. During this conference students are introduced to the areas of occupational medicine, rural health, and agricultural injuries and illnesses. As part of this orientation to clinical medicine, the medical students undertake a field trip to local farms or agribusinesses. Agricultural extension agents help select the site, with cooperation from farmers, and guide the students to potential hazards while on the site visit. They also explain and demonstrate the use of safety devices on farm equipment. Thus, first-year medical students are introduced to some of the hazards of agricultural employment that lead to potential injuries or illnesses that they may encounter during their clinical years.

During the family medicine clerkship in the third year, students are expected to visit a farm or agribusiness at their assigned rotation. This rotation involves practitioners in outlying counties throughout North Carolina who serve as preceptors for medical students during a 4-week period. Under the direction of an agricultural extension agent or their medical preceptor, students visit a farm or agribusiness to discuss agricultural health topics. Prior to the site visit, students are given a 1-hour didactic session on agricultural illnesses and injuries. The students are provided a check list that covers topics related to farm safety, and they are given instructions on how farmers may decrease their own risk of injury or illness. After the site visit, the students discuss with the farmer any concerns that they may have regarding farm safety. At the end of the rotation, all students are brought together to discuss their site visits and the usefulness of these visits to future patient care.

Agricultural professionals of the North Carolina Cooperative Extension Service have assisted physicians at two continuing medical education conferences in North Carolina. Participants at the 1990 Family Medicine Update on "Rural Health Care and Agrimedicine" heard the state associate director of agricultural extension discuss "The Agricultural Extension Agent—A Role in Rural Health."

Additionally, the CES assisted in presenting a model for university outreach to teachers of family medicine on "A Cooperative Extension Model for Serving the Rural Underserved."

The ECU–NCSU Agromedicine Program has involved cooperating physicians and agricultural professionals in several educational programs within the state. Farmers, agricultural extension agents, health department officials, and nurses have benefitted from attending educational programs having speakers from different disciplines such as family medicine, occupational medicine, and farm safety. The ECU–NCSU Agromedicine Program has stimulated coalition building with other groups in North Carolina interested in agricultural health. Examples of activities involving the CES include: conducting a workshop on agricultural health in conjunction with the North Carolina Department of Environment, Health and Natural Resources; participation in the 1991 Governor's Conference on Rural Health; and participation in the North Carolina Farm Workers Annual Conference sponsored by the North Carolina Primary Care Association and the Migrant Council. Additionally, farm safety specialists have participated in training emergency medical technicians in farm machinery extrication programs.

As noted from the above activities, the CES is playing a larger role in agricultural health education in North Carolina. The CES also is involved in research activities that not only affect the health of farm families but also benefit citizens in urban and rural areas.

Role of the Cooperative Extension Service: Service and Research

During 1990, North Carolina received two grants from the National Institute of Occupational Safety and Health (NIOSH) to evaluate agricultural health issues in the state. One grant was for the development of an Agricultural Health Promotion System through the CES of North Carolina. The second grant was to develop a reporting system for agricultural injuries and illnesses in North Carolina using health departments and nurses in selected counties.

The Agricultural Health Promotion System grant fosters the joint participation of the land grant universities (North Carolina State University and North Carolina Agricultural and Technical State University at Greensboro) and the CES as well as the East Carolina University School of Medicine, in the development of health educational material. Other goals of this program are to develop training programs in health promotion for agricultural extension agents, to provide continuing education on agricultural issues of importance to health professionals in North Carolina, and to conduct statewide training sessions on agricultural health awareness for farmers and their families through the CES. The second grant will employ nurses and local health departments to collect epidemiologic information on agricultural injuries and illnesses in several counties with strong agricultural bases. The nurses will spend several days with cooperative extension agents in order to learn more about farm equipment and farm operations. Extension agents will also report injuries or illnesses they may discover to the occupational health nurses. Accident investigations may also be conducted by both groups.

The long-term goals of both grants are to increase the awareness and knowledge of cooperative extension agents, students engaged in an agricultural field of study, medical students, practicing physicians, and farmers and their families in areas of hazard awareness, farm safety, and health promotion.

The North Carolina CES has recently entered into a cooperative relationship with the North Carolina Department of Environment, Health and Natural

Resources and the East Carolina University Community Health Advocacy Program (ECUCHAP). The goal of ECUCHAP is to improve the health and well-being of individuals in medically underserved areas. ECUCHAP helps identify and train community leaders to develop local community health advocacy programs. The ECUCHAP leaders advise their neighbors on local resources and services available in order to improve the health care within the community.

The CES and the local health departments serve as co-coordinators in development of local community health advocacy programs. The CES offers leadership skills, community program development and training materials, technical consultation, and support. Currently, approximately 30 of 100 counties in North Carolina are involved and the program is expanding. Local community health advocacy programs often choose health issues as community projects and thus contribute to the revitalization of the rural communities.

The CES is involved in research and service to local communities through its educational programs. Applied research may be in the form of a demonstration project to determine the practicality of a new technology before it is disseminated widely. The service component is usually the ability of CES agents to organize and mobilize local citizens to solve a particular community problem. Services through cooperative extension may involve water testing for agrichemicals, plant and insect identification for toxicity, plant disease identification, and economic and budgetary management assistance. These services enable the extension agents to educate their clients as well as assess results of the educational effort. They attempt to assess the appropriate use of biotechnology and ensure sound cultural practices.

COOPERATIVE EXTENSION IN INTERSTATE AGRICULTURAL HEALTH EDUCATION

North Carolina has been active in the development of an agromedicine consortium with other southeastern states. Led by the activities of the South Carolina Agromedicine Program, the Southeast Agromedicine Interuniversity Consortium (SEAMIUC) was formed in 1988. The East Carolina University School of Medicine and the North Carolina State University College of Agriculture and Life Sciences have been active participants since its inception. The CES has played an integral role in the organization's development. The SEAMIUC preamble describes itself as "an affiliation of faculty representing southeastern schools of agriculture, medicine, nursing, public health and veterinary medicine who have organized to share through a multidisciplinary approach their expertise and resources in public service, education and research for the enhancement of agricultural medicine within their states and region."

Meetings have been held biannually and alternate between medical and agricultural campuses to foster improved cooperation. The CES has been active in all phases of consortium development. Local agricultural extension agents are often invited to regional meetings to discuss perceived health problems. Roundtable discussions between physicians and agricultural professionals are common, and solutions often incorporate cooperative extension concepts.

Programs at the SEAMIUC meetings have highlighted agricultural and health issues of the host state. Common problems of southeastern agriculture allow other states to share proposed solutions. Bringing together the often divergent disciplines of agriculture and medicine forces participants to view problems from a different perspective. Solutions are often found in unexpected places.

One example is the epidemic of skin cancer among southeastern farmers. Skin cancer is frequently caused by overexposure to the sun's ultraviolet radiation. At a recent SEAMIUC meeting, physicians discussed the high incidence of this disease among farmers, especially of the face, head, neck, and ears. A discussion of the benefits of wide-brimmed hats to protect the skin ensued. Farmers wear minimal solar protection and are frequently not educated as to the risks of chronic sun exposure. Two state Cooperative Extension Services planned activities to ensure that agents were alerted to the problem. Many agents in these states now wear wide-brimmed straw hats and explain to farmers the benefits of their use, thus providing effective role models for healthful practices.

PROs AND CONs OF UTILIZING THE COOPERATIVE EXTENSION SERVICE

The North Carolina experience of health care professionals as equal partners in health education with the CES has demonstrated many benefits. It has opened lines of communication between two distinct scientific groups. This has fostered a sense of understanding and cooperation. It has provided an avenue to disseminate health-related education to agricultural workers. It has built credibility and trust between two professions that at times may have diverging agendas. It has provided avenues for education by adding credibility to health research among those who are engaged in production agriculture. It has demonstrated that distinct disciplines can work toward a common goal.

However, there may be barriers to working with any established organization such as the CES. It is important to understand these barriers so that more effective cooperation may result. First, tradition is often a problem with any established organization. However, the CES has been eager to assist in educating their constituents regarding safe agricultural practices. Many counties in North Carolina have incorporated within their 5-year plans topics on agromedicine.

A second potential barrier is the lack of specialized knowledge outside of one's area of training. Cooperation may be inhibited by emphasis on separate goals. Trust between the two groups must be built early by focusing on common goals. A third barrier is concern with documenting each organization's contributions. It is important to focus on problem-solving, involving all parties rather than fostering one side or another.

Finally, the most pressing barrier is the fear of loss of identity among constituents.[3] It is important for health care professionals to realize that the CES wears many hats and that health education is only one goal. By keeping in focus the organization's total agenda, appropriate cooperation and planning may be obtained.

SUMMARY

In summary, the North Carolina experience of cooperation and health education using the Cooperative Extension Service has been very successful. Agriculture and medicine have found a common ground where responsibilities can be shared. By discovering the special capabilities and contributions of the Cooperative Extension Service, medical professionals may more closely address preventive medicine in an agricultural setting.

Acknowledgements. The authors would like to thank Linda Loud, Mitch Smith, Barbara Garland, Ph.D., and Roger Crickenberger, Ph.D. for their assistance. Special thanks to Brenda Howard who assisted with manuscript preparation.

REFERENCES

1. Bernhardt J, Langley R: Farm Fatalities in North Carolina, 1984–1988. Journal of Rural Health 1991 (in press).
2. Crawford C, Johnston HL: Potentials for interstate, interagency cooperation. In D'Onofrio C, Wang VL (eds): Cooperative Rural Health Education. Thorofare, NJ, C.B. Slack, 1975, p 41.
3. Crawford C, Johnston HL: Potentials for interstate, interagency cooperation. In D'Onofrio C, Wang VL (eds): Cooperative Rural Health Education. Thorofare, NJ, C.B. Slack, 1975, p. 42.
4. Hildreth RJ: Preparing for tomorrow: Heritage horizons. Journal of Extension, 1976, p 230.
5. Johnston HL: Health education in the extension service: A historical perspective. In D'Onofrio C, Wang VL (eds): Cooperative Rural Health Education. Thorofare, NJ, C.B. Slack, 1975, pp 16–17.
6. Lilley S, Collender R, Schorman M, Lloyd J: North Carolina Farm Survey. Raleigh, NC, Agricultural Extension Publication, 1988.
7. National Safety Council: Accident Facts. Chicago, 1989.
8. National Traumatic Occupational Fatalities: 1980–1985. U.S. Dept. of Health & Human Services: CDC NIOSH. Cincinnati, OH, 1989.
9. Public Health Study Team: Pest control and public health. In Pest Control: An Assessment of Present and Alternative Technologies, Vol. V. Washington, D.C., National Academy of Sciences Press, 1976, pp 231–232.
10. Rasmussen WD: Taking the University to the People. Ames, IA, Iowa State University Press, 1989, p 3.
11. Research and Statistics Division, North Carolina Department of Labor: Occupational Injuries and Illnesses in North Carolina, 1988. Raleigh, NC, North Carolina Department of Labor, 1991.
12. Snyder LJ: Rural health education: An idea whose time has come. In D'Onofrio C, Wang VL (eds): Cooperative Rural Health Education. Thorofare, NJ, C.B. Slack, 1975, pp 2–3.
13. Vines CA: New thrust for the cooperative extension. In D'Onofrio C, Wang VL (eds): Cooperative Rural Health Education. Thorofare, NJ, C.B. Slack, 1975, pp 36–37.
14. Walden ML: Measuring the Economic Size of the North Carolina Agriculture/Life Sciences/ Food, Textile and Forestry Sectors. Economics Information Report #80. Raleigh, NC, Dept. of Economics and Business, College of Agriculture and Life Sciences, North Carolina State University. Sept, 1989.

JAMES A. MERCHANT, MD, DrPH

AGRICULTURAL INJURIES

From the Institute of Agricultural
  Medicine and Occupational
  Health
The University of Iowa
Iowa City, Iowa

Reprint requests to:
James A. Merchant, MD
Director, Institute of Agricultural
  Medicine and Occupational
  Health
The University of Iowa
Iowa City, IA 52242

The epidemic of agricultural injuries in the United States is an important part of a much larger increase in rural injury morbidity and mortality. It is now clear from the epidemiological data available that the risk of injury and traumatic death is significantly higher in rural areas than urban areas. Baker[1] analyzed death rates from unintentional injuries (population at risk was 51.6 million rural nonremote and 9.0 million remote) for the years 1977–1979 and found a combined mortality rate of 75 per 100,000 for rural areas, over twice the rate for the largest cities (37 per 100,000). The highest mortality rates, which were the same for motor vehicle and nonmotor vehicle deaths, were highest in the remote rural areas. Other national statistics come from National Safety Council estimates that are based on reports from city and state traffic authorities.[14] Of the 48,700 total motor vehicle deaths in 1987, 31,200 were classified as rural; many of these were the result of a noncollision. Analyses of the National Highway Traffic Safety Administration's Fatal Accident Reporting System (FARS) during the period 1979–1981 found that mortality was inversely associated with population density and per capita income ($p < .0001$).[2] These authors suggest that a variety of factors may explain this strong inverse correlation with population density and income—including higher travel speed in rural areas, poorer roads, less seat-belt use, more use of high-risk utility vehicles and travel in open pick up trucks, and poorer access to trauma care.

A disproportionate share of poor people live in rural areas and account for a third of America's poor.[17] Of the 45 million nonelderly rural residents, 8.3 million live in poverty with a family income of less than $11,600 for a family of four. One out of every five rural residents is poor. As a result, rural residents are less able to afford insurance coverage. Rural residents are also more likely to be employed in agriculture and small businesses, both of which are associated with higher injury rates and neither of which offers insurance coverage as often as urban industries. In addition, Medicaid coverage tends to be less prevalent in rural areas due to variations in coverage policy between states.[17] Lack of insurance contributes a further barrier to seeking medical care for rural injuries. Although good data are not available for nontransportation injury mortality in rural areas, it is likely that many of the factors that contribute to the high rate of rural motor vehicle deaths and injuries similarly contribute to the increase in nontransportation rural injury and death.

At particular risk to rural injury are farmers, farm family members who are exposed to agricultural production, and other agricultural workers. Because of varying definitions of agriculture and the current lack of complete 1990 U.S. Census statistics, the number and distribution of this population at risk is not precisely defined. It is estimated that this population is between 12 and 15 million and is divided among individuals with sole farm income, those with some farm income, additional farm family members, and hired farm workers.[12] This relatively small work force produces America's food and fiber for both domestic consumption and export, and provides the backbone of the rural community infrastructure. Culturally, America's farming population is regarded as independent, responsible, self-reliant, and industrious. Hence, America's farm families contribute significantly to both the economic and social fabric of rural America. Nevertheless, until recently the epidemic of rural and agricultural injuries had been largely ignored by both federal and state governments.[12]

EPIDEMIOLOGY

In addition to the several factors that place rural residents at increased risk are added the occupational risk factors of farming. The National Safety Council estimated farm resident deaths to be 56.2 per 100,000, 30.1 of which were motor vehicle related, 20.1 work related (18.1 in farm work), 8.0 home related, and 4.0 public nonmotor vehicle related deaths.[14] Available epidemiologic data show that agricultural work, relative to other occupations, is consistently associated with a high risk for traumatic death and injury. Mortality rates vary from those calculated by NIOSH from its National Traumatic Occupational Fatalities (NTOF) data base, which reports 20.7 deaths per 100,000 agricultural workers versus 7.9 deaths per 100,000 for the general private sector workforce, to that calculated by the National Safety Council (49 deaths per 100,000 agricultural workers versus 10 for all industries).[14] Based on these data, the mortality rate for agriculture is now the highest of any industrial sector. The 1987 rate for mining and quarrying was 38 per 100,000 and that for construction 35 per 100,000. Reasons for differences between the NIOSH and NSC rates relate to differences in definitions, differing sources of data, classification differences, differences in denominators, and questions of certainty as to whether the fatal injury occurred at work.

There are some National Center for Health Statistics (NCHS) mortality data that is based on the farm as the location of death. These data show that machinery-related deaths accounted for 26% of these deaths and were the most common cause of death. NCHS data for 1984 showed that 469 of 989 nontransport fatalities were machine-related and that the number of agricultural machinery deaths had risen to 693 by 1985 (the latest year available).[8] McKnight[11] analyzed farm equipment fatalities between 1975–1981 based on data from the Consumer Product Safety Commission, which collects fatality data related to various products. Of the 3,229 deaths on farms, three-fourths were associated with tractors, with one-half of these occurring when the tractor overturned. Another 800 deaths were associated with 30 other farm machines including auger-elevators, cornpickers, power take-offs, and manure spreaders. Most injuries were severe—crushing thoracic injuries, decapitation, and dismemberment. Children under 14 were found to be at higher risk than other age groups for nearly one-half of the study's 21 types of fatal injuries. A nearly linear increase was observed in the rate of all tractor fatalities, whereas a bimodal distribution showing higher rates among the very young and old was observed for both falls and those run over by farm tractors. These findings are supported by more contemporary data from the Olmstead County study, which found especially high rates of severe and fatal injuries among girls ages 1–4 (Fig. 1). Women were also found to have higher rates of severe and fatal injuries from falls and being hit by and being run over by tractors (Fig. 2).[7]

Assessment of state-based epidemiologic studies demonstrates continuity in the pattern of injury statistics over the past three decades, suggesting that efforts to intervene in this epidemic have been largely unsuccessful. Farm fatalities in Iowa were reported by Wardle and Hull[20] between the years 1947 and 1971. Although dated, this study illustrates this continuity in agricultural injury morbidity and mortality. It is also relevant, because much farm machinery still in use today is 20 years old, or older. Tractor fatalities in this study were the major cause of death and accounted for 1,326 deaths, of which 62% were caused by tractor overturns. About 20% of the deaths were accounted for by children under the age of 10. A recent state-wide analysis of farm deaths in Kentucky has been reported by Stallones for the years 1979–1985.[18] Distribution of fatalities in this study found 50.1% of the deaths to be unintentional, but high rates of intentional injuries were observed, with 11.7% arising from homicides and nearly a third (32.3%) from suicide. When analyzed by occupation, 64.9% were among farmers or farm workers, 21.4% were associated with another occupation, and 13.6% were accounted for by other family members. Thus, this study calls to attention rural violence as an important priority for further prevention research.

A comprehensive assessment of farm-related morbidity is not available, because the vast majority of farms in the United States employ fewer than 11 employees and are therefore not covered by the Department of Labor Bureau of Labor Statistics (BLS) injury and illness reports. However, based on larger agricultural operations, recent incident rates per 100 full-time employees for 1987 are higher for the agricultural sector (11.8—includes forestry and fishing in this classification) than any other industrial sector (mining 6.1, construction 8.0, and manufacturing 8.1).[14] Rates for agricultural production and crops (14.7) and for agricultural services (14.8) far exceed the rate for forestry (4.1).

The most comprehensive study of farm injury morbidity is based on the National Safety Council's survey of 127,169 farm family members, with 57,301 full- and part-time employees on 37,293 farms in 31 states. This data base covers more than 5,753 injuries, ranging from minor to crippling to fatal; 4,105 or 71% were occupational injuries.[8] Significantly higher injury rates were reported for those ages 5–24 than other age groups; smaller farms (49 acres or less) experienced the highest injury rates, and beef, dairy, and fruit farms reported significantly higher injury rates. Of the 4,105 work-related injuries, 30.2% were described as slight (no medical treatment other than first aid), whereas 65.4% were classified as

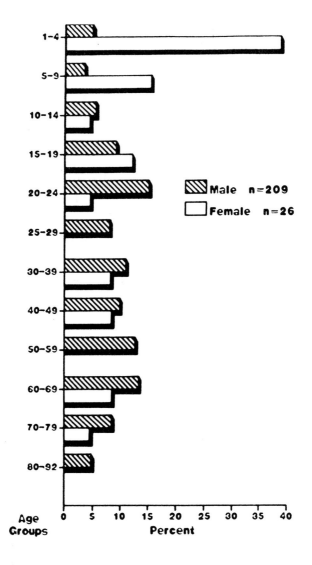

FIGURE 1. Severe and fatal farm-related injuries by age group and by gender, Minnesota, September 1981–August 1983. (From Gunderson P, et al: Injury surveillance in agriculture. Am J Ind Med 18:169–178, 1990, with permission.)

severe (requiring medical attention). Permanent injuries (loss of full use of body part) were reported in 1.9% of cases and fatal injuries in 0.7%. The distribution of fatal injuries from this cross-sectional study revealed higher fatality rates for those under age 15 and over age 64. Agricultural machinery was again the single leading cause of death (17.6%), followed by animal-related injuries (16.9%). Agricultural machinery was associated with 47.5% of injuries leading to permanent impairment, followed by power tools at 10%. Tractors were associated with 26.7% of all fatal injuries. The vast majority of these permanent injuries required medical care

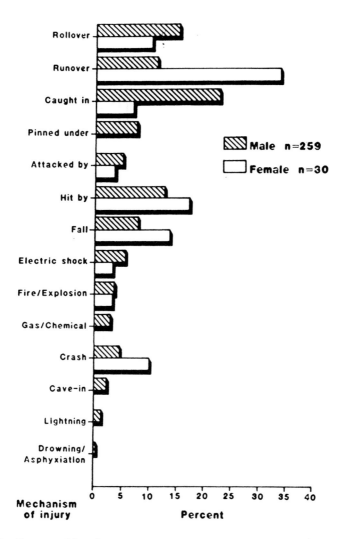

FIGURE 2.   Severe and fatal farm-related injuries by mechanism of injury and by gender, Minnesota, September 1981–August 1983. (From Gunderson P, et al: Injury surveillance in agriculture. Am J Ind Med 18:169–178, 1990, with permission.)

(93.9%), with 60.2% requiring more than one contact. About 45% of all injuries were treated at a doctor's office, 28% in an emergency room, and 9% required hospitalization. Most injuries (71%) involved 7 or fewer lost workdays, 11% involved lost time lasting 1 to 3 months, 3% reported a physical impairment following recovery from the injury, and 2.1% affected individuals who were unable to return to work.

A study of farm versus nonfarm injury hospitalizations in a random sample of 15 Iowa hospitals found that 14.7% of hospitalizations for trauma arose from work-related injuries.[5] Farmers were hospitalized for occupational injuries at a rate of 1,521 per 100,000, compared to nonfarmers who were hospitalized at a rate of 497 per 100,000. Farm and nonfarm patients were found to have similar types and mechanisms of injury, whereas the most common cause of farm injury was machine-related (61.3%) compared to nonfarm machine-related injuries (20.6%). Although there were no significant differences in the mean number of days per hospitalization for farmers versus nonfarmers (7.4 days for farmers and 6.7 days for nonfarmers), farmers reported significantly less time off from work, with a mean of 79 days compared to a mean of 289 for nonfarmers. Highly significant differences were reported regarding remuneration arising from the injury. Farmers were found to less frequently be covered by workers' compensation (9.2% vs. 74.8%), Social Security settlement (1.3% vs. 5.1%), and any type of remuneration (57% vs. 82.3%). Farmers were found to more frequently have other types of insurance settlements (41.8% vs. 25.9%). Despite the significantly higher rate of injury and significantly lower remuneration for injury among farmers, no farmer (of 75 respondents) in this study sought to switch to a job outside of farming, whereas 25% of the nonfarm patients (of 212 respondents) switched jobs because of injuries. This statistic raises the important question of the effect of a first injury as a risk factor for secondary injuries. Good data on this question are not available, but the rate of secondary injury is thought to be quite high.[21]

Several studies have documented an increased risk of injury among children on farms. An analysis of fatal and nonfatal farm injuries among children and adolescents have been reported by Rivara.[16] Data sources included 1979–1981 mortality statistics from the National Center for Health Statistics, emergency room reports to the National Electronic Injury Surveillance System (NEISS, 1979–1983), farm deaths investigated by the Consumer Product Safety Commission, and the 1980 Census. Based on these data, an estimated 300 children and adolescents were found to die each year from farm-associated injuries, while another 23,500 suffer nonfatal trauma. More than half (52.5%) were found to die without ever reaching a physician, 19.1% died in transit to a hospital, while only 7.4% lived long enough to receive inpatient care. Farm machinery was found to be the most common cause of death, with tractors accounting for one half of the machine-related deaths. Of nonfatal injuries, 10% required hospitalization. Based on these findings, a strong case is made by the author for evaluation of a number of preventive strategies, including legislation and improvement in acute medical care delivery to farm and rural areas.

SURVEILLANCE

Several existing national data bases, if analyzed systematically, could serve as very useful surveillance systems for national trends in agricultural injuries. These data bases, which have been used to conduct several epidemiologic studies of agricultural injuries, as reported above, include the National Center for Health Statistics (NCHS) Mortality Cause of Death Summary Tapes, the National Electronic Injury Surveillance System (NEISS) of the Consumer Product Safety Commission (CPSC), the Death Certificate Data Base of the CPSC, the National Institute for Occupational Safety and Health (NIOSH) National Traumatic Occupational Fatality Data Base (NTOF), the Department of Labor Bureau of Labor Statistics (BLS) Annual Survey of Occupational Injuries and Illnesses, the BLS Supplemental Data System, and the National Safety Council's (NSC) *Accident Facts,* which is based on data from NCHS, state vital statistics departments, the BLS, and other sources. Only the NSC has used these data to provide annual data to assess trends over time. Although each of these data bases is useful, they each have their limitations, especially in assessing the relationship between exposure and injury outcome.[9]

In order to develop surveillance systems that provide population-based injury morbidity and mortality data and that include improved assessment of exposure factors, a number of new state-wide or regional surveillance systems are now under development. One model to assess population-based agricultural injuries has been developed by a team from the University of Minnesota.[6,7] This Centers for Disease Control (CDC) model was developed as a part of the Olmstead Agricultural Trauma Study (OATS), which evaluated all farms in Olmstead County, Minnesota. The model is based on the United States Department of Agriculture's Master Sampling Frame to identify farms as the sampling unit. Demographic, exposure, and injury outcome data (ICD-9CM and E-Codes) are collected systematically via a computer-driven questionnaire by trained telephone interviewers. An injury is defined as "one which restricted normal activities for at least 4 hours, and/or resulted in loss of consciousness, loss of awareness, or amnesia for any length of time, and/or required professional medical care." Injuries included both farm and nonfarm related activities and are classified as intentional or nonintentional. Injured persons are then interviewed directly, except for those under age 18, in which case the female head of household is the preferred respondent. These interviews provide systematic assessment of type and severity of injury, and the source, mechanism, and contributing factors of injury. This data base has provided these investigators an opportunity to conduct case-control studies of specific types of injury to identify and quantify risk factors. Utilizing this surveillance methodology, the University of Minnesota has embarked on a five-state (Minnesota, Wisconsin, North Dakota, South Dakota, and Nebraska) Regional Rural Injury Study (RRIS) designed to provide regional and state-specific agricultural injury rates, to provide a data base for further case-control studies, and to provide the basis for regional injury prevention and control programs.

A regional surveillance approach is the NIOSH Farm Family Hazard and Health Survey (FFHHS), which is now underway in six states (Iowa, California, Colorado, Ohio, Kentucky, and New York). This approach is an outgrowth of the NIOSH National Occupational Hazard Surveys (NOHS) for both general industry and mining, both of which have provided very important profiles of occupational exposures and exposure-specific populations-at-risk estimates, which have been used to help prioritize NIOSH research and program development. While the NOHS surveys were limited to a systematic NIOSH assessment of exposures and estimates of numbers of workers exposed, the FFHHS will use a somewhat more flexible methodology and conduct the surveys in collaboration with six universities/health departments. These surveys will employ common definitions, questions, and exposure assessment methods wherever possible in order to assess regionally different types of agricultural production. The FFHHS will also collect limited medical data, including some assessment of injuries, respiratory disease, and noise-induced hearing loss. These initial surveys will provide the basis for estimating regional agricultural exposures, populations-at-risk, and priorities for further surveillance, research, and prevention program development.

A very promising surveillance approach is the Iowa statewide surveillance of acute farm injury system SPRAINS (Sentinel Project Researching Agricultural Injury Notification System). This CDC-sponsored system is based on voluntary reporting of farm-related injuries to the Iowa Department of Public Health. A standardized form has been developed that provides demographic, exposure information, and injury outcome data. Forms are mailed to the Health Department by any health care provider. Through the involvement of four regionally located nurses, special efforts are made to secure results from all Iowa hospitals. A number of physicians are regular reporters and a single county has been identified for active, systematic reporting of all farm-related injuries in order to estimate the degree of underreporting in other counties. This system began in early 1990 and has already produced some very useful surveillance data. Based on an incomplete first year of reporting, 2,143 injuries from 98 of 99 Iowa counties were reported.[3] Of these injuries, 83 were fatal (40.8/100,000 farming population), with children under 15 years and farmers over 65 years of age being disproportionately represented. While this number no doubt still represents underreporting of the actual number of farm-related deaths in 1990, it is significantly greater than the 54 deaths reported by the Iowa State University Agricultural Extension Service as based on newspaper clippings for 1989. Assessment of SPRAINS data found machinery-related incidents accounted for 32% of the injuries and 45% of the deaths. Tractor-related deaths (29) were the most common single cause; 16 of these deaths were from tractor roll-overs. Upon investigation, 15 of these deaths could have been prevented by roll-over protective structures (ROPS). Those injured included farmers (40%), farm-family members (27%), and employees/service personnel/visitors (33%).

A fourth approach to agricultural injury surveillance is based on the development of computerized hospital emergency room logs. Projects are now underway at the Injury Prevention Research Centers at the University of North Carolina and the University of Iowa. Both of these surveillance projects use computerization of the hospital emergency room log as a means for inexpensively involving community hospitals in systematic injury surveillance. This approach provides a computerized data base for data collection, which will provide health outcome data (ICD-9CM Codes and E-Codes), demographic information, some health care delivery data, and limited exposure data. In Iowa, this surveillance system (the Rural Injury Surveillance System or RISS) will develop a farm-injury surveillance module that will incorporate all of the data utilized by SPRAINS. Similar modules are being developed for head and neck injuries, for which the Iowa Department of Public Health also has a registry based on voluntary reporting. The Iowa Department of Public Health also requires (in addition to farm and head and neck injuries), through legislation and Health Department regulation, hospitals to report occupational lung diseases, toxic effects of chemical exposures, and carpal tunnel syndrome. These reporting requirements provide a substantial incentive for hospitals to participate in a system that will collect and assist in reporting the data to the Iowa Department of Public Health. Both the North Carolina and the Iowa IPRCs are now testing their systems in community hospitals. The goal of the Iowa RISS is to have these hospital data from all Iowa hospitals reported to the State Health Registry of Iowa, which is located at the University of Iowa and affiliated with the Iowa IPRC. The State Health Registry will assist the Iowa Department of Public Health in obtaining regulated injury and illness data. The data base arising from RISS will provide the basis for ongoing injury surveillance (and other health outcomes), and for the development of case-control studies to identify and quantitate the risk factors for specific types of injuries.

PREVENTION

The available data, which have been summarized above, document a sustained epidemic of agricultural injury in America. Much of this injury is related to the use of and exposure to farm machinery. A disproportionate amount of severe and permanent injury is attributable to farm machinery, especially to the tractor. A disproportionately high rate of injury is observed among children and the elderly, who participate in and are exposed to agricultural production. Unlike mining, construction, and general industry, which have all seen steady reductions in work-related injury, the rates for injury in agriculture have changed very little over the years.[14] In addition to the several hundred farm-related deaths, which are now well recognized to represent many fewer than the actual number of deaths, there are estimated to be some 170,000 farm injuries, many of which are severe.[12] Recent estimates of the costs of this epidemic are not available, but the hospital and rehabilitation costs were estimated to be 2.5 billion dollars annually in 1983.[15] Despite the numbers of those killed and injured and the associate costs, as of 1988 neither the federal government or state governments had mounted significant prevention initiatives.[12]

In 1988, the University of Iowa and Iowa State University, with support from agribusiness and foundations, sponsored a public policy conference "Agricultural Occupational and Environmental Health: Policy Strategies for the Future." This two-part conference sought to: (1) bring together national and international scientists for discussion and publication of state-of-the-art presentations on agricultural safety and health, environmental exposures and remediation, and rural health care delivery; and (2) bring together policy makers from agriculture, agribusiness, state and federal agencies, state and federal law makers, and academics to discuss issues and recommend public policy solutions. A brief summary of the scientific basis for mounting a major prevention campaign, and public policy recommendations to accomplish this mission are summarized in *Agriculture at Risk—A Report to the Nation*[12] and in a three-issue series of papers.[4] Recommendations from this conference encompassed five areas: (1) federal and state legislation for program development and funding; (2) research initiatives to guide priorities for data collection and prevention program development; (3) initiatives for the development of occupational health and safety delivery programs; (4) education and training recommendations for primary school children through university programs and for broad, community-based community education; and (5) initiatives to develop coalitions to carry these recommendations forward to implementation. Out of this conference came the development of the National Coalition for Agricultural Safety and Health (NCASH), which is composed of many participants from the conference, and now, in association with the National Rural Health Association, many others. NCASH was instrumental in taking the recommendations summarized in *Agriculture at Risk—Report to the Nation* to the U.S. Congress, the Centers for Disease Control, the National Institutes of Health, the Environmental Protection Agency, the Occupational Safety and Health Administration, the U.S. Department of Agriculture, the Office of Technology Assessment of the Congress, the National Governors' Association, to foundations concerned with public health, and to several state legislatures that expressed interest in this important public health problem.

In 1989 and 1990 the federal government, several state governments, and the W.K. Kellogg Foundation responded to these recommendations with substantial funding (over 30 million dollars in new monies from all sources) and multiple new programs targeting most of the recommendations arising from this public policy conference. Many of these federal and state initiatives focus on agricultural injuries as the highest priority for research and intervention program development. The Centers for Disease Control, through its National Institute for Occupational Safety and Health (NIOSH) and Center for Environmental Health and Injury Control, is sponsoring very significant new research, surveillance, education, training, and health promotion and prevention demonstration initiatives. The U.S. Department of Agriculture, through its Land Grand Universities, has begun a series of demonstration programs targeting education and rehabilitation of agricultural injuries. The W.K. Kellogg Foundation has begun an initiative for community-based programs to develop innovative models for providing agricultural safety and health care and prevention services. These programs, which are just beginning, will provide a very substantial research base, establish ongoing surveillance systems, provide testing of injury intervention models, and provide a scientific basis for developing long-range strategies to prevent agricultural injuries.

The single most compelling need at this time is to prevent the very substantial numbers of deaths and severe and often permanent injuries arising from tractor roll-overs. A model for prevention of this type of injury has been developed in Sweden, which has required installation of ROPS on both new and then used tractors.[19] Implementation of this strategy has virtually eliminated tractor roll-over deaths in Sweden (Fig. 3). The challenge to those now concerned with tractor and other agricultural injuries in the United States is to develop equally effective prevention programs for tractor roll-over, and other farm related injuries, in our diversified agricultural sector.

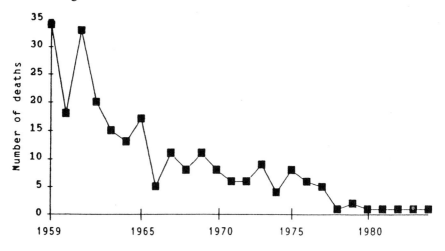

FIGURE 3. Number of deaths annually in Sweden according to roll-over accidents with tractors 1959–1984. (From Thelin A: Epilogue: Agricultural Occupational and Environmental Health Policy Strategies for the Future. Am J Ind Med 18:523–526, 1990, with permission.)

REFERENCES

1. Baker SP, O'Neill B, Karpf R: The Injury Fact Book. Lexington, MA, Lexington Books, 1984.
2. Baker SP, Whitfield MA, O'Neill B: Geographic variations in mortality from motor vehicle crashes. N Engl J Med 316:1384–1387, 1987.
3. Currier RW, Jones S: Iowa Statewide Surveillance of Acute Farm Injury. Proceedings of the National Conference on State-based Occupational Health and Safety Activities. Atlanta, GA, Centers for Disease Control, 1991.
4. Donham KJ: Agricultural, occupational, and environmental health: Policy strategies for the future—the scientific basis. Am J Ind Med 18(2, 3 & 4):105–237, 239–361, 363–527, 1990.
5. Fuortes LJ, Merchant JA, Van Lier SF, et al: 1983 occupational injury hospital admissions in Iowa: A comparison of the agricultural and non-agricultural sectors. Am J Ind Med 18:211–222, 1990.
6. Gerberich SG, Gibson RW, Gunderson PD, et al: Validity of trauma reporting in the agricultural community. J Occup Med 12:200, 1990.
7. Gunderson P, Gerberich S, Gibson R, et al: Injury surveillance in agriculture. Am J Ind Med 18:169–178, 1990.
8. Hoskin AF, Miller TA, Hanford WD, et al: Occupational Injuries in Agriculture: A 35-State Summary. Report No. DSR-87-0942. Morgantown, WV, National Institute for Occupational Safety and Health, 1988.
9. Layde PM: Beyond surveillance: Methodologic considerations in analytic studies in agricultural injuries. Am J Ind Med 18:193–200, 1990.
10. May JJ: Issues in agricultural health and safety. Am J Ind Med 18:121–132, 1990.
11. McKnight RH: U.S. Agricultural Equipment Fatalities, 1975–1981: Implications for Injury Control and Health Education. Doctor of Science Dissertation. Baltimore, MD, Johns Hopkins University, 1984.
12. Merchant JA, Kross BC, Donham KJ, et al: Agriculture at Risk—A Report to the Nation. Iowa City, IA, Institute of Agricultural Medicine and Occupational Health, The University of Iowa, 1988.
13. Myers JR: National surveillance of occupational fatalities in agriculture. Am J Ind Med 18:163–178, 1990.
14. National Safety Council: Accident Facts, 1988 Edition. Chicago, IL, National Safety Council, 1988.
15. Purschwitz MA, Field WE: Federal funding for farm safety relative to other safety programs. In Proceedings of the 1987 National Institute for Farm Safety Summer Meeting. Columbia, MO, NIFS, June 14–18, 1987.
16. Rivara FP: Fatal and nonfatal farm injuries to children and adolescents in the United States. Pediatrics 76:567–573, 1985.
17. Rowland D, Lyons B: Triple jeopardy: Rural, poor, and uninsured. HSR: Health Services Research 23:975–1004, 1989.
18. Stallones L: Surveillance of Fatal and Non-Fatal Injuries in Kentucky. Am J Ind Med 18:223–234, 1990.
19. Thelin A: Epilogue: Agricultural occupational and environmental health policy strategies for the future. Am J Ind Med 18:523–525, 1990.
20. Wardle NJ, Hull DO: Fatal Accidents of Iowa Farm People, 1947–1971. Ames, IA, Iowa State University Extension Service, 1975.
21. Willkomm T: Personal communication, 1991.

D. H. CORDES, MD, MPH
DOROTHY FOSTER REA, MA

PREVENTIVE MEASURES IN AGRICULTURAL SETTINGS

From the Section of Preventive
and Occupational Medicine
Department of Family and
Community Medicine
University of Arizona College
of Medicine
Tucson, Arizona

Reprint requests to:
D. H . Cordes, MD, MPH
Department of Family and
Community Medicine
University of Arizona College
of Medicine
Tucson, AZ 85724

The need for preventive measures to control death and injury in the agricultural work force is apparent. By their nature many farming tasks are hazardous endeavors; and although adequate protection in any dangerous job is important, foresight and planning for prevention can be more efficient safeguards against accidents and illnesses by effectively eliminating or significantly reducing exposures. The needs for preventive strategies exist in, but are not limited to, the areas of legislation, engineering and design, the environment, health care provider sensitization, and farmer education. It is important for practitioners with patients from rural areas to be cognizant of these needs in order to make farmers aware of the risks, to teach safety principles where possible, and to be an advocate for change.

LEGISLATION

Existing legislation affecting farm worker health, well-being, and safety is listed in Table 1. Most legislation has had an impact on the areas it governs, but in many cases there is more to be done. For example, whereas child labor laws restrict overall the age of children as workers, the laws do not adequately control child and adolescent labor in dangerous occupations. Children are a significant part of the farm work force and face the same risks for injury and illness as other workers. Laws in existence now allow children of any age to work on the family farm. The Fair Labor Standards Act only exempts children under 12 from working on other farms. Children aged 12 or older may work on other farms with permission of a parent.

TABLE 1.   State and Federal Legislation Affecting Farm Workers

Legislation	Provisions
1. 1966 Amendments to Fair Labor Standards Act	Minimum wage guarantees for some farm workers; child labor protection.
2. Federal Insecticide, Fungicide and Rodenticide Act (FIFRA) (1947)	Governs pesticides manufacturing, distribution, and use. States are granted authority to regulate sale and use. Created EPA in 1970 with responsibility for overseeing and regulating pesticides.
3. Federal Environmental Pesticide Control Act (FEPCA) (1972)	Amends FIFRA
4. State Reentry Intervals	California: reentry intervals from one to 70 days for approximately 80 pesticides. Physicians required to report pesticide-related illness. New Jersey, North Carolina, Texas: 24-hour reentry intervals for Category I chemicals (labeled "Danger").
5. Short-handled Hoe Legislation	The use of the short-handled hoe has been banned in Arizona, California, Texas, and Washington, thereby eliminating stoop labor in these states.
6. The Occupational Safety and Health Administration Hazard Communication Standard (1983)	Requires chemical manufacturers to place warning labels on containers of hazardous chemicals. Material Safety Data Sheets (MSDS) must be prepared giving safe use information. Workers must be given training and safety sheets (affects manufacturing only).
	States: May include MSDS, worker health and safety training, provision of protective clothing, posting of work areas, maintenance of employee health records, employee access to records. Farm workers specifically covered in Minnesota, Pennsylvania, Texas, Washington, and Wisconsin.
7. Occupational Safety and Health Act	Several standards apply to agriculture: a. Sanitation in temporary worker camps b. Storage and handling of anhydrous ammonia c. Fluorescent emblem on slow-moving vehicles d. Roll-over protective structures on tractors e. Safety for agricultural equipment (power take-off guards, operating instructions, electrical disconnect, etc.)
8. Agricultural Worker Protection Act (1983)	Provides regulations for farm labor contracts, including working and housing conditions, transportation, insurance and wage statements.
9. Migrant Health Act	Provides funding to clinics for migrant workers and their families.
10. U.S. Department of Transportation Act	Some provisions affect transport of farm workers: a. Driver of vehicle needs physical exam, valid driver's license, must be 21 years old, and understand English. b. Vehicles must be in good condition, equipment secured, passengers and cargo safely distributed. c. Meal stops and rest stops are required. d. Each passenger must have a seat and be protected from weather extremes. e. Drivers may not drive longer than 10 hours within any 24-hour period (excluding meal and rest stops).
11. State Field Sanitation Statutes	States with field sanitation (toilet and handwash) regulations: Arizona, California, Connecticut, Florida, Idaho, Illinois, Maine, New Jersey, Oregon, Pennsylvania, Texas. Water requirements only: Minnesota, New York, North Carolina. Others: California, Connecticut, Illinois, Maine, Massachusetts, New York, New Hampshire, Rhode Island; farm workers

(Table continued on next page.)

TABLE 1. State and Federal Legislation Affecting Farm Workers *(Cont.)*

Legislation	Provisions
11. State Field Sanitation Statutes *(continued)*	excluded in New Jersey and West Virginia. Some states adopted federal OSHA Hazard Communication Standard: Arizona, Alaska (excludes employers with residential businesses), Hawaii, Iowa (excludes farmers), Kentucky, Nevada, New Mexico, North Carolina, South Carolina, Tennessee, Utah, Vermont, Virginia, and Washington.
12. Workers' Compensation	About half the states provide coverage for farmers. Complete coverage: Arizona, California, Colorado, Connecticut, Hawaii, Massachusetts, Michigan, Montana, New Hampshire, New Jersey, Ohio, Oregon, Pennsylvania, Washington. Partial coverage: Alaska, Florida, Illinois, Iowa, Maryland, Minnesota, New York, North Carolina, Oklahoma, South Carolina, Texas, Utah, Vermont, Virginia, West Virginia, and Wisconsin.

Three hundred children and adolescents die each year of farm injuries. An additional 23,599 suffer nonfatal trauma.[24] These and other figures underscore the need for developing prevention programs on farms and for revision of farm safety legislation. The group most in need of protection is 15- to 19-year-old boys, with whom the accident rate is double that of younger children and 26 times higher than that for girls.[24] It is important to note that most family farms in this country are not within the jurisdiction of OSHA. To fall within the purview of that agency a farm must have more than 10 employees, and this number cannot include family members.

Certain regulations under the Federal Insecticide, Fungicide, and Rodenticide Act (FIFRA) applicable to farmers are the "Worker Protection Standards for Agricultural Pesticides," issued in 1974. The regulations prohibit exposing workers to pesticides directly or through drift, establish reentry intervals for 12 pesticides, require written or verbal warnings to farm workers in fields being sprayed, and require workers not wearing protective clothing to leave the field.[31] The Environmental Protection Agency (EPA) has proposed to revise its regulations and to provide greater protection of agricultural workers from pesticide exposure. The new regulations would require posted information of pesticide safety rules and the location of the nearest emergency medical facility, and would also establish additional reentry intervals for pesticide categories.[13]

The Texas Agriculture Hazard Communication Law was enacted in 1987. Texas could be a model for other states to pass similar stringent laws. It is the first state to require health and safety training for farm workers. Crop sheets must be read aloud to workers to inform them of pesticides in use, reentry intervals, symptoms of pesticide exposure, and emergency procedures. Training programs are provided statewide by the Texas Department of Agriculture and by the Texas Department of Agriculture District and Satellite Offices.[27] In cases of states with no workers' compensation coverage for farmers, medical costs are not paid for injured farmers, and work injury and illness statistics for agriculture may not be collected in those states. In states where workers' compensation does extend to agriculture, farmers must first enroll in the program, pay the necessary payroll tax or have it paid on workers' behalf, and then be aware of the mechanics of filing claims to collect medical expenses and lost wages due to them. In the case of migrant and seasonal workers, claims might never be filed or collected.

In Canada, workers' compensation is available in 9 of the 11 provinces. However, few farmers insure themselves. In Saskatchewan, 3% of eligible farmers are enrolled with the workers' compensation board, and this enrollment is often for employed farm laborers.[8]

That legislated changes can be effective has been demonstrated in Sweden, where a 1958 law mandated all new tractors be equipped with rollover protection, and a 1978 law stated that no tractor could be used without rollover protection.[28] While the number of deaths annually in Sweden due to rollover accidents declined significantly between 1958 and 1959, since 1978 these deaths have been nearly eliminated. Also in Sweden, 3,000 chain saw accidents occurred annually during the 1960s. An improved chain saw was developed through engineering changes, and it became illegal to sell a chain saw without protective equipment. In 1981, reported chain saw accidents numbered less than 500 annually.

Most tractors manufactured in the United States after 1976 have offered the option of rollover protective structures (ROPS), but it is not illegal to use tractors that do not have this feature. Since the inception of ROPS, the number of deaths in the U.S. due to rollovers has dropped to 4.0 per 100,000 from 7.3 annually.[20] However, in 1970, 49% of tractor-related deaths were due to rollovers, and in 1989 this figure was 55%.[20] An estimated 3 million tractors still lack the devices. Tractors must be equipped with power take-off guards and electrical disconnect devices, and they must be sold with complete operating instructions. But there is no law against taking off these protective devices, and some farmers think machines operate better without them. Older machinery simply does not have protective equipment.

ENGINEERING AND DESIGN

Since most farm work involves machinery, and accidents occur as a result of machine use, the design and engineering of the mechanics of farm machines need to be scrutinized and, when possible, modified to make safer equipment. The farmer often works alone, out of sight of family, neighbors, or any co-workers. Adding this to the difficulties of working outdoors in conditions of frequently inclement weather increases risks of unattended accidents.

Proper ergonomic placement of controls, instruments, and the operator's seat on tractors has long been studied.[18] But additional approaches are being considered to reduce postural stresses and distraction that occur when the driver must frequently turn to observe machinery behind the tractor. Alternate approaches, such as rear view mirrors or a swiveling seat, have been proposed.[18]

A driver's cab on tractors has several advantages. It protects the driver from severe weather, dust, and chemical exposures, and it is designed to prevent the driver from being crushed if the vehicle overturns. While early cabs in the 1960s were found to increase noise levels and presented a severe risk to the hearing threshold of farmers, further research led to the development of tractor cabs with improved acoustics.[18] Cabs now provide lower noise environments with antivibrational mounting, an acoustic barrier to external noise, and internal acoustic absorption to prevent reverberation. However, tractor drivers often use the tractor for more than an 8-hour day on successive days, and noise levels vary depending upon the task being performed. So although decibel levels may be kept at or below the maximum noise level limit, the intensity and duration of exposure may exceed that of other occupations.

In Great Britain, research has shown[18] that by isolating the driver's platform from vibration, combined with acoustic screening, the noise level of a smaller tractor can be reduced from 101 to 89 decibels, a reduction of 95% in sound energy. Work on other engineering designs for tractors is necessary, such as suspension seats to reduce vibration and more efficient climate-controlled cabs. The latter are necessary due to radiant heat load in summer and lack of heating from the motor in the winter due to the physical separation of the cab. Ergonomic design changes and improved safety features should continue to be part of the tractor's evolution.

Historically, gases and dusts in silos have created a safety hazard. Not only should prevention procedures continue to be taught, but new engineering designs should be pursued to eliminate the development of toxic gas conditions. Test strips to indicate the presence of NO_2 or insufficient oxygen should be developed.[11] And an example could be taken from Austria, where signs indicating the possible existence of hazardous gases are painted on the silos.[11] A warning sign would at least be a start at control of this deadly problem.

Control of organic dusts in stock-raising buildings is a problem that might be best solved by improved design of confinement buildings. Conventional ventilation systems do not control dust to a significant degree,[4] and good ventilation systems must be part of engineering control in the design of these buildings. Systems for handling animals, bedding, feed, and manure should have efficient dust controls in their design.[4] Reducing the decay of feeds and bedding and controlling animal movement should also be an aim in dust-reduction methods. Ventilation control during handling and inhibition of growth of microbes are preventive measures to be considered in design and engineering changes. The technology to control dust is present in industry[30] and has been shown to reduce dust levels in agricultural settings.[12]

Personal protective equipment should not be a substitute for dust control.[4] Respirators should be a part of an overall plan of protective measures. That is, respirators should be employed in addition to adequate work practices. Respirators must be fitted individually to be airtight[4] and must be properly maintained.[7] Protective clothing worn during the application and handling of pesticides offers protection only when worn correctly.[23] Workers resist wearing clothing that is not comfortable or that restricts movement. Currently, research is being done to improve the design and comfort of such clothing. Evidence shows that cotton or a cotton blend fabric offers equal protection to rubberized suits, unless the worker becomes drenched with pesticides during handling. Studies done in California indicate that gloves can significantly reduce exposure when properly worn.[23] Regardless of the material, gloves placed on hands already contaminated only increase dermal penetration.

A challenge to health practitioners is to inform workers of the dangers and thereby convince them to use protective equipment and to take other preventive measures. An ongoing goal is to design comfortable, effective equipment.[23] Practitioner organizations can be influential in bringing about legislative and engineering changes.

ENVIRONMENT

Use of agricultural chemicals, specifically fertilizers and pesticides, can result in human health effects beyond those implied by occupational exposures accompanying their handling and application.[17] Nitrates from fertilizers are of concern for groundwater contamination. Other environmental sources of nitrates on the farm are animal manures, human wastes, nitrogen-fixing bacteria and plants, and other natural sources.[17] Data from the monitoring of rural drinking water wells in a number of states show nitrate concentrations in excess of safe drinking water standards for nitrates.[17] The health concern is the formation of nitrosamines from secondary amines in the body. Many nitrosamines are known to be cancer-causing agents and mutagens. Studies indicate an association between nitrates and non-Hodgkin's lymphoma, stomach cancer, and possibly birth defects.[17]

A panel of scientists, agricultural specialists, industry leaders, health professionals, government agency leaders, elected officials, and public policy analysts, recently convened to study environmental health strategies for agriculture, showed concern over these possible chronic effects in the report generated as a result of their meetings.[17] The same panel indicated that evidence is lacking on the effects of pesticide residues in food and in drinking water. However, concerns about data gaps, synergistic effects, and lack of knowledge of food consumption patterns, particularly those of infants or children, decrease the level of confidence that food and water supplies are without risks from their current level of pesticide residue.[17] Pesticides occur in drinking water by way of groundwater from farm and commercial spills, waste dumps, and from handling and application areas. In citrus-growing areas, for example, pesticides are delivered to the fields in irrigation water. The report recommended that all sources of groundwater contamination be identified to develop prevention and cleanup strategies.[17]

The panel believes prevention of groundwater contamination at the source is the least costly and most effective control strategy. It advocates improved agriculture management practices to reduce the amount of pesticides available to run off into surface water or groundwater. Specifically, it recommends that farm-management decisions be guided by environmental factors and not economic factors alone. Choices of less toxic or less persistent chemicals would reduce the risk of environmental damage. On the legislative level, the panel suggests the development of drinking water standards by the federal government using information from the EPA's health advisories or maximum contaminant level goals. States would have the option of setting stricter standards, if desired. As an example, the state of Wisconsin has recently established groundwater protection approaches. Other states could follow its model. The federal role would be to set standards, to evaluate health effects data, and to oversee state management plans.[17]

In the future, if genetically improved plants resistant to destruction by pests become a reality, farmers will not have to spray as abundantly with pesticides to protect their crops. The risks from exposure to pesticides, both to individuals and to the environment, will be reduced. However, at this time genetically modified plants are infertile, and there are still public health concerns about the potential adverse health effects of the expression of foreign protein in food.[5] This research should be encouraged in the hope that biotechnologic progress will result in a safer environment.

HEALTH PROVIDER EDUCATION

An important step in implementing preventive strategies to persuade farmers to observe sound safety practices for themselves and their families is to improve physician awareness of health and safety problems in rural areas and their corresponding preventive approaches. This stand has been taken by the American Medical Association (AMA), regarding pesticides, in its Resolution 94(1-86). The resolution calls for the AMA, "through its scientific journals and publications, to alert physicians to the potential hazards of agricultural pesticides, to provide physicians with advice on such hazards for their patients, and to urge that these substances be appropriately labeled."[6] This same resolve could be applied to all other agricultural hazards.

Such education could address not only pesticide use but tractor safety; protection from dust, noise, and vibration; precautions for silo workers; the importance of careful supervision of children; and proper training for all who work on the farm, particularly the high-accident risk group of young males. Avenues for physicians and nurses to reach farmers are personal contact with patients, local newspapers and other media, and rural hospitals and clinics. Health care providers can also advocate additional or expanded health services in rural areas where needed, as well as training of local individuals.

The Surgeon General's Conference on Agricultural Safety and Health, which took place from April 30 through May 3, 1991 in Des Moines, Iowa, was intended to promote consciousness, build coalitions, disseminate information, and encourage action to prevent injury and disease in relation to agricultural activities. The theme for the conference was "Farm Safe 2000: A National Coalition for Local Action." The conference was planned to cover all aspects of surveillance, chemical and biological hazard research, physical and mechanical hazard research, health promotion and behavior interventions, and health protection interventions as they relate to agricultural activities.

Physician education concerning health problems related to agriculture should begin during medical school[14] and should be emphasized in certain specialty residency training programs, especially family practice residencies, but also in pediatrics and emergency medicine. A report on pediatric cardiopulmonary arrests in a rural population remarks on the importance of training people responsible for pediatric emergencies.[29] While accident prevention is most important, the ability to treat these trauma patients with multiple organ problems is extremely important. Recognition and management of respiratory embarrassment, trauma, and accidental injuries should be a high priority in training programs. The ability to recognize possible respiratory problems, intervene appropriately, and prevent cardiac arrest could alter the outcome and should be a priority in teaching rural health care providers.[29]

Of family medicine residency graduates, 10% to 14% each year begin practice in communities with a population size of fewer than 2,500 people, and 45% begin practice in communities with fewer than 25,000 people.[1] Thus, a sizable portion of the resident cohorts is in need of concentrated training in agricultural health. For this purpose community-based rotations are recommended. Rural health care training is partly represented in family medicine curricula by the Area Health Education Centers (AHEC), which are part of a system of curricula reform to promote careers for physicians in rural health care. While the AHECs are a viable method for training, it has been suggested that the AHEC plan has remained at the model stage and has not attracted physicians permanently to rural areas.[16] Rural areas remain underserved. But recruiting physicians and attracting them to settle and stay to provide needed health care is just part of the problem. Intensive training and the technical and financial assistance to carry out this training are also needed as a component of producing physicians well-trained in prevention in agricultural settings.

FARMER EDUCATION

The National Institute for Occupational Safety and Health (NIOSH) has designed special programs to address the problem of the high mortality rate among agricultural workers. The programs, called the 1990 Agricultural Initiative, are both interventional and academic.[2] The initiative will use as a network the land-grant universities and their extension services. Agricultural workers are a difficult population to reach because of the scattered nature of the worksites. The network will reduce some of the difficulties of reaching these workers, because the extension services provide referrals and disseminate information to farmers. Each county has such a unit, and they are all connected to a state extension service. Several of the programs are:

1. To distribute injury and illness prevention messages to farmers;
2. To assign nurses to rural areas to talk about prevention in farming communities and to assess the incidence of injury and illness among farmers;
3. To provide cancer screening and to assess cancer rates in farming communities;
4. To evaluate farms for safety hazards and determine the incidence of illness among farm family members; and
5. To award academic grants: (a) to establish new Agricultural Health and Safety Centers; and (b) for applied research in intervention methods.

These programs began in the fall of 1990, and funds were awarded for the research grants in late September. Other possible sites for dissemination of information suggested by a NIOSH survey[21] are: businesses serving agricultural communities, such as farm equipment sales, agricultural chemical dealers (pesticides and fertilizers), seed and feed dealers, and suppliers of farm tools and electrical supplies; state and county health departments; and farm organizations, such as Cattleman's Association, 4-H, Future Farmers of America, the Grange, Farm Bureau commodity groups, and the Dairyman's Association. An attempt to involve these businesses and entities was attempted in Colorado. While attempts to involve agribusinesses met with limited success, contact with ranch and community groups resulted in a positive trend in interest in health and safety services provided by the program.[26]

Some methods like those proposed by NIOSH have been used in this country and others. A Salinas Valley, California medical center uses a slide show with narration and music to present information on pesticides, routes of exposure, symptoms of poisoning, first aid, methods of minimizing exposure, and government protection, including workers' compensation.[3]

A University of Minnesota group[19] has used OSHA funding to develop a program designed to increase farmers' awareness of health and safety hazards on the farm. Units of the program consist of slides and audiotape and deal with hazards such as noise, airborne substances, and farm machinery repair. They are used by vocational-agricultural teachers and county agents.

The Marshfield Clinic in Marshfield, Wisconsin has organized health surveys and medical screening for that rural area over the past 30 years,[10] including serological testing for farmer's lung disease and studies of organic dust levels, pulmonary response to organic dust exposure, hearing loss, noise production by agricultural equipment, arthritis, Lyme disease, skin cancer, accident and injury data, herbicide and pesticide exposure, and groundwater contamination from fuel supplies.

In Sweden, a nationwide health service for farmers began in 1977.[15] An occupational health care program takes care of 35,000 farmers on a volunteer basis. The program offers biennial health checkups, in addition to educational activities for farmers and farm visits. Nurses, physicians, and physiotherapists deal with work-related symptoms and disease. Farm inspections are conducted by safety engineers. Twenty-six local health centers serve 1,000 to 2,000 farmers each. In remote areas agricultural health services are provided through other occupational health centers to provide outreach services for farmers. In addition to health care, centers carry out research and development projects in cooperation with hospitals and universities, with grant financing.

In Canada, the goal of the Ontario Farm Safety Association[22] is to reduce injuries and fatalities. It provides safety education services to the agricultural community. Services include health and safety seminars, farm inspections, technical consulting, and agricultural safety publications and audiovisual materials. The association also conducts statistical gathering and analysis. An elementary school program called "Rural Ontario Safety Kit" is available to country and regional schools. The association has also developed credit level instruction in agricultural occupational safety and health for community colleges and colleges of agricultural technology, thereby reaching all levels of school education.

CONCLUSION

Keys for improving occupational health in agricultural settings are federal leadership, health care provider education, and farmer education, and the three are closely linked.

Federal interest has been demonstrated by the Surgeon General's Conference and by the recent funding of NIOSH programs and research awards. Federal leadership should also be demonstrated in strengthening safety legislation. Stricter child labor laws for agriculture are needed. For example, the tractor-driving age of children should be limited. Government should also influence the farm work activities and safety training of adolescent males. ROPS and other existing safety features of tractors should be mandatory for operation of the equipment. The environment must be protected from pesticides and other agricultural chemicals. Groundwater protection legislation is needed. Workers' compensation coverage for farmers should be expanded to all states, along with provider, farm owner, and farm worker education in the working of the system. Educational and other materials for farm workers should be written in English and Spanish, and warning labels, reentry periods, and other safety materials should be read aloud for the benefit of illiterate workers.

Physician education should begin in medical school and carry through the pertinent residency programs. Resolutions such as the AMA position on pesticides have applications for other potential hazards of agricultural work. New NIOSH agricultural projects are an encouraging sign that farmer education in work safety will result in strong outreach programs.

Physicians are the undeveloped resource—the link to the farmer, federal and state governments, and agricultural safety. Through direct contact by health care providers, farmers can be encouraged to use protective clothing and equipment, and preventive principles can be reinforced. It is important to be aware of major hazards and health risks of agriculture when dealing with individuals. But it is also important to appreciate the broader issues: (1) the need for engineering changes to bring about a safer environment; (2) the role of legislation in farm and environmental safety, and (3) current needs for legislative changes. Heightened awareness on the part of physicians and other practitioners can lead to a powerful coalition to improve farmers' education and bring about needed reforms to reduce morbidity and mortality on the farm.

REFERENCES

1. American Academy of Family Physicians: American Academy of Family Physicians Residency Completion Survey. Kansas City, American Academy of Family Physicians. Reprint No. 155.
2. And on the farm . . . JAMA 263:2600, May 16, 1990.
3. Barnett P, Midtling J, Velasco A, et al: Educational intervention to prevent pesticide-induced illness of field workers. J Fam Prac 19:123–125, 1984.
4. Clark S: Report of prevention and control. Am J Ind Med 10:267–273, 1986.
5. Council on Scientific Affairs: Council Report: Biotechnology and the American agricultural industry. JAMA 265:1429–1436, 1991.
6. Council on Scientific Affairs: Council Report: Cancer risk of pesticides in agricultural workers. JAMA 260:959–966, 1988.
7. Cuthbert OD, Gordon MF: Ten-year follow-up of farmers with farmer's lung. Br J Ind Med 50:173–176, 1983.
8. Dosman JA, Cockcroft DW (eds): Principles of Health and Safety in Agriculture. Boca Raton, FL, CRC Press, 1989, Introduction, n.p.
9. Douglas WW, Hepper NG, Colby TV: Silo-filler's disease. Mayo Clin Proc 64:291–304, 1989.
10. Emanuel D: A case for medical, environmental, and safety screening. Am J Ind Med 18:413–419, 1990.
11. Epler GR: Silo-filler's disease: A new perspective (editorial). Mayo Clin Proc 64:368–370, 1989.
12. Feddes JJR: The influence of selected management practices on heat moisture and air quality in swine housing. Can Agric Eng 25:175–179, 1983.
13. Federal Register 40 CFR. Parts 156 and 170. July 8, 1988.
14. Hartye J: Physicians as the weak link in agricultural health services: Defining the agenda for action. Am J Ind Med 18:421–425, 1990.
15. Hoglund S: Occupational health service for farmers in Sweden. J Occup Med 31:767–770, 1989.
16. Kindig DA: Commentary: Policy priorities for rural physician supply. Academic Med 65:515–517, 1990.
17. Kross BC: Technical Workshop Report: Working Group III: Environmental health strategies for agriculture. Am J Ind Med 18:517–522, 1990.
18. Mathews J: Ergonomics and farm machinery. J Soc Occup Med 33:126–136, 1983.
19. McJilton CE, Aherin RA: Getting the message to the farmer. Am Ind Hyg Assoc J 43:469–471, 1982.
20. National Safety Council: Accident Facts, 1990 Edition. National Safety Council, Chicago, IL, 1990.
21. Occupational Health and Safety for Agricultural Workers. US Department of Health, Education, and Welfare. National Institute for Occupational Safety and Health. Publication No. 77-150, Cincinnati, OH, 1976.
22. Ontario Farm Safety Association: Safety programs of the Farm Safety Association in Ontario, Canada. Am J Ind Med 18:409–411, 1990.
23. Ritter L: Assessment of pesticide toxicity: Regulatory viewpoints. In Dosman JA, Cockcroft DW (eds): Principles of Health and Safety in Agriculture. Boca Raton, FL, CRC Press, 1989, pp 214–216.
24. Rivera FP: Fatal and nonfatal farm injuries to children and adolescents in the United States. Pediatrics 76:567–573, 1985.
25. Salmi LR, Weiss HB, Peterson PL, et al: Fatal farm injuries among young children. Pediatrics 83:267–271, 1989.
26. Sandfort D: Reaching the difficult audience: An experiment to provide occupational health services to farmers and ranchers in Colorado, U.S.A. Am J Ind Med 18:395–403, 1990.
27. Texas Department of Agriculture: A Guide to the Texas Agricultural Hazard Communication Law: Right-to-Know. Austin, TX, Texas Department of Agriculture, 78711.
28. Thelin A: Epilogue: Agricultural occupational and environmental health policy strategies for the future. Am J Ind Med 18:523–526, 1990.
29. Thompson JE, Bonner B, Lower GM: Pediatric cardiopulmonary arrests in rural populations. Pediatrics 86:302–306, 1990.
30. Watson RD: Prevention of dust exposure. Am J Ind Med 10:299, 1986.
31. Wilk VA: The Occupational Health of Migrant and Seasonal Farmworkers in the United States. Washington, D.C., Farmworkers Justice Fund, 1986.

INDEX

Entries in **boldface type** indicate complete chapters.

551